AF180558

# Essentials in Arthroplasty

# Essentials in Arthroplasty

Edited by **Robert Berry**

hayle medical

New York

Published by Hayle Medical,
30 West, 37th Street, Suite 612,
New York, NY 10018, USA
www.haylemedical.com

**Essentials in Arthroplasty**
Edited by Robert Berry

© 2015 Hayle Medical

International Standard Book Number: 978-1-63241-218-8 (Hardback)

This book contains information obtained from authentic and highly regarded sources. Copyright for all individual chapters remain with the respective authors as indicated. A wide variety of references are listed. Permission and sources are indicated; for detailed attributions, please refer to the permissions page. Reasonable efforts have been made to publish reliable data and information, but the authors, editors and publisher cannot assume any responsibility for the validity of all materials or the consequences of their use.

The publisher's policy is to use permanent paper from mills that operate a sustainable forestry policy. Furthermore, the publisher ensures that the text paper and cover boards used have met acceptable environmental accreditation standards.

**Trademark Notice:** Registered trademark of products or corporate names are used only for explanation and identification without intent to infringe.

Printed in China.

# Contents

# Preface

This book is a sequel of all the successful volumes dedicated to one of the rapidly progressing fields in orthopedics - arthroplasty. The method of enhancing care for patients and standards of treatment requires straightforward approach. Novel technologies, advancements in implant design and developments in surgical technique have better results after joint substitution and have led to a declined rate of difficulties. It is no surprise that the number of arthroplasties grows constantly every year; and nowadays, more than one million people go through the procedure annually worldwide. Focusing at dissemination of scientific research this book offers a thorough sketch of the current advancement of technology and surgical techniques. Novel advancements of implant design and current treatment strategies have also been analytically examined by the contributing authors. Also, the result of arthroplasty by etiology is analyzed. This book is a valuable source of reference for students and practitioners.

This book is a result of research of several months to collate the most relevant data in the field.

When I was approached with the idea of this book and the proposal to edit it, I was overwhelmed. It gave me an opportunity to reach out to all those who share a common interest with me in this field. I had 3 main parameters for editing this text:

1. Accuracy - The data and information provided in this book should be up-to-date and valuable to the readers.
2. Structure - The data must be presented in a structured format for easy understanding and better grasping of the readers.
3. Universal Approach - This book not only targets students but also experts and innovators in the field, thus my aim was to present topics which are of use to all.

Thus, it took me a couple of months to finish the editing of this book.

I would like to make a special mention of my publisher who considered me worthy of this opportunity and also supported me throughout the editing process. I would also like to thank the editing team at the back-end who extended their help whenever required.

**Editor**

Section 1

# Decision Making for Arthroplasty

Chapter 1

# Surgical Approaches to the Hip Joint and the It's Clinical Implications in Adult Hip Arthroplasty

Hiran Amarasekera

Additional information is available at the end of the chapter

## 1. Introduction

The Hip joint can be approached in many ways and therefore many different exposures have been described. The choice of which approach to use depend on the type of surgery, what part of the hip needs to be exposed, age of the patient and surgeon's preference and expertise.

When approaching the hip it is also important to consider whether the surgery is done for trauma or elective surgery, whether the patient is an adult or a child whether it is conservative hip surgery or replacement surgery and what part needs to be accessed for the specific surgery such as the acetabulum, femoral head or whether both need equal access as in total hip arthroplasty.

The main aim of this chapter is to discuss the available surgical approaches in the adult hip when elective reconstructive surgery is done such as total hip resurfacing and revision hip arthroplasty.

The advantages and dis-advantages and the clinical relevance of these approaches to each surgery and basic surgical steps are discussed including the traditional approach and the modification of these approaches.

For completion of the chapter most approaches and classifications are mentioned but the emphasis is mainly on the common approaches used in hip arthroplasty. A good approach to the hip should have good access to both femoral head and acetabulum, should have minimal dissection of soft tissues, leading to reduced operative time and blood loss, less post operative pain and early mobilisation, least risk of damage to neurovascular bundles muscles and tendons with minimal risk of infection thrombosis and dislocation. However in practice there is no one ideal approach hence many approaches have been described and used among orthopaedic surgeons over the years.

## 2. Classification of different surgical approaches

Surgical approaches to the hip joint can be classified in many ways. One simple classification is based on the direction of approach. (Fig 1) The common approaches used based on this classification are the anterior, antero-lateral and posterior. Some of the different ways of classifying surgical approaches to the hip is given below. [1]

a. **Based on the direction**

1. Anterior type
2. Lateral and antero lateral type
3. Posterior type
4. Medial type
5. Combined e.g. anterior and posterior

b. **Based on incision and invasiveness**

1. Standard incision e.g. Posterior
2. Mini incision posterior (MIS)

c. **Based on type od surgery**

1. Open surgical e.g. anterior
2. Arthroscopic

It is also important to know that certain new approaches described are essentially a modification of an existing approach. E.g. Trochanteric flip approach is a modification of an anterior type approach. [2]

## 3. Surgical approaches to the hip joint

Before performing any surgical approach it is important understand the anatomical principles that lie behind the surgical dissection.

Like in all orthopaedic surgeries positioning the patient, draping and preparing the area, identification of landmarks and making the incision along skin creases, are important to remember. It is also important to note that all incisions should be made along the identified line of incision but the initial incision is best made within the middle half of the incision line so that if needed this can be extended in either direction. Previous concept of "Big surgeons make big incisions" does not hold true in modern day practice as the demand is for mini incisions and key hole surgery as they give a better cosmetic outcome.

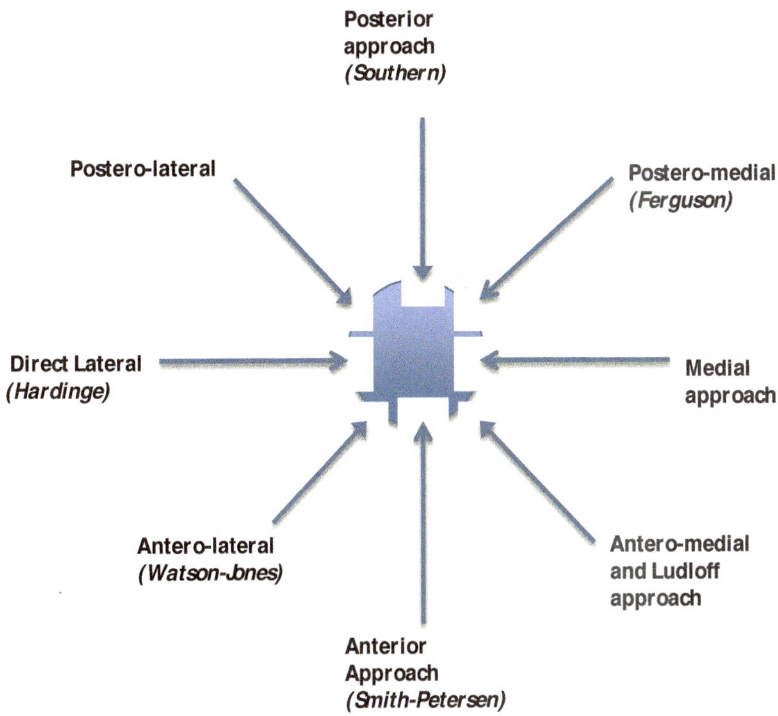


**Figure 1.** All directions the hip can be approached.

Another principle in operative orthopaedic surgery is the attempt to go directly to the operative area whether it is a bone or a joint. This minimises the lateral dissection thus avoiding damage to soft tissues such as nerves and vessels.

The concept of *"internervous plane"* is important to understand before any surgical approach is done. This means that all deep dissection should be done by dissecting and separating the muscles between two nervous planes so that all muscles supplied by one nerve and it's branches are retracted towards one side to avoid damage and denervating the muscles. (Fig 2)

It is not always possible to dissect along the internervous plane. Sometimes dissection planes are developed by splitting the muscles. (Fig 3) The principles of muscle splitting incision are

1. Always muscles are split longitudinally along the line of the fibres.
2. Splitting is done away from the neuromuscular junction to avoid denervation.
3. Bulk of the muscle is retracted along with the nerve-so that most of the muscle will retain the nerve supply.

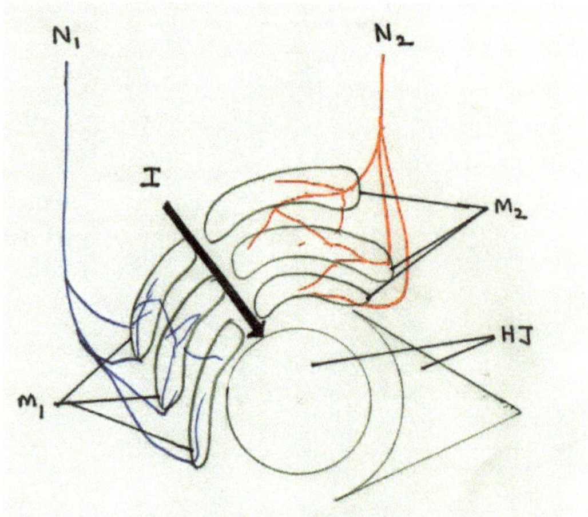


**Figure 2.** Concept internervous plane, (HJ, Hip Joint; N1Nerve supplying the muscle group M1; N2 nerve supplying the muscle groupM2; I internervous plane)

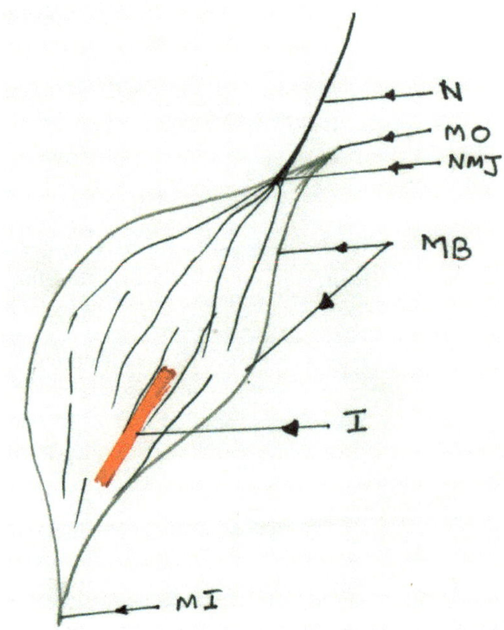


**Figure 3.** Muscle splitting incisions *(I)* are made along the line of the fibres, away from the Neuro-muscular junction *(NMJ) MO: Muscle Origin, MB: muscle Belly, MI: Muscle Insertion, N: Nerve*

In the next few paragraphs the following approaches are described in relation to the clinical implications.

1. **Anterior approaches**

a. Anterior type approach is Smith Peterson approach

b. Mini incision anterior approach

2. **Lateral approaches**

a. Direct Lateral /Hardinge

b. Antero-Lateral /Watson Jones

3. **Posterior approach**

a. Southern Approach [3]

4. **Medial approaches**

a. Antero medial

b. Postero-medial (Ferguson Approach)

c. Ludloff's approach

5. **Modern**

a. Arthroscopic

b. Minimally invasive

6. **Modified and combined approaches**

a. Trochanteric Flip Ganz [2]

b. Antero –lateral minimally invasive [4]

c. Mini incision posterior approach [5]

d. Modified antero-lateral [6]

e. Combined approaches [7]

Out of these approaches it is important understand that the medial approaches are rarely used in hip arthroplasty due to poor access to acetabulum and femoral head.

Even though a detailed description of each surgical approach is beyond the scope of this chapter all the salient features of above approaches are discussed with regard to their key steps, key advantages, key limitations, specific complications, common surgical procedures done through the approach, modifications of the traditional approach and other key issues.

The approaches described in depth below are the surgical approaches used commonly in hip arthroplasty.

## 4. The anterior approach *(Smith-Petersen)*

**a.** Key steps

This approach initially described by Smith-Peterson [8] is one of the approaches but not a very popular approach used by arthroplasty surgeons as the femoral exposure is limited. It is mainly used for arthrotomies to drain the hip in presence of infection. The key steps and the details are given below.

*Position:* Supine with a pillow under the pelvis on the operating side

*Incision*: Longitudinal incision lies between anterior iliac crest towards upper thigh curving over anterior superior iliac spine.

*Soft tissue dissection:* This is between sartorius and the tensor fasciae lata and rectus femoris and gluteus medius.

*Internervous plane:* Lies between the sartorius (Femoral nerve) and the tensor fasciae latae (Superior gluteal nerve)

*Arthrotomy:* Adduct and externally rotate the leg and incise the capsule longitudinally or with W or T shape incision.

Dislocation: by external rotation

Closure: In layers capsule rarely closed. Fascial planes are closed and skin

**b.** Key advantages

The advantages of this approach include preservation of the vascularity, stability following the procedure with less chance of dislocation. Limited morbidity, high stability and with good access to the acetabulum are key advantages of this approach. [9] The approach limits muscle cutting and separation, reduce chance of dislocations, and makes it easier to take intra-operative radiographs as the patient is supine in position. Key muscle groups the extensors and the abductors are kept intact the along with the medial circumflex femoral artery and it's branches. [10], [11]

c. Key Limitations

The key limitation of this approach is the limited access making it technically demanding to place components in arthroplasty. Even though the approach to the acetabulum is good approach to proximal femur is limited through this approach. Some encourage to use a fracture table to get a better approach to the femur [12] while others use the standard operating table. [13]

Even though many total hip arthroplasties and even resurfacing hip replacements are done using this approach [10] due to limited access and technical demanding nature [14] this may not be a popular approach among arthroplasty surgeons.

**d.** Specific complications, [15]

Damage to lateral cutaneous nerve and the anterior cutaneous nerve should be kept in mind. [16]

**e.** Common surgical procedures

Even though hip arthroplasty is not commonly done some surgeons still prefer to do total hip arthroplasty [17] and hip resurfacing [10] through an anterior approach.

**f.** Modifications to the approach

The modification of this approach includes two incision direct anterior approach and minimally invasive direct anterior approaches. [18], [19] Low blood loss, early recovery, early mobilisation reduced operating time are the advantages of the minimally invasive anterior approach. [20]

## 5. Antero-lateral approach *(Watson-Jones)*

Described initially by Watson-Jones [21] approaches the hip between tensor fascia lata and the gluteus medius muscle planes.

**a.** Key Steps:

*Position:* The patient can be positioned supine or laterally on the table

In the supine position a sand bag may be placed under the pelvis on the operating side.

*Incision:* Longitudinal incision is made while flexing the hip slightly extending over the centre of the greater trochanter running posteriorly along the shaft of the femur.

*Soft tissue dissection:* This is done by identifying the plane between the tensor fasciae latae and the gluteus medius taking care not to damage the inferior branch of the superior gluteal nerve as it supplies the former muscle.

Vastus lateralis is identified and the muscle is detached from the origin and the capsule identified.

*Internervous plane:* Since the superior gluteal nerve supply both gluteus medius and tensor fasciae latae it is difficult to define a true internervous plane for this approach. However as long as the plane between these muscles are not dissected superiorly up to the origin the nerve will remain intact.

*Arthrotomy:* The capsule is divided longitudinally over the anterior superior femoral neck.

*Dislocation:* This is done by applying external rotation, traction and adduction to dislocate the hip.

*Closure:* The wound is closed in layers starting with the capsule. If a trochanteric osteotomy is performed it has to be re attached.

**b.** Key advantages

The key advantages of the approach include stability, less chance of posterior dislocation, less risk to sciatic nerve damage unless during dislocation where traction can stretch the nerve. Precautions should also be taken not to damage the superior gluteal nerve.

c. Key limitations

One of the key limitations is that possibility of abductors getting weak during dissection or by denervation of the nerve supply. [22]

d. Specific complications

Damage to superior gluteal nerve and lateral circumflex femoral artery (LCFA) should be kept in mind.

Damage to the femoral nerve and vessels are a relatively rare complication.

e. Modifications

Mueller modified the approach to avoid trochanteric osteotomy.

Another recent modification for this approach is the minimally invasive approach.[4] Antero lateral minimally invasive approach (ALM) has been described as a good alternative [23] to traditional approaches as it reduces hospital stay, surgical time, blood loss, morbidity, and encourages early mobilisations, and recovery. Even though some report high complication rates [24] with this approach over all this is an approach with many advantages in the modern day practice. However this is a technically demanding procedure that needs expertise.

Trochanteric flip approach developed by Ganz et al is can be considered as a modification or combined type approach where steps of posterior approach is used but the hip is dislocated anteriorly by performing a trochanteric flip osteotomy.[2]

f. Advantages

The key advantage of this approach is the protection of medial circumflex femoral artery thus preserving the main blood supply to the hip. Therefore this becomes an important approach to use in conservative hip surgery and the surface replacement of the hip joint as this can protect the femoral head and neck from developing avascular necrosis (AVN). [25] The key step of this approach is the trochanteric flip osteotomy where a bony flip of around 1.5cm made over the greater trochanter and reflected anteriorly along with vastus lateralis, gluteus medius and minimus and the hip is dislocated anteriorly thus avoiding and dissection of short external rotators.

g. Key limitations

The key limitations include the patient need to be non-weight bearing for six weeks or until the trochanteric osteotomy is healed. Non-union and separation of the osteotomy are other potential complications. [6] (Fig 4)

## 6. Direct lateral approach

Direct lateral approach also called as the trans-gluteal approach initially described by Kocher in 1903 [26] popularised by Hardinge in the modern age [27] gives good exposure to the hip

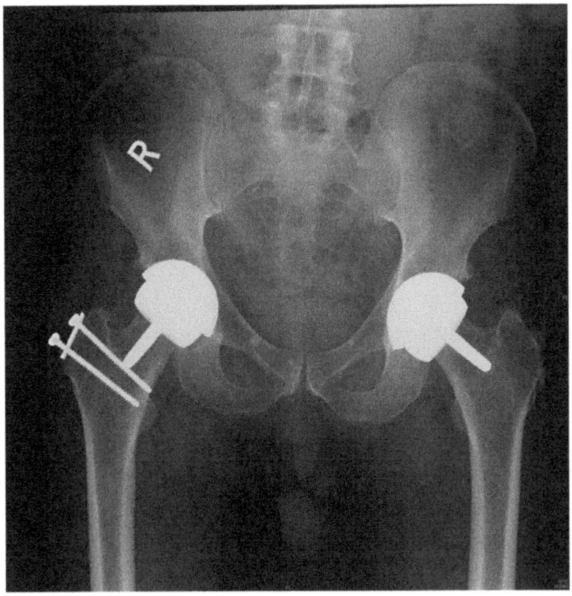


**Figure 4.** Post-operative X ray of patient showing Hip resurfacing done through Posterior approach (Left Hip) and Trochanteric flip approach (Right hip), note the re-attachment of the osteotomy with screws and loosening of the lower screw.

joint preserving most of gluteus medius minimus and vastus lateralis, and the vascularity. It exposes the femur well with good access to the joint.

a. Key steps

*Position:* This can either be done on lateral or supine position

*Incision:* from mid point of greater trochanter longitudinally along the femoral shaft extending around 8-10 cm with proximal extension up to anterior superior iliac spine. [27]

*Incision:* Usually it is made about 7-10 cm below the tip of the greater trochanter along the anterior border of the femur.

*Soft tissue dissection:* Gluteal fascia and illio tibial band divided and plane between tensor facia late and gluteus maximus is identified. Gluteus medius incised and approach via gluteus medius and vastus muscles.

*Internervous plane:* As the gluteus medius tendon and muscle fibres and the vastus lateralis muscles are split there is no true internervous plane. However it is important are split protect the superior gluteal nerve by making the incision distal to the point which it enters the muscle.

*Dislocation:* Leg can be externally rotated and abducted for dislocation [27].

*Closure:* Illio tibial ligament initially re attached followed by gluteus medius suturing.

b. Key advantages

This approach gives good access to the hip and yet preserves vascularity and minimise risk of damage to sciatic nerve as compared to the posterior approach.

c. Key limitations

Damage to gluteal muscle mainly medius can increase recovery time,

d. Specific complications

Complications are relatively rare with low dislocation rates. Heterotopic ossification may be a problem in selected cases. [28]

e. Common surgical procedures

Total hip replacements, hip resurfacing, [29] trauma, and many procedures can be done via this.

f. Modifications

Modifications include the trans gluteal approach. [30] This has been compared with Watson Jones approach and appear to be a good alternative to the traditional approach. [31] According to some authors the surgical exposure can be improved by modifying the way muscle fibres are split, fascia is cut retractors are placed and closing the wound. [32]

Lateral trans trochanteric approach was initially described in 1881 by Ollier and popularised by Sir John Charnley provide a good exposure hip joint is mainly used in revision arthroplasties. [33]

## 7. Posterior approach

Also called, as the Southern approach is one of the commonest approaches used by the orthopaedic surgeons at present.

a. Key Steps

*Position*: Mostly done in lateral position

*Incision*: standard incision is 10-15 cm long curve-linear extending from posterior superior iliac spine to greater trochanter and extending down in a variable distance along the shaft of the femur. The modern incisions are shorter than the standard. As this can be extended if needed it is sensible to initially make a smaller incision and extend if needed.

*Soft tissue dissection:* Initially fascia lata and vastus lateralis is cut. The gluteus maximus fibres are split. Then the hip is internally rotated and short external rotators are cut after holding them with stay sutures.

Obturator internus and piriformis is detached and reflected backwards to protect the sciatic nerve.

*Internervous plane*: As we split through the fibres of gluteus maximus rather than between muscle planes it is difficult to find a true internervous plane. How ever as the nerve enters the muscle medial to the split the muscle denervation is unlikely.

*Arthrotomy:* Capsule is incised with a T shaped incision

*Closure:* Capsular closure is described but the practicality is an issue mainly following hip arthroplasty procedures.

It is important re-attached the external rotators and obturator internus and piriformis.

**b.** Key advantages

This is a good approach that provides excellent exposure to both acetabulum and the femoral head and neck equally making it easier to surgical procedures well.

c. Key Limitations

Due to the possibility that blood supply may get damaged resulting in AVN has limited it's used in conservative hip surgery such as open hip debridement, open surgery for hip impingement and use of this in paediatric population is not recommended.

**d.** Specific Complications

The posterior approach has specific complications these are

1. Damage to sciatic nerve, which could be either stretching which recover usually, or permanent damage, which will result in a foot drop.
2. Damage to inferior gluteal vessels, branches of profunda femoris vessels and rarely femoral vessels.
3. Invariably branches of medial circumflex femoral artery are cut during this approach, which can theoretically give rise to AVN of femoral head and neck. This does not matter in total hip replacement as the head and neck is removed but in conservative procedures including hip resurfacing arthroplasty. Many authors have challenged however the clinical implications of this blood flow drop. [34]- [37] Some argue the blood supply drop is transient which may recover during post-operative period. [38]

e. Common surgical procedures

This is in an approach commonly used to do Primary and revision total hip replacements, hip resurfacings, and other procedures such as open reduction of hip dislocations and fixation of acetabular fractures.

**f.** Modifications

Minimally invasive (MIS) posterior approach is a modification. This approach when compared with standard lateral approach has similar outcomes during early post-operative period such as surgical duration, blood loss and hospital stay but long term results such as Harris Hip score is higher in the MIS. [39] Similar results have been achieved when compared with postero-lateral approaches. [40] When compared with the standard posterior approach it was found to be less blood loss, less post-operative pain and early recovery. [41] Gibson approach [42] is another modification and can be considered a poster-lateral type of approach.

## 8. Postero-lateral approach

Initially described by Langenback in 1874 [43] is another approach that can be used in hip arthroplasty surgery. Compared with trans trochanteric approach it is believed that this has less blood loss and shorter hospital stay. [44]

6.Medial approaches are mainly used developmental dysplasia of the hip, in young patients and children as it protects most soft tissues and blood supply to the hip joint.

The medial approaches can be further sub classified to antero-medial, postero-medial (Ferguson) and Ludloff's approach

a. Antero-medial approach,

b. Postero-medial approach

c. Ludloff's approach

These approaches are mainly used in children to treat DDH and open reduction of CDH and other conservative procedures. [45], [46]

The minimally invasive approaches to the hip joint used in hip arthroplasty.

Due to ion crease blood loss, slow recovery increase intra operative time, and delay in discharge more and more orthopaedic surgeons have been keen to develop minimally invasive approaches. These are usually modifications of existing approaches so that a surgeon preferring a certain standard approach can try the minimally approaches. The commonest minimally invasive approaches are minimally invasive antero lateral, minimally invasive direct lateral [24] minimally invasive posterior, minimally invasive anterior

The principles include shorter skin incision either single or multiple, minimal soft tissue dissection, without compromising the access or the quality of the surgery.

Optimal incision is around 8-9 cm either used as single or two separate incisions. [47] [48]

The results suggests better immediate outcomes and similar long term out comes in total hip arthroplasty for antero lateral MIS [23], postero-lateral MIS [49]

The reasons for developing Modified and modern approaches to the hip joint was mainly driven by the concept of minimal invasive surgeries being developed through out the surgical fields as they are supposed to be less invasive with low intra-operative complications such as low blood loss, less tissue dissection and less operative time, with early recovery, early mobilisation and early discharge from hospital. With development of smaller implants better instrumentation, better pre-operative planning, use of navigation, and better intra-operative imaging it has been possible to develop and use minimally invasive approaches to major surgeries like total hip arthroplasty or revision hip surgery. How ever at present there is debate over the long term out comes quality of surgery including implant positioning and learning curve for minimally invasive approaches over standard surgical approach. The answers to these questions will come from the research done comparing minimally invasive approaches versus the standard surgical approaches.

## 9. Conclusion

In conclusion it is important note that there are multiple surgical approaches to the hip joint and some better suited for arthroplasty and some for more conservative hip surgery. A checklist of factors one should consider before an approach is selected is,

1. What type of surgery? Is it conservative or hip arthroplasty?
2. If is arthroplasty, is it Total hip replacement, Hip resurfacing or a Revision hip replacement?
3. Age of patient? Adult young adult or a child
4. What part of the hip do you need the best exposure to? Acetabular socket, Femoral head and neck or both
5. Surgeon's preference and competence in doing the approach.
6. Whether the surgery is elective or trauma/emergency.

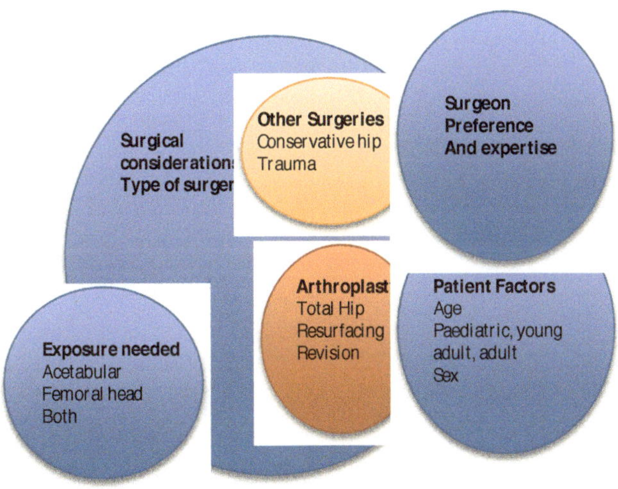


**Figure 5.** Show different factors that has to be taken to consideration when selecting

The relationship between the outcome of surgery and the surgical approach is still less understood, even though many comparison studies have been done. [50] [51] The final decision on what surgical approach to use is a clinical decision that has to be made by the operating surgeon.

## Author details

Hiran Amarasekera

Orthopaedic Research Fellow/ PhD Student, Warwick Medical School, University of Warwick, And University Hospital of Coventry and Warwickshire, UK

## References

[1] Gerdesmeyer, L, Gollwitzer, H, Bader, R, & Rudert, M. Surgical approaches in hip resurfacing]. *Orthopade* (2008).

[2] Ganz, R, Gill, T. J, Gautier, E, Ganz, K, Krugel, N, & Berlemann, U. Surgical dislocation of the adult hip: A TECHNIQUE WITH FULL ACCESS TO THE FEMORAL HEAD AND ACETABULUM WITHOUT THE RISK OF AVASCULAR NECROSIS. *J Bone Joint Surg Br* (2001). B-, 8, 1119-24.

[3] Hunter, S. C. Southern hip exposure. *Orthopedics* (1986).

[4] Jerosch, J, Theising, C, & Fadel, M. E. Antero-lateral minimal invasive (ALMI) approach for total hip arthroplasty technique and early results. *Arch Orthop Trauma Surg* (2006).

[5] Mcminn, D. J, Daniel, J, Pynsent, P. B, & Pradhan, C. Mini-incision resurfacing arthroplasty of hip through the posterior approach. *Clin Orthop Relat Res* (2005). *441*, 91-8.

[6] Khan, R. M, Cooper, G, & Hull, J. B. Hip resurfacing through a modified anterolateral approach, as compared with the Ganz trochanteric flip osteotomy: a two year follow-up study. *Hip Int* (2009).

[7] Lusskin, R, Goldman, A, & Absatz, M. Combined anterior and posterior approach to the hip joint in reconstructive and complex arthroplasty. *J Arthroplasty* (1988).

[8] Smith-petersen, M. N. Approach to and exposure of the hip joint for mold arthroplasty. *J Bone Joint Surg Am* (1949). A-, 1, 40-6.

[9] Light, T. R, & Keggi, K. J. Anterior approach to hip arthroplasty. *Clin Orthop Relat Res* (1980).

[10] Kreuzer, S, Leffers, K, & Kumar, S. Direct anterior approach for hip resurfacing: surgical technique and complications. *Clin Orthop Relat Res* (2011).

[11] Judet, J, & Judet, H. Anterior approach in total hip arthroplasty]. *Presse Med* (1985).

[12] Horne, P. H, & Olson, S. A. Direct anterior approach for total hip arthroplasty using the fracture table. *Curr Rev Musculoskelet Med* (2011).

[13] Lovell, T. P. Single-incision direct anterior approach for total hip arthroplasty using a standard operating table. *J Arthroplasty* (2008). Suppl:64-8., 23-7.

[14] Goytia, R. N, Jones, L. C, & Hungerford, M. W. Learning curve for the anterior approach total hip arthroplasty. *J Surg Orthop Adv* (2012).

[15] Barton, C, & Kim, P. R. Complications of the direct anterior approach for total hip arthroplasty. *Orthop Clin North Am* (2009).

[16] Bhargava, T, Goytia, R. N, Jones, L. C, & Hungerford, M. W. Lateral femoral cutaneous nerve impairment after direct anterior approach for total hip arthroplasty. *Orthopedics* (2010).

[17] Bender, B, Nogler, M, & Hozack, W. J. Direct anterior approach for total hip arthroplasty. *Orthop Clin North Am* (2009).

[18] Oinuma, K, Eingartner, C, Saito, Y, & Shiratsuchi, H. Total hip arthroplasty by a minimally invasive, direct anterior approach. *Oper Orthop Traumatol* (2007).

[19] Rachbauer, F. Minimally invasive total hip arthroplasty. Anterior approach]. *Orthopade* (2006).

[20] Hallert, O, Li, Y, Brismar, H, & Lindgren, U. The direct anterior approach: initial experience of a minimally invasive technique for total hip arthroplasty. *J Orthop Surg Res* (2012).

[21] Watson-JonesFractures of the neck of femur. *British Journal of surgery* (1936). 23, 787-808.

[22] Pawlowski, Z, Bohatyrewicz, A, Czajkowski, A. A, Kominiak, P, & Gusta, A. Early abductor muscle strength after total hip replacement performed by antero-lateral approach]. *Chir Narzadow Ruchu Ortop Pol* (2002).

[23] Walde, T. A, Blattgerste, D, Sehmisch, S, Kuttler, W, Walde, H. J, & Koster, G. Early results and patient satisfaction after total hip arthroplasty using a minimally invasive anterolateral approach. *Hip Int* (2009).

[24] Spaans, A. J. van den Hout JA, Bolder SB. High complication rate in the early experience of minimally invasive total hip arthroplasty by the direct anterior approach. *Acta Orthop* (2012).

[25] Amarasekera Surface Replacement of the Hip Joint. In: K.Fokter S, ed. *Recent Advances in Hip and Knee Arthroplasty*, 1 ed. Croatia: Intech, (2012)., 2012, 181-90.

[26] Kocher, T. In: *Text book of operative surgery*. London: Adams and Charles Blac, (1903).

[27] Hardinge, K. The direct lateral approach to the hip. *J Bone Joint Surg Br* (1982).

[28] Foster, D. E, & Hunter, J. R. The direct lateral approach to the hip for arthroplasty. Advantages and complications. *Orthopedics* (1987).

[29] Gerdesmeyer, L, Gollwitzer, H, Diehl, P, Buttgereit, B, & Rudert, M. The minimally invasive anterolateral approach combined with hip onlay resurfacing. *Oper Orthop Traumatol* (2009).

[30] Bauer, R, Kerschbaumer, F, Poisel, S, & Oberthaler, W. The transgluteal approach to the hip joint. *Arch Orthop Trauma Surg* (1979).

[31] Eyb, R. Clinical results following the transgluteal and anterolateral (Watson-Jones) approach to hip prosthesis implantation]. *Z Orthop Ihre Grenzgeb* (1985).

[32] Warren, P. J, Jennings, G. J, & Fletcher, M. D. Improvement in surgical exposure of the hip using the direct lateral approach. *Ann R Coll Surg Engl* (2002).

[33] Mulliken, B. D, Rorabeck, C. H, Bourne, R. B, & Nayak, N. The surgical approach to total hip arthroplasty: complications and utility of a modified direct lateral approach. *Iowa Orthop J* (1995). *15*, 48-61.

[34] Amarasekera, H. W, Costa, M. L, Foguet, P, Krikler, S. J, Prakash, U, & Griffin, D. R. The blood flow to the femoral head/neck junction during resurfacing arthroplasty: A COMPARISON OF TWO APPROACHES USING LASER DOPPLER FLOWMETRY. *J Bone Joint Surg Br* (2008).

[35] Amarasekera, H. W, Costa, M. L, Parsons, N, Achten, J, Griffin, D. R, Manktelow, S, & Williams, N. R. SPECT/CT bone imaging after hip resurfacing arthroplasty: is it feasible to use CT attenuation correction in the presence of metal implants? *Nucl Med Commun* (2011).

[36] Campbell, P, Mirra, J, & Amstutz, H. C. Viability of femoral heads treated with resurfacing arthroplasty. *J Arthroplasty* (2000).

[37] Amarasekera, H, Costa, M, Prakash, U, Krikler, S, Foguet, P, & Griffin, D. FEMORAL BLOOD FLOW DURING HIP RESURFACING: A COMPARISON OF TWO APPROACHES USING LASER DOPPLER FLOW MEASUREMENT. *Journal of Bone & Joint Surgery, British 2012*B-SUPP III:148.

[38] Amarasekera, H, Roberts, P, Costa, M, Parsons, N, Achten, J, Griffin, D, & Williams, N. Scintigraphic assessment of bone status at one year following hip resurfacing: comparison of two surgical approaches using SPECT-CT scan. *Bone and Joint Research* (2012).

[39] Schleicher, I, Haas, H, Adams, T. S, Szalay, G, Klein, H, & Kordelle, J. Minimal-invasive posterior approach for total hip arthroplasty versus standard lateral approach. *Acta Orthop Belg* (2011).

[40] Fink, B, & Mittelstaedt, A. Minimally invasive posterior approach for total hip arthroplasty]. *Orthopade* (2012).

[41] Fink, B, Mittelstaedt, A, Schulz, M. S, Sebena, P, & Singer, J. Comparison of a minimally invasive posterior approach and the standard posterior approach for total hip arthroplasty A prospective and comparative study. *J Orthop Surg Res* (2010).

[42] Gibson, A. Posterior exposure of the hip joint. *J Bone Joint Surg Br* (1950). B-, 2, 183-6.

[43] Pellegrini VJaECM. Surgical approaches to the hip. In: Evarts C, ed. *Surgery of the Musculoskeletal system*. NewYork: Churchil Livingstone, (1990).

[44] Aglietti, P, & Salvati, E. The postero-lateral approach for total hip prosthesis. *Ital J Orthop Traumatol* (1981).

[45] Di Mascio LCarey-Smith R, Tucker K. Open reduction of developmental hip dysplasia using a medial approach: a review of 24 hips. *Acta Orthop Belg* (2008).

[46] Broughton, N. S, Graham, H. K, Nattrass, G. R, Torode, I. P, Marshall, P. D, Sullivan, O, & Ludloff, M. s medial approach for open reduction of congenital dislocation of the hip. *J Bone Joint Surg Br* (1997).

[47] Noble, P. C, Pfluger, G, Junk-jantsch, S, Thompson, M. T, Alexander, J. W, & Mathis, K. B. The optimal skin incision for minimally invasive total hip arthroplasty performed via the anterolateral approach. *J Arthroplasty* (2012).

[48] Wetzel, R, & Dorsch, M. Minimally invasive approach to implantation of a hip endoprosthesis]. *Orthopade* (2006).

[49] Varela Egocheaga JRSuarez-Suarez MA, Fernandez-Villan M, Gonzalez-Sastre V, Varela-Gomez JR, Murcia-Mazon A. [Minimally invasive posterior approach in total hip arthroplasty. Prospective randomised trial]. *An Sist Sanit Navar* (2010).

[50] Barber, T. C, Roger, D. J, Goodman, S. B, & Schurman, D. J. Early outcome of total hip arthroplasty using the direct lateral vs the posterior surgical approach. *Orthopedics* (1996).

[51] Jolles, B. M, & Bogoch, E. R. Posterior versus lateral surgical approach for total hip arthroplasty in adults with osteoarthritis. *Cochrane Database Syst Rev* (2006). CD003828.

Chapter 2

# Predictors of Pain and Function Following Total Joint Replacement

Michelle M. Dowsey and Peter F. M. Choong

Additional information is available at the end of the chapter

## 1. Introduction

Osteoarthritis (OA) is one of the most disabling diseases in developed countries and is responsible for significant disability in over 43 million people worldwide, 27 million of whom are 60 years of age or older [1]. Age is the strongest predictor of the development and progression of osteoarthritis, as such the number of people suffering with OA is expected to continue to increase over the coming years due to the ageing population [2]. Other predictors associated with OA include; gender, obesity, physical inactivity, smoking, excess alcohol and injuries [2].

Total joint replacement is the treatment of choice (among suitably 'fit' candidates) for end-stage OA [3]. It is a high-cost and high-volume procedure, which dominates surgical waiting lists and this is expected to become critical with the rapidly ageing population [4]. The number of hip and knee replacement being performed each year has risen markedly over the past decade in most OECD countries [2]. On average, the rate of hip replacement has increased by over 25% and the rate of knee replacement has nearly doubled. While joint replacement surgery is mainly carried out in people aged 60 and over, the rate of surgery is also increasing in younger people due to the increasing prevalence of obesity, advances in surgery and greater patient demand.

Many studies have confirmed the beneficial impact of TJR on pain, disability and quality of life [5, 6]. However, surgery is not without risk. In the immediate post-operative period, there is a small but important risk of severe complications [7-9] and in the longer term there is the risk of prosthesis failure, primarily through loosening, resulting in the need for complex revision surgery [10]. While the majority can expect improvements in pain and function in the intermediate period, there is a minority who remain dissatisfied after TJR and this is despite procedurally excellent outcomes. There are a number of risk factors for continuing pain and disability after surgery and given the increasing demand for TJR, understanding more about the determinants of good and bad outcomes has become an imperative.

This chapter provides an overview of baseline patient characteristics and predictors associated with pain and function following total joint replacement.

## 2. Incidence

The incidence of dissatisfaction or suboptimal outcome following total joint replacement varies in the literature. Quantifying the influence of a single patient factor on the functional and quality of life outcomes in joint replacement is a complex process. Variations in reporting may in part be due to the range of instruments used to measure patient centred outcomes and the lack of consensus and consistency amongst health professionals in how these tools are used [11-14]. Furthermore, to understand the complexities of what contributes to a suboptimal outcome, large data sets with samples representative of the total study population and extensive follow-up are essential, however this is a labour intensive and challenging process.

In 1998 our institution established a joint replacement registry to respond to this issue and to contribute to our understanding of what constitutes and predicts a good versus poor outcome following TJR. The St Vincent's Total Joint Replacement Registry (SVHM JRR) currently contains over 8000 procedures undertaken in over 7000 consecutive patients, and grows by approximately 800 procedures each year. Data include patient demographics, diagnoses, and type of surgery, prostheses, co-morbidities and peri-operative interventions, and an extensive range of outcomes including death, re-hospitalisation and complications. The registry includes marginalised and disadvantaged groups and is characterised by i) cultural and linguistic diversity (15% from a non-English speaking background representing over 20 languages); ii) 15% rural representation; and iii) socio-economic diversity (20% are ranked as living in the most "disadvantaged" socio-economic areas (Australian Bureau of Statistics [15]). Since 2006, we have obtained near complete (> 99%) 12 month follow-up of our cohort. Pain and functional outcomes as well as quality of life (QoL) are measured using validated surveys including; the Harris Hip Score [13, 16], the International Knee Society Score[17, 18] and Short Form Health Survey[12, 13, 19].

From our registry and that of the literature, dissatisfaction (variously measured) is as high as 50% among patients undergoing total joint replacement [20-25]. The level of dissatisfaction amongst recipients of hip and knee replacement is considerably different with a much higher rate of satisfaction reported amongst patients undergoing hip than knee replacement.

### 2.1. Pain

Chronic pain is a major global health care problem reported in 1 in 5 adults. The major causes of non-cancer chronic pain are; arthritis (40%) and surgery or injury (25%). For many, chronic pain substantially impairs daily physical activities, social activities and ability to enjoy life [26]. It carries a major economic burden with estimated costs running into billions in many OECD countries; US$635 billion in America [27], EUR$32 billion in Sweden [28] and AU$34 billion in Australia [29].

Chronic disabling pain is the primary indicator for recommending TJR in those with radiographic evidence of arthritis. For those that present with early disease, conservative treatment modalities including physical and pharmacological therapies are the first line of treatment [30, 31] however arthritis is a progressive disease and non-surgical modalities can effectively delay but not negate the need for eventual surgical intervention. Surgical interventions such as arthroscopy, bone marrow stimulation or osteotomy, may be recommended in carefully selected patients, however TJR remains the most effective and cost effective intervention for relieving pain and restoring function in suitably fit patients [32, 33]

Total joint replacement is a major surgical procedure that requires multidisciplinary input prior to and after surgery to ensure the best possible outcome. Recovery from surgery is optimized with the inclusion of rehabilitation programs which are tailored to restore mobility and independence [34]. Time to recovery can vary following TJR and most patients will report substantial gains between 3 to 6 months after surgery. Patients undergoing THR report faster recovery in terms of both pain and function, with significant improvements occurring within the first 3 months of surgery [35]. In comparison patients undergoing TKR are more likely to report improvement between 3 to 6 months [36, 37]. Overall a continuing pattern of improvement can be observed up to 12 months following surgery [5, 38].

While on average a majority of patients report an improvement in pain following total joint replacement [39, 40] for a substantial number of individuals the level of improvement is suboptimal or does not meet expectation at 12 months or more after surgery. In total knee replacement ongoing pain has been reported in as many as 53% of patients and for hip replacement the incidence is as high as 38% (Table 1).

The causes of ongoing pain following TJR are not clearly understood. Recent literature reports a high prevalence of features of pain sensitisation in knee OA patients. Wylde et al (2011) identified 70% of patients as having various somatosensory abnormalities in a study of 117 knee OA patients [44]. Hochman et al (2011) reported neuropathic symptoms in 28% of older adults with chronic symptomatic knee OA [52]. Ohtori et al (2012) reported similar findings with neuropathic symptoms in as many as 20.6% of patients with radiographically confirmed knee OA [53]. These mechanisms of pain are not necessarily addressed by undergoing joint replacement.

Recent trials of the use of second-generation antiepileptic drugs (AED's), which are commonly used to treat neuropathic pain however, report mixed results in TJR studies. Both Gabapentin and Pregalbin use are associated with a reduction in post-operative opioid consumption following knee replacement [54, 55]. A randomized controlled trial comparing pre-operative Pregalbin to placebo has also reported a significant reduction in neuropathic pain at 6 months post TKR [54]. In contrast, Gabapentin had no effect on post-operative opioid consumption or pain scores at 6 months following total hip replacement [56]. While pre-operative Pregalbin has shown to reduce post-operative opioid consumption following THR, the longer term effects on post surgery pain have not been reported.

Overall higher rates of persistent pain are reported after knee replacement as compared to hip replacement (Table 1). Features of pain sensitisation and neuropathic type symptoms are also predominately reported in knee OA patients. This may explain the differences in response to AED's between hip and knee replacement recipients and is an indication that the underlying mechanisms of persistent pain following surgery differ according to the surgical site.

| Author | Cohort | Follow-up | Pain Measure | Incidence of Ongoing Pain |
|---|---|---|---|---|
| Liu et al 2012 [41] | TJR = 1030 | Minimum 1 year<br>32% response rate | McGill Pain Questionnaire [42] | Persistent pain<br>THR = 38.0%<br>TKR = 53.0% |
| Dowsey et al 2012 [40] | TKR = 478 | 99.4% at 1 year<br>93.5% at 2 years | IKSS [43] pain | Moderate to severe pain<br>29.5% at 12 months<br>30.6% at 2 years |
| Wylde et al 2011 [44] | THR = 909<br>TKR = 860 | 3 to 4 years<br>73.0% hip and knee | WOMAC [45] pain | Persistent pain<br>THR = 27.0%<br>TKR = 44.0% |
| Singh & Lewallen 2010 [46] | THR =<br>9,154 (2yrs)<br>6,243 (5yrs) | 62.3% at 2 years<br>52.7 at 5 years | Mayo [47] Hip Score | Moderate to severe pain<br>8.1% at 2 years<br>10.6% at 5 years |
| Czurda et al 2010 [5, 48] | TKR = 411 | 18 to 42 months<br>80.3% | WOMAC [45] pain | Knee pain<br>13.9% |
| Wylde et al 2009 [49] | THR = 1,534<br>TKR = 857 | 5 to 8 years<br>72.5% hip<br>71.5% knee | Oxford [50] pain | Moderate to severe pain<br>THR = 13.0%<br>TKR = 26.0% |
| Baker et al 2007 [51] | TKR = 9417 | 87.4% at 1 year | Oxford [50] pain | Persistent pain<br>19.8% at 1 year |

(IKSS – International Knee Society Score, WOMAC – Western Ontario and McMaster Universities Arthritis Index)

**Table 1.** Incidence of self reported pain > 12 months following TJR

## 2.2. Function

While arthritis accounts for 40% of non-cancer chronic pain it is the leading cause of disability in most developed countries. [57-59]. For many sufferers of arthritis even the most basic daily activities such as dressing, walking and stair climbing are substantially restricted. Pain and deformity associated with the progression of arthritis are the main contributors to impeding function and activity. As such joint replacement surgery that results in amelioration of pain and correction of deformity should lead to improved function and activity participation. However poor function and difficulty with daily activities have been reported up to 51% of TJR recipients, (Table 2).

A decrease in activity participation outside those required for basic daily functioning has also been noted in a proportion of patients who have undergone TJR. Wylde et.al interviewed 56 hip and 60 knee replacement patients about their leisure activities [60]. They reported that THR patients participated in 209 leisure activities but rated 82% of these activities as difficult to perform prior to surgery and TKR patients participated in 171 leisure activities 86% of which were rated as difficult to perform prior to surgery due to joint problems. At 1 year post surgery THR patients still rated 25% of leisure activities as difficult to perform and TKR patients rate 32% of leisure activities difficult to perform. In a larger study Groen et.al measured adherence to an activity regimen recommended to maintain health in patients who underwent total knee replacement and found that 42% of patients were not active enough to maintain their health and fitness [61].

| Author | Cohort | Follow-up | Functional Measure | Incidence of Functional Impairment |
|---|---|---|---|---|
| Dowsey et al 2012 [40] | TKR = 478 | 99.4% at 1 year<br>93.5% at 2 years | IKSS [43] function | Poor function<br>48.9% at 12 months<br>50.7% at 2 years |
| Wylde et al 2009 [49] | THR = 1,534<br>TKR = 857 | 5 to 8 years<br>72.5% hip<br>71.5% knee | Oxford [50] function | Extreme difficulty with individual activities<br>THR = 5% to 17%<br>TKR = 7% to 24% |
| Franklin et al 2008 [175] | TKJR = 17270 | 46.6% at 1 year | SF12 PCS [12] function | Function score worse than baseline = 19.0% |
| Lubbeke et al 2007 [62] | THR = 435 | 4 to 6 years<br>80.2% | HHS [16] function | Fair or poor function<br>9.0% |
| Nilsdotter et al 2003 [25] | THR = 211 | 26 to 65 months<br>94% | OARSI Criteria [63] | No improvement in function = 8.7% |
| Singh & Lewallen 2010 [64] | THR =<br>9,154 (2yrs)<br>6,243 (5yrs) | 62.3% at 2 years<br>52.7% at 5 years | Mayo [47] Hip Score | Moderate to severe activity limitation<br>30% at 2 years<br>35% at 5 years |
| Singh et al (2010) [126] | TKR =<br>10,957 (2 yrs)<br>7,404 (5yrs) | 65.0% at 2 years<br>57.0% at 5 years | IKSS [43] function | Moderate to severe activity limitation<br>20.7% at 2 years<br>27.1% at 5 years |

(SF-12 PCS – Short Form 12 Physical Component Summary, HHS – Harris Hip Score, OARSI – Osteoarthritis Research Society International

**Table 2.** Incidence of self reported functional impairment > 12 months following TJR

As function and activity levels depends on all other joints and systems, not just the joint being replaced, improvements may not be achieved as a result of joint replacement alone in patients who have multiple joint arthropathy or systemic health issues. Functional outcomes also seem to be dependent on the site of joint replacement (Table 2). Consistent with pain outcomes, a higher proportion of patients undergoing TKR report poor function or difficulty with activities than do patients undergoing THR. Demographic and patient characteristics are of predictive value in determining barriers to functional gain and activity participation following TJR recipients.

## 3. Predictors of pain and function

Intuitively, those who present with the "worst" symptoms might be those who should be prioritized for TJR. However, the literature reports a mismatch between patient reported symptom severity and response to surgery and it is becoming clearer that TJR outcomes are influenced by a multitude of factors. Recent work has identified a number of baseline risk factors for continuing pain and disability after TJR and these can be stratified into those which are modifiable and non-modifiable. Non-modifiable risk factors include; age, gender, socio-economic status, aetiology and culture and ethnicity. Modifiable risk factors include; psychological state, co-morbidities, obesity, baseline symptom severity and patient expectation.

Importantly, our work to date has demonstrated that a majority of baseline patient characteristics (obesity, mental health, co-morbidities, radiographic OA severity, baseline pain and function) associated with sub-optimal outcome following TJR are those that could be "modified" with appropriate intervention [8, 39, 40, 65]; hence there is opportunity to alter patient outcomes. Appreciating the nature of patient pre-operative risk factors and the impact of different outcomes is critical for improving response rates to surgery.

### 3.1. Patient demographics

#### *3.1.1. Age*

As age is the strongest predictor of the development and progression of osteoarthritis the ageing population has no doubt contributed to the world wide increase in TJR numbers. However, TJR in younger patients is also on the rise particularly for knee replacement [66], and this is likely due in part to the rising incidence of obesity in patients presenting for surgery [8, 39]. The median age at presentation for joint replacement demonstrates a downward trend over the past 10 years at our institution (Figure 1)

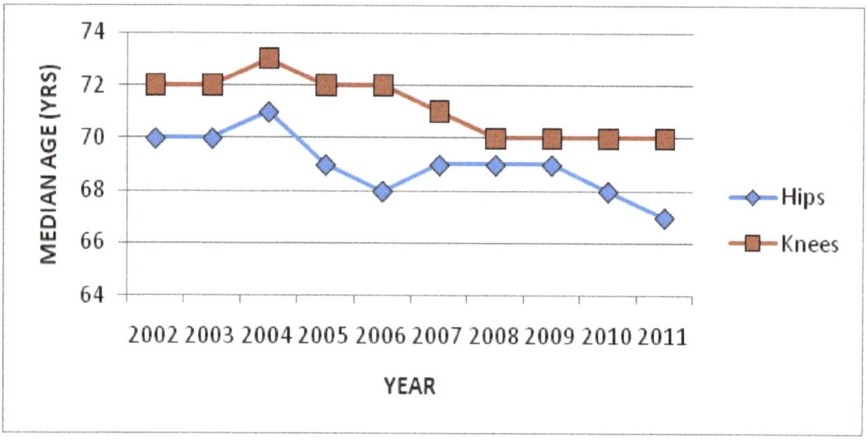


**Figure 1.** Median age at presentation for primary elective TJR (SVHM JRR)

Total joint replacement in the elderly carries a higher risk of peri-operative complication, requires a longer recovery time and is associated with a significant mortality rate in the longer term [67, 68]. However advancing age is not a barrier to pain and functional improvements after TJR surgery [67, 68] and excellent pain relief has been reported in individuals in their 80's and 90's [69-71]. While advancing age is associated with poorer function and activity levels following TJR [40] higher satisfaction with activity levels have been reported in those older than 70 years when compared to their younger counterparts [72].

*3.1.2. Gender*

Worldwide more females than males undergo joint replacement each year, with the greatest difference being for knee replacement. Various National Joint Replacement Registries report the ratio of females to males undergoing knee replacement as high as 2:1 and this concurs with gender patterns at our institution (Figure 2), [73-76]. Despite these figures inequities in referral patterns and reluctance in women to undergo joint replacement, resulting in late presentation have been reported [77, 78]. A gender bias in physician referral for knee replacement was identified in one study, with family physicians twice as likely and orthopaedic surgeons 22 times more likely to recommend knee replacement to male patients [79]. However it has also been identified that women delay seeking joint replacement until a later point in their functional decline [77].

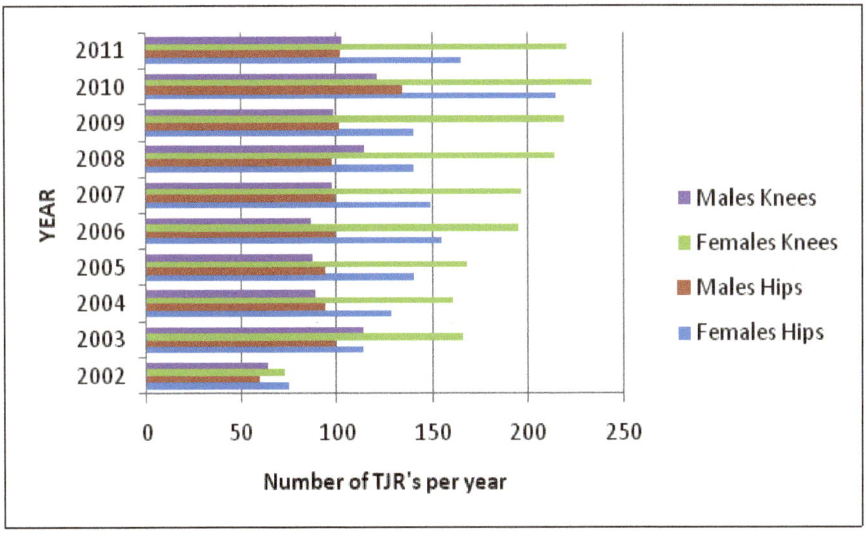


**Figure 2.** Gender breakdowns at presentation for primary elective TJR (SVHM JRR)

Females generally present with worse self-reported pain and functional impairment compared to males at the time hip and knee replacement [80-83], as such females do not tend to achieve the same level of physical function after surgery as males [84, 85]. However when taking into account baseline pain and function, women generally demonstrate greater improvements in pain and function scores after surgery than men [84-86]. Faster recoveries in terms of pain and function have also been reported in females undergoing total knee replacement when compared to males [87]. Despite this a significantly higher odds of poor function at 12 months (OR 1.81; 95% CI 1.08-3.03) and 2 years (OR 2.06; 95% CI 1.20 – 3.53) post knee replacement have been reported by women undergoing TKJR [40]. Impairment with specific activities such as stair climbing, despite achieving greater improvements in knee flexion, have also been reported in females compared to males [86]. These data suggest women may benefit from tailored rehabilitation programs following joint replacement surgery.

### *3.1.3. Socio-economic status*

Differences among nations in their socio-economic fabric, ethnic composition, health care systems and cultural expectations, may confound studies examining the importance of socioeconomic status as a predictor of outcome following TJR. Variations in classifications of socio-economic status also require that caution should be exercised in making direct comparisons between studies. To date studies have largely focused on socio-economic status in patients undergoing total hip replacement, with most data derived from cohorts in Western countries.

A large UK study by Jenkins et.al (2009) reported significant differences in SF-36 physical improvement between the least and most "deprived groups" 18 months post THR [88]. A study based in Scotland by Clement et.al (2011) reported similar findings. In a cohort of 1312 patients who underwent primary THR a significant improvement in Oxford scores across all socioeconomic categories was noted, however social deprivation predicted a poorer functional outcome [89]. In a smaller study based in the US, Allen-Butler et.al (2011) conducted a secondary analysis of a prospective randomised study originally comparing 2 different hip stems. They also concluded that individual socioeconomic parameters such as education level, household income, as well as being African American were associated with lower Harris Hips Scores up to 2 years post THR [90]. Finally a German based study by Schafer et.al (2010) also concluded that socioeconomic parameters independently predicted response to THR as measured using the WOMAC [91]. An increased risk for "non-response" to surgery at 6 months was demonstrated in widowed patients, those who lived alone, those on a disability pension and those who had a shorter duration of school education.

Only one study reported outcomes according to socioeconomic status in patients undergoing total knee replacement. In a multicentre study conducted in several countries (USA, UK, AU, Canada) socio-economic status did not appear to affect the outcome of knee replacement [92]. Socioeconomic data were derived from a pre-operative questionnaire regarding education, income, working status and living arrangements, to allow for direct comparison between countries. Despite reporting a correlation between lower income and worse pre-operative pain and function, there were no differences in post-operative pain and function at 24 months.

Despite variations in definitions and study designs, patient reported outcomes following THR are consistently poorer for disadvantaged groups. In contrast there is a dearth of literature on TKR with only one study that reported no differences in patient reported outcomes. Poorer outcomes in socioeconomically disadvantaged groups may occur as a result underutilization of health services [93] and this has important implications in relation to preparing disadvantaged patients for joint replacement surgery.

#### *3.1.4. Culture and ethnicity*

Racial and ethnic TJR utilization disparities exist and are likely due to a lower willingness to undergo surgery amongst ethnic minorities rather than lower disease prevalence [78, 94, 95]. Poor health literacy, financial constraints, cultural influences and concerns about possible outcomes are amongst reported reasons for a lower willingness to undergo surgery and delayed presentation [96-100]. As such self-reported baseline pain and function are worse amongst ethnic minorities presenting for total joint replacement surgery [100-103].

Substantial improvements in pain and function have been reported following primary total joint replacement irrespective of race and ethnicity however ethnic minorities do report worse outcomes following both hip and knee replacement surgery. Lavernia et al (2011) studied patient reported outcomes in a large cohort of hip and knee replacements (739 hips and 1010 knees) and found that ethnic minorities had worse pain, function and well-being scores 2 years after surgery compared to Whites and worse outcomes was most pronounced for African Americans [103]. Kamath et al (2010) reported similar findings for African-Americans undergoing TKJR [100]. In an Australian study of 237 TKR's, 41 were non-English speaking patients, Dowsey et al (2009) reported poorer International Knee Society pain and function scores at 12 months after surgery in those who required Interpreters compared to their English speaking counterparts[104]. A Swedish study analysed 1216 patients' pre and 1 year after THR, comparing those who were born inside and outside the country. Krupic et al (2012) reported lower self care and activity scores and more pain amongst those born abroad [102].

Promoting greater dialogue with health care providers and understanding the health literacy needs of ethnic minorities may help to address willingness to undergo joint replacement surgery and lead to better patient reported outcomes [105, 106].

### 3.2. Patient characteristics

#### *3.2.1. Aetiology*

Osteoarthritis is the principle diagnosis for a majority of total joint replacements performed each year [73-76]. In Australia it accounted for 88% of primary elective total hip replacement and 97% of primary elective knee replacement in 2010 [73]. The remaining diagnoses for elective THR included avascular necrosis (3.7%), dysplasia (1.3%) and rheumatoid arthritis (1.3%) and for TKR; rheumatoid arthritis (1.7%), inflammatory arthritis (0.5%) and necrosis (0.4%) [73].

Despite the worldwide increase in TJR numbers in recent years, the rate of joint replacement surgery in patients with rheumatoid arthritis has remained relatively stable and for some countries a decrease in numbers has been noted [107-110]. Contemporary treatment of rheumatoid arthritis now includes disease modifying medications or biologics, anti-tumour necrosis factor drugs and corticosteroids are proving to be more effective in the management of this immune disease when taken in combination as opposed to mono-therapy [111]. Despite advances in conservative management of rheumatoid arthritis, joint replacement remains a viable treatment option for those with significant joint pain and stiffness although joint destruction, osteoporosis and severe deformity make surgery technically challenging in this group [110]. Nevertheless rheumatoid patients demonstrate substantial improvements in pain, function and quality of life following TJR [112-115]. Although functional outcomes after surgery are inferior, rheumatoid patients report equivalent pain relief from TJR when compared to OA patients[110].

Aside from rheumatoid arthritis total hip replacement in young adults is generally reserved for those with developmental dysplasia (DDH) and slipped upper femoral epiphysis (SUFE). Anatomical abnormalities including acetabular or femoral deformity, leg length discrepancy and the age at which joint replacement is performed can contribute to higher failure rates observed in these patient compared to patients with osteoarthritis [73, 116, 117]. Setting aside the higher likelihood of revision surgery for patients who have hip replacement for DDH or SUFE in the longer term, post-operative outcome scores for these patients are comparable to patients with OA in the short term. No significant differences in Oxford hips scores at 6 months have been observed in THR patients with either DDH or SUFE when compared OA patients [118, 119]. Excellent functional outcomes have also been reported in patients with DDH under the age of 30 years with an average Harris Hips score of 90.6 at 9 [3-14] years follow-up [117]. Similar Harris Hip Scores (average 93) have been reported in THR for SUFE at 15 years follow-up [120].

### *3.2.2. Co-morbidities*

Individual comorbidities such as diabetes, cardiovascular and respiratory disease are commonly reported in patients undergoing TJR and many patients carry multiple comorbidities [7, 8, 39, 40, 121]. When reported as a composite, self-reported functional outcomes are poorer in patients with multiple comorbidities for both hip and knee replacement. Lingard et al (2004) reported an association with higher comorbidity and poorer SF-36 physical function scores at 1 year after knee replacement [122] and Gandhi et al (2010) reported similar findings at 3 [1–8] years [123]. In total hip replacement Young et al (2008) reported better functional outcomes following hip replacement in those had no comorbid disease [124].

Deyo-Charlson comorbidity index, a validated clinical comorbidity index [125] is an independent predictor of functional outcome in TJR. Singh & Lewallen (2010) studied activity limitation and dependence on walking aids in both hip and knee replacement patients 2 and 5 years after surgery. Deyo-Charlson comorbidity index independently predicted a greater reliance on walking aids at 2 and 5 years after both total hip and knee replacement and higher odds of moderate to severe activity limitation at 2 years after knee replacement [64, 126]. We have reported similar findings in patients undergoing TKR using an Age-Adjusted Charlson Comorbidity Index [127], demonstrating higher odds of reporting poor function at 2 years in those with a higher comorbidity index [40].

Very little is known about the effect of individual comorbidities on patient reported outcomes in TJR. A recent study of 677 consecutive primary knee and 547 consecutive primary hip replacements, demonstrated an association between metabolic syndrome risk factor and 1 year WOMAC scores [128]. Metabolic syndrome risk factors were self-reported and defined as body mass index >30kg/m$^2$, hypercholesterolemia, hypertension and diabetes. While increasing number of metabolic risk factors were associated with higher (worse) WOMAC scores, individual risk factors were found to better predict outcome. Obesity predicted higher WOMAC scores in both total hip and total knee replacement and hypertension also predicted higher WOMAC scores in total hip replacement only.

### *3.2.3. Obesity*

Obesity features prominently in the patho-physiological mechanisms underpinning OA especially end-stage OA requiring TJR [129]. Obesity affects 1 in 4 members of the community, but our data indicate a 2-3 fold over-representation of obesity in patients presenting for TJR (Figure 3). The economic impact of obesity-related OA in Australia was estimated to be $221.3 million in 2005 [130]. While the real costs of treating obese patients with TJR remain unknown, we have demonstrated higher episode of care costs for TKR in the first 12 months

(+$1,821[95% CI $245, $3,398]; p=0.024) in a comparative cohort of 520 patients [131]. The cost of THR is also estimated to be higher for obese ($523) and morbidly obese patients, ($1,432) patients [132]. In addition to the increasing overrepresentation of obese patients presenting for TJR (Figure 3) our data demonstrates that the severity of obesity is also increasing over time (Figure 4), as such developing strategies to reduce the burden of obesity-related joint disease should be an imperative [133].

Weight loss in obese patients awaiting TJR is a problem because the symptoms of disabling arthritis may limit an individual's ability to exercise. Patients often identify this as the reason for the inability to lose weight, and believe that joint replacement would be critical for weight loss. However, numerous studies have confirmed that undergoing total joint replacement does not result in clinically significant weight loss and as many as one-third of patients gain weight at 12 months after surgery [8, 39, 134-140]. It has also been demonstrated that weight gain continues to increase over time after joint replacement [141].

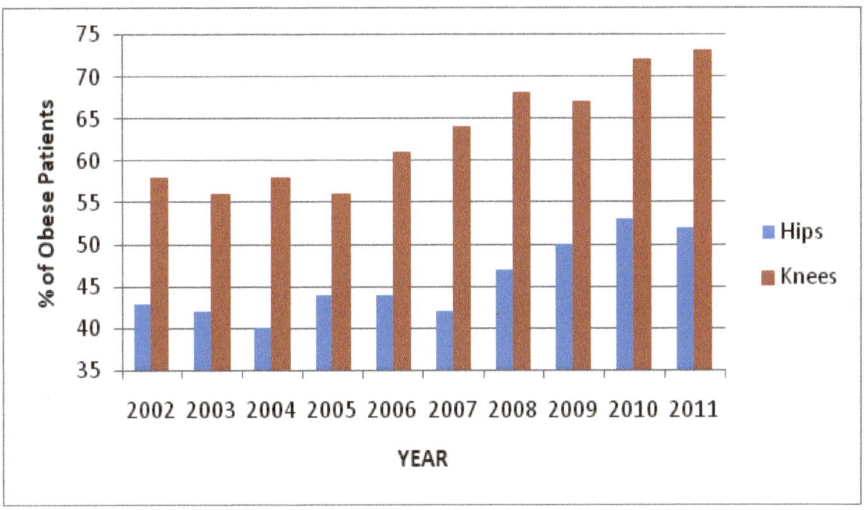


**Figure 3.** Obesity rates in OA patients at presentation for primary elective TJR (SVHM JRR)

Data from our registry demonstrates that both the number of obese patients presenting for joint replacement (Figure 3) and the average BMI of patients is increasing over time, particularly in the past 5 years. Of note there are higher rates of obesity and a more rapid rise in average BMI demonstrated amongst recipients of knee replacement compared to recipients of hip replacement, with females undergoing knee replacement recording the highest BMI average.

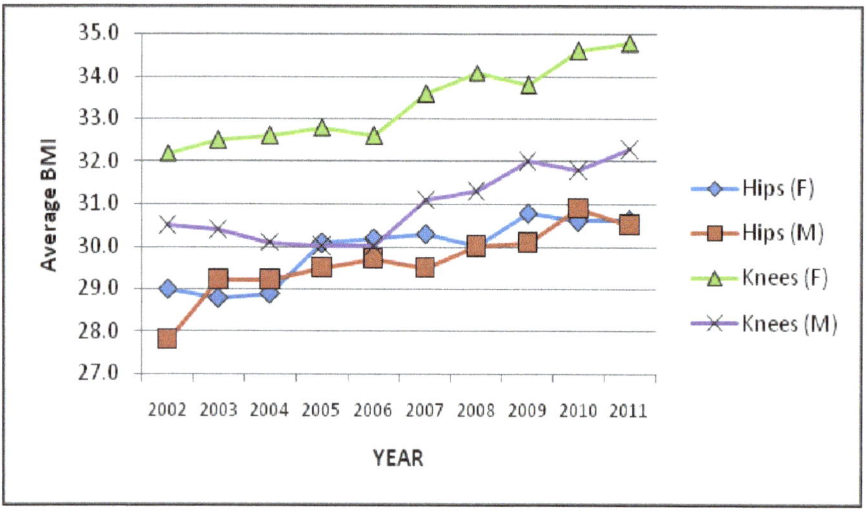


**Figure 4.** Mean BMI of OA patients at presentation for primary elective TJR (SVHM JRR)

Although widely reported there remains disagreement in the literature as to the impact of obesity on patient reported outcomes following TJR. Numerous reviews confirm that obese patients report substantial improvements in pain and function following joint replacement surgery [142-145]. However when limited to level 1 studies [146], the evidence does suggests that obese and particularly morbidly obese patients may not achieve the same level of functional improvement after TJR when compared to non-obese patients in both the short and longer term.

*3.2.3.1. Outcomes for primary THR*

Obesity and advancing BMI have been shown to have a negative impact on pain and more so function after primary elective total hip replacement in both the short and longer term. Functional gains and activity levels after THR remain poorer for obese when compared to non-obese individuals. Obese groups also report worse pain and higher usage of pain medication after THR. A review of level 1 large cohort studies is presented.

Moran et al (2005) compared functional and QoL outcomes using the Harris Hip Score (HHS) and Short-Form-36 (SF-36) in 800 patients undergoing total hip replacement, pre surgery (100% follow-up) and at 6 (97% follow-up) and 18 months (86% follow-up) [147]. BMI was found to be a significant predictor of poorer function at both 6 and 18 months. The authors concluded that the difference between obese and non-obese scores were small and therefore not clinically significant, however this was based on comparing post-operative scores only and the change in scores between groups was not provided.

Gandhi et al (2010) investigated the influence of self-reported metabolic syndrome risk factors defined as obesity, hypertension, hypercholesterolemia and diabetes on patient function in a consecutive cohort of 547 primary hip replacements [128]. As measured using the WOMAC obesity was associated with higher odds (2.4; 95% CI 1.4 – 4.2) of less functional improvement at 12 months after surgery.

Dowsey et al (2010) compared pain, function (HHS) and quality of life (SF-12) in a consecutive cohort of 471 primary THR's with 98.5% follow-up. Function and physical health scores were worse at baseline and 12 months after surgery for obese and morbidly obese patients. Baseline mental health scores were also worse in obese and morbidly obese patients, however were comparable at 12 months with obese patients demonstrating a significantly greater improvement in scores compared to non-obese patients [39].

Lubbeke et.al (2007) reported significantly poorer functional outcomes in obese patients (n=182), who underwent primary THR compared to non-obese patients (n=635), at 5 years follow-up, as measured using the Harris Hip Score [148]. Eighty-one percent of hips in the non obese group and 70% in the obese group had a good to excellent results according to their HHS. When broken down by gender it was obese females who demonstrated significantly poorer outcomes compared to non-obese females with very little differences in outcomes demonstrated between obese and non obese males.

Singh & Lewallen (2010) measured activity limitation and dependence on walking aids in 5,707 patients at 2 years and 3,289 patients at 5 years after primary total hip replacement [64]. Predictors of moderate to severe activity limitation (defined as limitation in 3 or more activities), included BMI > 30kg/m$^2$ at both time intervals. Obese (BMI > 30kg/m$^2$) patients had higher odds of complete dependence on a walking aid at 2 years and severely obese (BMI >35kg/m$^2$) had a higher odds of complete dependence on a waking aid at 5 years.

Singh & Lewallen (2010) also examined pain as measured by the Mayo Hip Score and the use of pain medications at 2 and 5 years following primary total hip replacement in the same cohort of patients [46]. The odds of reporting ongoing moderate to severe pain at 2 years after surgery were higher in those with a BMI 35-39.9kg/m$^2$ (OR 1.8; 95% CI 1.2 – 2.4) and BMI > 40kg/m$^2$ (1.7; 95% CI 1.0 – 2.9) compared to those with a BMI < 25kg/m$^2$. At 5 years the odds of reporting ongoing moderate to severe pain was higher for all weight groups compared to the baseline group; BMI 25 – 29.9kg/m$^2$, (OR 1.5; 95% CI 1.1 – 2.1); BMI 30-34.9kg/m$^2$, (OR 1.8; 95% CI 1.2 – 2.6); BMI 35-39.9kg/m$^2$, (OR 1.9; 95% CI 1.2 – 3.1); and BMI > 40kg/m$^2$, (OR 3.1 95% CI 1.7 – 5.7). BMI 35-39kg/m$^2$ was also a predictor of non-steroidal anti-inflammatory use at 2 years and BMI 30-34.9kg/m$^2$ predicted use of opioid medication at 5 years after THR.

*3.2.3.2. Outcomes for primary TKR*

Obesity and advancing BMI have been shown to have a negative impact on function after primary elective total knee replacement in both the short and longer term. Functional gains and activity levels after TKR are poorer for obese when compared to non-obese individuals.

Obese groups however do report comparable pain outcomes compared to non-obese patients after surgery. A review of level 1 large cohort studies is presented.

Gandhi et al (2010) investigated the influence of self-reported metabolic syndrome risk factors defined as obesity, hypertension, hypercholesterolemia and diabetes on patient function in a consecutive cohort of 677 primary knee replacements with 83% follow-up [128]. As measured using the WOMAC, obesity (BMI > 30kg/m$^2$) was associated with higher odds (3.6; 95% CI 0.02 – 7.2) of less functional improvement at 12 months after surgery.

Rajgopal et al (2008) compared functional outcomes between morbidly obese (BMI > 40kg/m$^2$) and non-morbidly obese (BMI < 40kg/m$^2$) patients 12 months after total knee replacement in a series of 550 patients; of which 69 patients were classified as morbidly obese [149]. BMI ≥ 40 predicted 12 month WOMAC scores (coefficient −5.188, 95% CI −9.771 −0.606), however no differences in the change in WOMAC or SF-12 scores were demonstrated when comparing morbidly obese to non-morbidly obese patients.

We also measured improvement in pain, function and quality of life from baseline to 12 months following elective primary knee replacement in consecutive series of 529 patients with 98% follow-up [8]. The change in IKSS function scores were 10 points lower for both obese (BMI > 30kg/m$^2$) and morbidly obese (BMI > 40kg/m2) patients compared to non-obese (BMI <30kg/m$^2$), (p=0.002). No significant difference in IKSS pain scores was noted between the 3 groups at baseline or 12 months and there was no significant difference in SF-12 scores between the 3 groups at baseline or 12 months.

Singh et al (2010) measured activity limitation in 4,701 patients at 2 years and 2,395 patients at 5 years after primary knee replacement [126]. Predictors of moderate to severe activity limitation (defined as limitation in 3 or more activities), included all BMI groups > 30 compared to BMI < 25kg/m$^2$ at 2 years after surgery; BMI 30-34.9kg/m$^2$, (OR 1.5; 95% CI 1.0 – 2.0); BMI 35-39.9kg/m$^2$, (OR 1.8; 95% CI 1.3 – 2.7); and BMI > 40kg/m$^2$, (OR 3.0 95% CI 2.0 – 4.5). Higher BMI also predicted moderate to severe activity limitation at 5 years; BMI 35-39.9kg/m$^2$, (OR 2.1; 95% CI 1.4 – 3.3); and BMI > 40kg/m$^2$, (OR 3.9 95% CI, 2.3 – 6.5).

Sing et al (2011) also examined whether BMI was associated with pain as measured using the IKSS after primary knee replacement at 2 and 5 years after surgery [150]. Patients were classified into BMI groups as above for comparison. In contrast to their study on activity limitation, there was no association demonstrated between BMI and ongoing moderate to severe pain at either 2 or 5 years after TKR.

Our findings mirror that of Singh et al (2010 & 2011). We reported pain and function outcomes in a cohort of 478 consecutive primary elective total knee replacements at 1 and 2 years post surgery with 99% and 94% follow-up respectively [40]. Each incremental increase in BMI significantly increased the odds of poor function as measured using the IKSS at 12 months (OR 1.07, 95% CI 1.03 – 1.12) and at 2 years (OR 1.09, 95% CI 1.05 – 1.14). However we found no association between advancing BMI and ongoing moderate to severe pain at either time point.

### 3.2.4. Psychosocial state

Psychological distress leading to patient dissatisfaction after TJR is an important cause for TJR failure. Pre-operative psychological distress is associated with excessive analgesic intake and higher rates of hospital readmission and long term mortality [151]. Our research has also drawn a link between poorer pre-operative mental health and weight gain after TJR [39]. Published results from the SVHM TJR cohort and that of others have i) identified a high rate (30-60%) of self-reported psychological distress in TJR patients [152-154] and ii) determined that pre-operative psychological distress is an independent risk factor for poorer post-operative outcomes after surgery [8, 65]. A number of recent comprehensive literature reviews have found pre-operative psychological distress to be an independent predictor of pain and function after TKR in a majority of published studies [155, 156].

Psychological co-morbidities and traits reported in TJR patients include; anxiety, depression, neuroticism, catastrophising and poor self-esteem. These individual traits and poorer pre-operative mental health scores in general are associated with poorer function and/or greater pain after TJR in the short and longer term.

In general pre-operative psychological distress is associated with poorer pain and worst function 1 year after total joint replacement. We have reported an association between lower SF-12 MCS scores and risk for ongoing moderate to severe pain and poor function at 12 months and 2 years following TKR. Lingard et al (2004) also reported an association between lower SF-36 MCS scores and worse WOMAC pains scores at 1 and 2 years after TKR [122]. An analysis of pre-operative and one-year post-operative data in 6,158 patients from the Swedish Hip Arthroplasty Register, also demonstrated that anxiety/depression measured on the EQ-5D [157] was a strong predictor of pain after THR [158].

Anxiety is a psychological and physiological state characterized by somatic, emotional, cognitive, and behavioural components [159]. Anxiety can occur as a result of transient negative stimuli such as in a threatening situation and this is referred to as state anxiety. In contrast trait anxiety is referred to as a general tendency to experience anxiety [160]. In patients undergoing total hip replacement trait anxiety has shown to correlate with impaired health related quality of life 3 to 6 months after surgery [161, 162]. In contrast state anxiety had no effect on outcome suggesting pre-existing anxiety disorder rather than anxiety induced by fear of surgery predicts poorer outcomes form joint replacement.

Pre-existing depression has been shown to predict greater pain and poorer function in patients undergoing total knee replacement at 1 year and it has also been demonstrated that worse outcomes persist at 5 years [20, 163]. However this finding is not consistent, with some studies suggesting that there is no association between depression measured prior to surgery and pain and function outcomes following TJR. Of note Riddles et al (2010) measured the association between a range of psychological comorbidities including depression, anxiety and panic disorders, self efficacy and fear of movement and found that only pain catastrophising predicted poorer pain outcomes after total knee replacement [164],

Pain catastrophising has been described as a tendency to magnify or exaggerate the threat value or seriousness of pain sensations [165]. Pre-operative pain catastrophising is a predictor of worse post-surgical pain following TKR in the short (6 weeks and 6 months) term, but does not correlate with function [164, 166]. The correlation between catastrophising and poorer post-operative pain has also been shown to persist at 24 months following TKR [167]. To date the link between pain catastrophising and post operative pain after TJR seems to be unique to knee replacement, with no evidence of pain catastrophising in total hip replacement patients.

Neuroticism is a personality trait described as an enduring tendency to experience negative emotional states [168]. There is a dearth of literature examining the association between neuroticism and TJR, however one study on total hip replacement did report that neuroticism was amongst a number of psychological traits that predicted poorer quality of life outcomes at 6 months after surgery [162].

### 3.3. Baseline symptom severity

Total joint replacement is most often performed for the management of "end-stage' arthritis characterised by retractable pain, loss of function and deformity [30]. According to the NIH statements for both hip and knee replacement, candidates for elective TJR should have radiographic evidence of joint damage, moderate-to-severe persistent pain that is not adequately relieved by an extended course of nonsurgical management, and clinically significant functional limitation resulting in diminished quality of life [32, 33]. However there is discordance between radiographic changes and patient reported symptom severity at presentation for surgery, with some people receiving joint replacement reporting severe preoperative symptoms of pain and disability and mild radiographic changes [80, 83].

#### *3.3.1. Baseline clinical symptoms*

Baseline symptom severity is a predictor of outcome for both total hip and knee replacement. Several studies have concluded that those with worse pain and poor function at the time of surgery also report comparatively worse pain and function after surgery, suggesting that surgery could be prioritized based on clinical symptom severity [169].

In a multicentre study involving more than 200 hip and knee replacements Fortin et al (1999] reported that lower preoperative physical function scores predicted worse WOMAC pain and function at 6 months compared to those with higher baseline function scores [170]. Fortin et al (2002) continued to follow the cohort up at 2 years post surgery and confirmed that their initial findings at 6 months persisted [169], concluding that undergoing surgery earlier in the course of functional decline may be associated with better outcome.

In a larger study involving 860 recipients of primary TKR from 3 different countries, Lingard et al (2004) reported that worse baseline WOMAC pain scores were a strong determinant of worse pain at 1 and 2 years after surgery. Pre-operative WOMAC function was also the strongest predictor of worse function at both 1 and 2 years after surgery [122].

### *3.3.2. Baseline radiographic characteristics*

In contrast to clinical symptoms emerging literature suggests that those with the worst radiographic OA symptoms report better outcomes after total joint replacement.

We recently evaluated the association between pre-operative radiographic changes and outcomes after primary total knee replacement for osteoarthritis. We reported that pain relief was unsatisfactory in about 30% and functional improvement suboptimal in about 50% of patients [40]. In this study radiographic OA severity was measured using a modified version of the Kellgren-Lawrence Classification system [80]. We noted that radiographic OA severity was an independent predictor of pain and function at 12 months following TKR. Patients with evidence of mild radiographic OA changes were 5 times more likely (OR 5.39, 95% CI 1.23 – 15.69) to report moderate to severe pain at 12 months post TKR than those with severe radiographic changes.

Merle-Vincent et al (2011) examined predictors of satisfaction in 299 patients undergoing primary TKR and reported an association between radiographic OA severity and outcome 2 years after surgery [171]. Those with severe pre-operative joint space narrowing were nearly 4 times more likely to report satisfaction with surgery at 2 years compared to those with mild to moderate narrowing, (OR 3.9, 95% CI 1.1 – 14.3).

Valdes et al (2012) examined predictors of chronic pain using the WOMAC in 860 patients who had undergone TKR and 928 patients who had undergone THR with an average of 3.2 years follow-up [172]. They reported an OR 1.56 (95% CI 1.04 – 2.36) of ongoing pain in TKR patients with a Kellgren-Lawrence grade <3 and in THR patients with minimal joint space narrowing (>2mm width).

Cushnaghan et al (2007) reported on long term (approximately 8 years) functional outcomes following THR in a series of 282 patients matched with 295 community controls [173]. Radiographic OA severity defined as Croft grade 5 OA[174] was a predictor of greater functional improvement in cases as measured using the SF-36 physical function scores (19.4, 95% CI 7.7 – 31.2), when compared to cases with Croft grade < 3.

These findings suggest an inverse relationship between baseline radiographic OA and outcome up to 8 years following total joint replacement. More severe radiographic changes predict worse pain and to a lesser degree suboptimal function after surgery, providing important implications for timing of joint replacement.

## 4. Conclusion

Total joint replacement is the most effective and cost effective treatment for end-stage osteoarthritis. Most patients derive substantial benefits from joint replacement surgery; however those that don't are subject to chronic pain and disability and a higher risk for revision surgery. The causes of poor outcomes of surgery are multifactorial but almost certainly patient selection is a key determinant. While those who present with the "worst" symptoms might be those who should be prioritized for TJR, the literature reports a mismatch between patient reported symptom severity and response to surgery. Although many risk factors are recognised, their individual or combined contributions to the *absolute risk* of suboptimal outcome after TJR remains poorly quantified. Importantly a majority of baseline patient characteristics (obesity, mental health, co-morbidities, radiographic OA severity, baseline pain and function) associated with sub-optimal outcome following TJR are those that could be "modified" with appropriate intervention. However baseline risk factors tend to remain unidentified or identified and managed at the point of surgery, which is too late. Hence there remains a need for exploring early interventions where there is opportunity to alter patient outcomes.

## Acknowledgements

Dr Dowsey holds an NHMRC Early Career Australian Clinical Fellowship (APP1035810)

## Author details

Michelle M. Dowsey[1] and Peter F. M. Choong[2]

1 University of Melbourne, Department of Surgery, St. Vincent's Hospital Melbourne, Australia

2 Department of Orthopaedics, St. Vincent's Hospital Melbourne, Australia

## References

[1] World Health Organization. World Report on Disability. Malta: WHO; 2011 [cited 06/08/2012. Available from: http://www.who.int/disabilities/world_report/2011/en/index.html.

[2] Organization for Economic Co-operation and Development. Health at a Glance 2011: OECD Indicators. Heatlh Care Activities: 47 Hip and Knee Replacement [serial on the Internet]. 2011 06/08/2012]: Available from: http://www.oecd-ilibrary.org.

[3] Wang Y, Simpson JA, Wluka AE, Teichtahl AJ, English DR, Giles GG, et al. Relationship between body adiposity measures and isk of primary knee and hip replacement for osteoarthritis: a prospective cohort study. Arthritis Res Ther. 2009;11(2):R31.

[4] Productivity Commission. Economic implications of an aging Australia. Austrtalian Government Research Report (Canberra, 2005).

[5] Nilsdotter AK, Toksvig-Larsen S, Roos EM. A 5 year prospective study of patient-relevant outcomes after total knee replacement. Osteoarthritis Cartilage. 2009 May; 17(5):601-6.

[6] Santaguida PL, Hawker GA, Hudak PL, Glazier R, Mahomed NN, Kreder HJ, et al. Patient characteristics affecting the prognosis of total hip and knee joint arthroplasty: a systematic review. Can J Surg. 2008 Dec;51(6):428-36.

[7] Dowsey MM, Choong PF. Obese diabetic patients are at substantial risk for deep infection after primary TKA. Clin Orthop Relat Res. 2009 Jun;467(6):1577-81.

[8] Dowsey MM, Liew D, Stoney JD, Choong PF. The impact of pre-operative obesity on weight change and outcome in total knee replacement: a prospective study of 529 consecutive patients. J Bone Joint Surg Br. 2010 Apr;92(4):513-20.

[9] Malviya A, Martin K, Harper I, Muller SD, Emmerson KP, Partington PF, et al. Enhanced recovery program for hip and knee replacement reduces death rate. Acta Orthop. 2011 Oct;82(5):577-81.

[10] Australian Orthopaedic Association. National Joint Replacement Registry. Annual Report. Adelaide:AOA. 2010; Available from: www.dmac.adelaide.edu.au/aoanjrr/publications.jsp..

[11] Ashby E, Grocott MP, Haddad FS. Outcome measures for orthopaedic interventions on the hip. J Bone Joint Surg Br. 2008 May;90(5):545-9.

[12] Dunbar MJ, Robertsson O, Ryd L, Lidgren L. Appropriate questionnaires for knee arthroplasty. Results of a survey of 3600 patients from The Swedish Knee Arthroplasty Registry. J Bone Joint Surg Br. 2001 Apr;83(3):339-44.

[13] Ostendorf M, van Stel HF, Buskens E, Schrijvers AJ, Marting LN, Verbout AJ, et al. Patient-reported outcome in total hip replacement. A comparison of five instruments of health status. J Bone Joint Surg Br. 2004 Aug;86(6):801-8.

[14] Pollard B, Johnston M, Dieppe P. What do osteoarthritis health outcome instruments measure? Impairment, activity limitation, or participation restriction? J Rheumatol. 2006 Apr;33(4):757-63.

[15] Australian Bureau of Statistics. Postal Area (POA) Index of Relative Socio-economic Advantage and Disadvantage. Canberra: Commonwealth of Australia; 2008 [Accessed 1/2/2011]; Available from: www.abs.gov.au.

[16] Harris WH. Traumatic arthritis of the hip after dislocation and acetabular fractures: treatment by mold arthroplasty. An end-result study using a new method of result evaluation. J Bone Joint Surg Am. 1969 Jun;51(4):737-55.

[17] Bach CM, Nogler M, Steingruber IE, Ogon M, Wimmer C, Gobel G, et al. Scoring systems in total knee arthroplasty. Clin Orthop Relat Res. 2002 Jun(399):184-96.

[18] Davies AP. Rating systems for total knee replacement. Knee. 2002 Dec;9(4):261-6.

[19] Sanderson K, Andrews G. The SF-12 in the Australian population: cross-validation of item selection. Aust N Z J Public Health. 2002 Aug;26(4):343-5.

[20] Brander VA, Stulberg SD, Adams AD, Harden RN, Bruehl S, Stanos SP, et al. Predicting total knee replacement pain: a prospective, observational study. Clin Orthop Relat Res. 2003 Nov(416):27-36.

[21] Dickstein R, Heffes Y, Shabtai EI, Markowitz E. Total knee arthroplasty in the elderly: patients' self-appraisal 6 and 12 months postoperatively. Gerontology. 1998;44(4): 204-10.

[22] Jones CA, Beaupre LA, Johnston DW, Suarez-Almazor ME. Total joint arthroplasties: current concepts of patient outcomes after surgery. Rheum Dis Clin North Am. 2007 Feb;33(1):71-86.

[23] Jones CA, Voaklander DC, Johnston DW, Suarez-Almazor ME. Health related quality of life outcomes after total hip and knee arthroplasties in a community based population. J Rheumatol. 2000 Jul;27(7):1745-52.

[24] Mancuso CA, Salvati EA, Johanson NA, Peterson MG, Charlson ME. Patients' expectations and satisfaction with total hip arthroplasty. J Arthroplasty. 1997 Jun;12(4): 387-96.

[25] Nilsdotter AK, Petersson IF, Roos EM, Lohmander LS. Predictors of patient relevant outcome after total hip replacement for osteoarthritis: a prospective study. Ann Rheum Dis. 2003 Oct;62(10):923-30.

[26] European Federation of ISAP chapters. EFICF's declaration on pain as a major health problem, a disease in its own right: Available from: http://www.iasp-pain.org/AM/Template.cfm?Section=Press_Release&Template=/CM/ContentDisplay.cfm&ContentID=2908.

[27] (IOM) Institute of Medicine. Relieving pain in America: A Blueprint for Transforming Prevention, Care, Education and Research. Washington DC, 2011.

[28] Gustavsson A, Bjorkman J, Ljungcrantz C, Rhodin A, Rivano-Fischer M, Sjolund KF, et al. Socio-economic burden of patients with a diagnosis related to chronic pain--register data of 840,000 Swedish patients. Eur J Pain. 2012 Feb;16(2):289-99.

[29] Access Economics. The high price of pain: the economic impact of persistent pain in Australia: MBF Foundation in conjunction with the University of Sydney, 2007.

[30] Choong PF, Dowsey MM. Update in surgery for osteoarthritis of the knee. Int J Rheum Dis. 2011 May;14(2):167-74.

[31] Sinusas K. Osteoarthritis: diagnosis and treatment. Am Fam Physician. 2012 Jan 1;85(1):49-56.

[32] NIH consensus conference: Total hip replacement. NIH Consensus Development Panel on Total Hip Replacement. JAMA. 1995 Jun 28;273(24):1950-6.

[33] NIH Consensus Statement on total knee replacement December 8-10, 2003. J Bone Joint Surg Am. 2004 Jun;86-A(6):1328-35.

[34] Jones CA, Beaupre LA, Johnston DW, Suarez-Almazor ME. Total joint arthroplasties: current concepts of patient outcomes after surgery. Clin Geriatr Med. 2005 Aug;21(3): 527-41, vi.

[35] Laupacis A, Bourne R, Rorabeck C, Feeny D, Wong C, Tugwell P, et al. The effect of elective total hip replacement on health-related quality of life. J Bone Joint Surg Am. 1993 Nov;75(11):1619-26.

[36] Shields RK, Enloe LJ, Leo KC. Health related quality of life in patients with total hip or knee replacement. Arch Phys Med Rehabil. 1999 May;80(5):572-9.

[37] Rissanen P, Aro S, Sintonen H, Slatis P, Paavolainen P. Quality of life and functional ability in hip and knee replacements: a prospective study. Qual Life Res. 1996 Feb; 5(1):56-64.

[38] Huang NF, Dowsey MM, Ee E, Stoney JD, Babazadeh S, Choong PF. Coronal Alignment Correlates With Outcome After Total Knee Arthroplasty: Five-Year Follow-Up of a Randomized Controlled Trial. J Arthroplasty. 2012 Aug 3.

[39] Dowsey MM, Liew D, Stoney JD, Choong PF. The impact of obesity on weight change and outcomes at 12 months in patients undergoing total hip arthroplasty. Med J Aust. 2010 Jul 5;193(1):17-21.

[40] Dowsey MM, Nikpour M, Dieppe P, Choong PF. Associations between pre-operative radiographic changes and outcomes after total knee joint replacement for osteoarthritis. Osteoarthritis Cartilage. 2012 Jul 16.

[41] Liu SS, Buvanendran A, Rathmell JP, Sawhney M, Bae JJ, Moric M, et al. A Cross-Sectional Survey on Prevalence and Risk Factors for Persistent Postsurgical Pain 1 Year After Total Hip and Knee Replacement. Reg Anesth Pain Med. 2012 Jul;37(4):415-22.

[42] Melzack R. The McGill Pain Questionnaire: major properties and scoring methods. Pain. 1975 Sep;1(3):277-99.

[43] Insall JN, Dorr LD, Scott RD, Scott WN. Rationale of the Knee Society clinical rating system. Clin Orthop Relat Res. 1989 Nov(248):13-4.

[44] Wylde V, Hewlett S, Learmonth ID, Dieppe P. Persistent pain after joint replacement: prevalence, sensory qualities, and postoperative determinants. Pain. 2011 Mar;152(3): 566-72.

[45] Bellamy N, Buchanan WW, Goldsmith CH, Campbell J, Stitt LW. Validation study of WOMAC: a health status instrument for measuring clinically important patient relevant outcomes to antirheumatic drug therapy in patients with osteoarthritis of the hip or knee. J Rheumatol. 1988 Dec;15(12):1833-40.

[46] Singh JA, Lewallen D. Predictors of pain and use of pain medications following primary Total Hip Arthroplasty (THA): 5,707 THAs at 2-years and 3,289 THAs at 5-years. BMC Musculoskelet Disord. 2010;11:90.

[47] Kavanagh BF, Fitzgerald RH, Jr. Clinical and roentgenographic assessment of total hip arthroplasty. A new hip score. Clin Orthop Relat Res. 1985 Mar(193):133-40.

[48] Czurda T, Fennema P, Baumgartner M, Ritschl P. The association between component malalignment and post-operative pain following navigation-assisted total knee arthroplasty: results of a cohort/nested case-control study. Knee Surg Sports Traumatol Arthrosc. 2010 Jul;18(7):863-9.

[49] Wylde V, Blom AW, Whitehouse SL, Taylor AH, Pattison GT, Bannister GC. Patient-reported outcomes after total hip and knee arthroplasty: comparison of midterm results. J Arthroplasty. 2009 Feb;24(2):210-6.

[50] Dawson J, Fitzpatrick R, Murray D, Carr A. Questionnaire on the perceptions of patients about total knee replacement. J Bone Joint Surg Br. 1998 Jan;80(1):63-9.

[51] Baker PN, van der Meulen JH, Lewsey J, Gregg PJ. The role of pain and function in determining patient satisfaction after total knee replacement. Data from the National Joint Registry for England and Wales. J Bone Joint Surg Br. 2007 Jul;89(7):893-900.

[52] Hochman JR, Gagliese L, Davis AM, Hawker GA. Neuropathic pain symptoms in a community knee OA cohort. Osteoarthritis Cartilage. 2011 Jun;19(6):647-54.

[53] Ohtori S, Orita S, Yamashita M, Ishikawa T, Ito T, Shigemura T, et al. Existence of a neuropathic pain component in patients with osteoarthritis of the knee. Yonsei Med J. 2012 Jul 1;53(4):801-5.

[54] Buvanendran A, Kroin JS, Della Valle CJ, Kari M, Moric M, Tuman KJ. Perioperative oral pregabalin reduces chronic pain after total knee arthroplasty: a prospective, randomized, controlled trial. Anesth Analg. 2010 Jan 1;110(1):199-207.

[55] Clarke H, Pereira S, Kennedy D, Gilron I, Katz J, Gollish J, et al. Gabapentin decreases morphine consumption and improves functional recovery following total knee arthroplasty. Pain Res Manag. 2009 May-Jun;14(3):217-22.

[56] Clarke H, Pereira S, Kennedy D, Andrion J, Mitsakakis N, Gollish J, et al. Adding gabapentin to a multimodal regimen does not reduce acute pain, opioid consumption or chronic pain after total hip arthroplasty. Acta Anaesthesiol Scand. 2009 Sep;53(8): 1073-83.

[57] Dunlop DD, Manheim LM, Yelin EH, Song J, Chang RW. The costs of arthritis. Arthritis Rheum. 2003 Feb 15;49(1):101-13.

[58] Mathers CD, Vos ET, Stevenson CE, Begg SJ. The Australian Burden of Disease Study: measuring the loss of health from diseases, injuries and risk factors. Med J Aust. 2000 Jun 19;172(12):592-6.

[59] Yelin E, Murphy L, Cisternas MG, Foreman AJ, Pasta DJ, Helmick CG. Medical care expenditures and earnings losses among persons with arthritis and other rheumatic conditions in 2003, and comparisons with 1997. Arthritis Rheum. 2007 May;56(5): 1397-407.

[60] Wylde V, Livesey C, Blom AW. Restriction in participation in leisure activities after joint replacement: an exploratory study. Age Ageing. 2012 Mar;41(2):246-9.

[61] Groen JW, Stevens M, Kersten RF, Reininga IH, van den Akker-Scheek I. After total knee arthroplasty, many people are not active enough to maintain their health and fitness: an observational study. J Physiother. 2012;58(2):113-6.

[62] Lubbeke A, Katz JN, Perneger TV, Hoffmeyer P. Primary and revision hip arthroplasty: 5-year outcomes and influence of age and comorbidity. J Rheumatol. 2007 Feb;34(2):394-400.

[63] Escobar A, Gonzalez M, Quintana JM, Vrotsou K, Bilbao A, Herrera-Espineira C, et al. Patient acceptable symptom state and OMERACT-OARSI set of responder criteria in joint replacement. Identification of cut-off values. Osteoarthritis Cartilage. 2012 Feb;20(2):87-92.

[64] Singh JA, Lewallen DG. Predictors of activity limitation and dependence on walking aids after primary total hip arthroplasty. J Am Geriatr Soc. 2010 Dec;58(12):2387-93.

[65] Paulsen MG, Dowsey MM, Castle D, Choong PF. Preoperative psychological distress and functional outcome after knee replacement. ANZ J Surg. 2011 Oct;81(10):681-7.

[66] A WD, Robertsson O, Lidgren L. Surgery for knee osteoarthritis in younger patients. Acta Orthop. 2010 Apr;81(2):161-4.

[67] Hamel MB, Toth M, Legedza A, Rosen MP. Joint replacement surgery in elderly patients with severe osteoarthritis of the hip or knee: decision making, postoperative recovery, and clinical outcomes. Arch Intern Med. 2008 Jul 14;168(13):1430-40.

[68] Stroh DA, Delanois R, Naziri O, Johnson A, Mont M. Total knee arthroplasty in patients over 80 years of age. J Knee Surg. 2011 Dec;24(4):279-83.

[69] Joshi AB, Gill G. Total knee arthroplasty in nonagenarians. J Arthroplasty. 2002 Sep; 17(6):681-4.

[70] Joshi AB, Markovic L, Gill G. Knee arthroplasty in octogenarians: results at 10 years. J Arthroplasty. 2003 Apr;18(3):295-8.

[71] Pagnano MW, McLamb LA, Trousdale RT. Primary and revision total hip arthroplasty for patients 90 years of age and older. Mayo Clin Proc. 2003 Mar;78(3):285-8.

[72] Dahm DL, Barnes SA, Harrington JR, Sayeed SA, Berry DJ. Patient-reported activity level after total knee arthroplasty. J Arthroplasty. 2008 Apr;23(3):401-7.

[73] Australian Orthopaedic Association. National Joint Replacement Registry Annual Report. Adelaide2011.

[74] Swedish Hip Arthroplasty Register. Annual Report 2010 Göteborg, 2011: Available from: http://www.shpr.se/en/default.aspx.

[75] The Swedish Knee Arthroplasty Register Annual Report 2010 Lund, 2011: Available from: http://www.knee.nko.se/english/online/thePages/contact.php.

[76] National Joint Replacement Registry for England and Wales. 8th Annual Report 2011 Hertfordshire, 2011: Available from: www.njrcentre.org.uk.

[77] Karlson EW, Daltroy LH, Liang MH, Eaton HE, Katz JN. Gender differences in patient preferences may underlie differential utilization of elective surgery. Am J Med. 1997 Jun;102(6):524-30.

[78] Mujica-Mota RE, Tarricone R, Ciani O, Bridges JF, Drummond M. Determinants of demand for total hip and knee arthroplasty: a systematic literature review. BMC Health Serv Res. 2012 Jul 30;12(1):225.

[79] Borkhoff CM, Hawker GA, Kreder HJ, Glazier RH, Mahomed NN, Wright JG. The effect of patients' sex on physicians' recommendations for total knee arthroplasty. CMAJ. 2008 Mar 11;178(6):681-7.

[80] Dieppe P, Judge A, Williams S, Ikwueke I, Guenther KP, Floeren M, et al. Variations in the pre-operative status of patients coming to primary hip replacement for osteoarthritis in European orthopaedic centres. BMC Musculoskelet Disord. 2009;10:19.

[81] Ackerman IN, Graves SE, Wicks IP, Bennell KL, Osborne RH. Severely compromised quality of life in women and those of lower socioeconomic status waiting for joint replacement surgery. Arthritis Rheum. 2005 Oct 15;53(5):653-8.

[82] Hoogeboom TJ, van den Ende CH, van der Sluis G, Elings J, Dronkers JJ, Aiken AB, et al. The impact of waiting for total joint replacement on pain and functional status: a systematic review. Osteoarthritis Cartilage. 2009 Nov;17(11):1420-7.

[83] Dowsey MM, Dieppe P, Lohmander S, Castle D, Liew D, Choong PF. The association between radiographic severity and pre-operative function in patients undergoing primary knee replacement for osteoarthritis. Knee. 2012 Mar 23.

[84] Lavernia CJ, Alcerro JC, Contreras JS, Rossi MD. Patient perceived outcomes after primary hip arthroplasty: does gender matter? Clin Orthop Relat Res. 2011 Feb; 469(2):348-54.

[85] O'Connor MI. Implant survival, knee function, and pain relief after TKA: are there differences between men and women? Clin Orthop Relat Res. 2011 Jul;469(7):1846-51.

[86] Ritter MA, Wing JT, Berend ME, Davis KE, Meding JB. The clinical effect of gender on outcome of total knee arthroplasty. J Arthroplasty. 2008 Apr;23(3):331-6.

[87] Liebs TR, Herzberg W, Roth-Kroeger AM, Ruther W, Hassenpflug J. Women recover faster than men after standard knee arthroplasty. Clin Orthop Relat Res. 2011 Oct; 469(10):2855-65.

[88] Jenkins PJ, Perry PR, Yew Ng C, Ballantyne JA. Deprivation influences the functional outcome from total hip arthroplasty. Surgeon. 2009 Dec;7(6):351-6.

[89] Clement ND, Muzammil A, Macdonald D, Howie CR, Biant LC. Socioeconomic status affects the early outcome of total hip replacement. J Bone Joint Surg Br. 2011 Apr; 93(4):464-9.

[90] Allen Butler R, Rosenzweig S, Myers L, Barrack RL. The Frank Stinchfield Award: the impact of socioeconomic factors on outcome after THA: a prospective, randomized study. Clin Orthop Relat Res. 2011 Feb;469(2):339-47.

[91] Schafer T, Krummenauer F, Mettelsiefen J, Kirschner S, Gunther KP. Social, educational, and occupational predictors of total hip replacement outcome. Osteoarthritis Cartilage. 2010 Aug;18(8):1036-42.

[92] Davis ET, Lingard EA, Schemitsch EH, Waddell JP. Effects of socioeconomic status on patients' outcome after total knee arthroplasty. Int J Qual Health Care. 2008 Feb; 20(1):40-6.

[93] Dixon A, Le Grand J, Henderson J, Murray R, Poteliakhoff E. Is the British National Health Service equitable? The evidence on socioeconomic differences in utilization. J Health Serv Res Policy. 2007 Apr;12(2):104-9.

[94] Irgit K, Nelson CL. Defining racial and ethnic disparities in THA and TKA. Clin Orthop Relat Res. 2011 Jul;469(7):1817-23.

[95] Ang DC, James G, Stump TE. Clinical appropriateness and not race predicted referral for joint arthroplasty. Arthritis Rheum. 2009 Dec 15;61(12):1677-85.

[96] Dunlop DD, Song J, Manheim LM, Chang RW. Racial disparities in joint replacement use among older adults. Med Care. 2003 Feb;41(2):288-98.

[97] Hanchate AD, Zhang Y, Felson DT, Ash AS. Exploring the determinants of racial and ethnic disparities in total knee arthroplasty: health insurance, income, and assets. Med Care. 2008 May;46(5):481-8.

[98] Ibrahim SA. Racial and ethnic disparities in hip and knee joint replacement: a review of research in the Veterans Affairs Health Care System. J Am Acad Orthop Surg. 2007;15 Suppl 1:S87-94.

[99] Dunlop DD, Manheim LM, Song J, Sohn MW, Feinglass JM, Chang HJ, et al. Age and racial/ethnic disparities in arthritis-related hip and knee surgeries. Med Care. 2008 Feb;46(2):200-8.

[100] Kamath AF, Horneff JG, Gaffney V, Israelite CL, Nelson CL. Ethnic and gender differences in the functional disparities after primary total knee arthroplasty. Clin Orthop Relat Res. 2010 Dec;468(12):3355-61.

[101] Joshy S, Datta A, Perera A, Thomas B, Gogi N, Kumar Singh B. Ethnic differences in preoperative function of patients undergoing total knee arthroplasty. Int Orthop. 2006 Oct;30(5):426-8.

[102] Krupic F, Eisler T, Garellick G, Karrholm J. Influence of ethnicity and socioeconomic factors on outcome after total hip replacement. Scand J Caring Sci. 2012 May 23.

[103] Lavernia CJ, Alcerro JC, Contreras JS, Rossi MD. Ethnic and racial factors influencing well-being, perceived pain, and physical function after primary total joint arthroplasty. Clin Orthop Relat Res. 2011 Jul;469(7):1838-45.

[104] Dowsey MM, Broadhead ML, Stoney JD, Choong PF. Outcomes of total knee arthroplasty in English- versus non-English-speaking patients. J Orthop Surg (Hong Kong). 2009 Dec;17(3):305-9.

[105] Schonberg MA, Marcantonio ER, Hamel MB. Perceptions of physician recommendations for joint replacement surgery in older patients with severe hip or knee osteoarthritis. J Am Geriatr Soc. 2009 Jan;57(1):82-8.

[106] Suarez-Almazor ME, Souchek J, Kelly PA, O'Malley K, Byrne M, Richardson M, et al. Ethnic variation in knee replacement: patient preferences or uninformed disparity? Arch Intern Med. 2005 May 23;165(10):1117-24.

[107] Hekmat K, Jacobsson L, Nilsson JA, Petersson IF, Robertsson O, Garellick G, et al. Decrease in the incidence of total hip arthroplasties in patients with rheumatoid arthritis--results from a well defined population in south Sweden. Arthritis Res Ther. 2011;13(2):R67.

[108] Skytta E, Honkanen P, Eskelinen A, Huhtala H, Remes V. Fewer and older patients with rheumatoid arthritis need total knee replacement. Scand J Rheumatol. 2012 Jul 24.

[109] Sokka T, Kautiainen H, Hannonen P. Stable occurrence of knee and hip total joint replacement in Central Finland between 1986 and 2003: an indication of improved long-term outcomes of rheumatoid arthritis. Ann Rheum Dis. 2007 Mar;66(3):341-4.

[110] Clement ND, Breusch SJ, Biant LC. Lower limb joint replacement in rheumatoid arthritis. J Orthop Surg Res. 2012;7:27.

[111] Donahue KE, Gartlehner G, Jonas DE, Lux LJ, Thieda P, Jonas BL, et al. Systematic review: comparative effectiveness and harms of disease-modifying medications for rheumatoid arthritis. Ann Intern Med. 2008 Jan 15;148(2):124-34.

[112] Borstlap M, Zant JL, Van Soesbergen M, Van der Korst JK. Effects of total hip replacement on quality of life in patients with osteoarthritis and in patients with rheumatoid arthritis. Clin Rheumatol. 1994 Mar;13(1):45-50.

[113] Kageyama Y, Miyamoto S, Ozeki T, Hiyoshi M, Kushida K, Inoue T. Outcomes for patients undergoing one or more total hip and knee arthroplasties. Clin Rheumatol. 1998;17(2):130-4.

[114] Kirwan JR, Currey HL, Freeman MA, Snow S, Young PJ. Overall long-term impact of total hip and knee joint replacement surgery on patients with osteoarthritis and rheumatoid arthritis. Br J Rheumatol. 1994 Apr;33(4):357-60.

[115] March LM, Barcenilla AL, Cross MJ, Lapsley HM, Parker D, Brooks PM. Costs and outcomes of total hip and knee joint replacement for rheumatoid arthritis. Clin Rheumatol. 2008 Oct;27(10):1235-42.

[116] Tabutin J, Cambas PM. Hip arthroplasty up to the age of 30 and considerations in relation to subsequent revision. Hip Int. 2009 Jul-Sep;19(3):201-5.

[117] Dudkiewicz I, Salai M, Ganel A, Blankstein A, Chechik A. Total hip arthroplasty in patients younger than 30 years of age following developmental dysplasia of hip (DDH) in infancy. Arch Orthop Trauma Surg. 2002 Apr;122(3):139-42.

[118] Boyle MJ, Frampton CM, Crawford HA. Early results of total hip arthroplasty in patients with slipped upper femoral epiphysis compared with patients with osteoarthritis. J Arthroplasty. 2012 Jun;27(6):1003-7.

[119] Boyle MJ, Frampton CM, Crawford HA. Early results of total hip arthroplasty in patients with developmental dysplasia of the hip compared with patients with osteoarthritis. J Arthroplasty. 2012 Mar;27(3):386-90.

[120] Pietrzak K, Strzyzewski W, Pucher A, Kaczmarek W. [Total hip replacement after Legg-Calve-Perthes disease]. Chir Narzadow Ruchu Ortop Pol. 2011 May-Jun;76(3): 129-33.

[121] Dowsey MM, Choong PF. Obesity is a major risk factor for prosthetic infection after primary hip arthroplasty. Clin Orthop Relat Res. 2008 Jan;466(1):153-8.

[122] Lingard EA, Katz JN, Wright EA, Sledge CB. Predicting the outcome of total knee arthroplasty. J Bone Joint Surg Am. 2004 Oct;86-A(10):2179-86.

[123] Gandhi R, Dhotar H, Razak F, Tso P, Davey JR, Mahomed NN. Predicting the longer term outcomes of total knee arthroplasty. Knee. 2010 Jan;17(1):15-8.

[124] Young NL, Cheah D, Waddell JP, Wright JG. Patient characteristics that affect the outcome of total hip arthroplasty: a review. Can J Surg. 1998 Jun;41(3):188-95.

[125] Deyo RA, Cherkin DC, Ciol MA. Adapting a clinical comorbidity index for use with ICD-9-CM administrative databases. J Clin Epidemiol. 1992 Jun;45(6):613-9.

[126] Singh JA, O'Byrne M, Harmsen S, Lewallen D. Predictors of moderate-severe functional limitation after primary Total Knee Arthroplasty (TKA): 4701 TKAs at 2-years and 2935 TKAs at 5-years. Osteoarthritis Cartilage. 2010 Apr; 18(4):515-21.

[127] Hall WH, Ramachandran R, Narayan S, Jani AB, Vijayakumar S. An electronic application for rapidly calculating Charlson comorbidity score. BMC Cancer. 2004 Dec 20;4:94.

[128] Gandhi R, Razak F, Davey JR, Mahomed NN. Metabolic syndrome and the functional outcomes of hip and knee arthroplasty. J Rheumatol. 2010 Sep;37(9):1917-22.

[129] Lementowski PW, Zelicof SB. Obesity and osteoarthritis. Am J Orthop (Belle Mead NJ). 2008 Mar;37(3):148-51.

[130] Access-Economics. The economic costs of obesity. (Commissioned by Diabetes Australia, 2006).

[131] Leung A, Liew D, Lim J, Page C, Boukris-Sayag V, Mundae M, et al. The effect of joint aspiration and corticosteroid injections in osteoarthritis of the knee. Int J Rheum Dis. 2011 Oct;14(4):384-9.

[132] Kim SH. Morbid obesity and excessive hospital resource consumption for unilateral primary hip and knee arthroplasty. J Arthroplasty. 2010 Dec;25(8):1258-66.

[133] Kouris-Blazos A, Wahiqvist M. Health economics of weight management: evidence and cost. Asia Pac J Clin Nutri. 2007;16 (Suppl.1):329-38.

[134] Aderinto J, Brenkel IJ, Chan P. Weight change following total hip replacement: a comparison of obese and non-obese patients. Surgeon. 2005 Aug;3(4):269-72, 305.

[135] Donovan J, Dingwall I, McChesney S. Weight change 1 year following total knee or hip arthroplasty. ANZ J Surg. 2006 Apr;76(4):222-5.

[136] Heisel C, Silva M, dela Rosa MA, Schmalzried TP. The effects of lower-extremity total joint replacement for arthritis on obesity. Orthopedics. 2005 Feb;28(2):157-9.

[137] Jain SA, Roach RT, Travlos J. Changes in body mass index following primary elective total hip arthroplasty. Correlation with outcome at 2 years. Acta Orthop Belg. 2003 Oct;69(5):421-5.

[138] Lachiewicz AM, Lachiewicz PF. Weight and activity change in overweight and obese patients after primary total knee arthroplasty. J Arthroplasty. 2008 Jan;23(1):33-40.

[139] Middleton FR, Boardman DR. Total hip arthroplasty does not aid weight loss. Ann R Coll Surg Engl. 2007 Apr;89(3):288-91.

[140] Woodruff MJ, Stone MH. Comparison of weight changes after total hip or knee arthroplasty. J Arthroplasty. 2001 Jan;16(1):22-4.

[141] Zeni JA, Jr., Snyder-Mackler L. Most patients gain weight in the 2 years after total knee arthroplasty: comparison to a healthy control group. Osteoarthritis Cartilage. 2010 Apr;18(4):510-4.

[142] Vincent HK, Horodyski M, Gearen P, Vlasak R, Seay AN, Conrad BP, et al. Obesity and long term functional outcomes following elective total hip replacement. J Orthop Surg Res. 2012 Apr 25;7(1):16.

[143] Gillespie GN, Porteous AJ. Obesity and knee arthroplasty. Knee. 2007 Mar;14(2):81-6.

[144] Samson AJ, Mercer GE, Campbell DG. Total knee replacement in the morbidly obese: a literature review. ANZ J Surg. 2010 Sep;80(9):595-9.

[145] Dowsey MM, Choong PF. Early outcomes and complications following joint arthroplasty in obese patients: a review of the published reports. ANZ J Surg. 2008 Jun; 78(6):439-44.

[146] Wright JG, Swiontkowski MF, Heckman JD. Introducing levels of evidence to the journal. J Bone Joint Surg Am. 2003 Jan;85-A(1):1-3.

[147] Moran M, Walmsley P, Gray A, Brenkel IJ. Does body mass index affect the early outcome of primary total hip arthroplasty? J Arthroplasty. 2005 Oct;20(7):866-9.

[148] Lubbeke A, Stern R, Garavaglia G, Zurcher L, Hoffmeyer P. Differences in outcomes of obese women and men undergoing primary total hip arthroplasty. Arthritis Rheum. 2007 Mar 15;57(2):327-34.

[149] Rajgopal V, Bourne RB, Chesworth BM, MacDonald SJ, McCalden RW, Rorabeck CH. The impact of morbid obesity on patient outcomes after total knee arthroplasty. J Arthroplasty. 2008 Sep;23(6):795-800.

[150] Singh JA, Gabriel SE, Lewallen DG. Higher body mass index is not associated with worse pain outcomes after primary or revision total knee arthroplasty. J Arthroplasty. 2011 Apr;26(3):366-74 e1.

[151] Burg MM, Benedetto MC, Soufer R. Depressive symptoms and mortality two years after coronary artery bypass graft surgery (CABG) in men. Psychosom Med. 2003 Jul-Aug;65(4):508-10.

[152] Lingard EA, Riddle DL. Impact of psychological distress on pain and function following knee arthroplasty. J Bone Joint Surg Am. 2007 Jun;89(6):1161-9.

[153] Walton MJ, Newman JH. Pre-operative mental wellbeing and the outcome of knee replacement. Knee. 2008 Aug;15(4):277-80.

[154] Caracciolo B, Giaquinto S. Self-perceived distress and self-perceived functional recovery after recent total hip and knee arthroplasty. Arch Gerontol Geriatr. 2005 Sep-Oct;41(2):177-81.

[155] Paulsen M, Dowsey M, Castle D, Choong P. Pre-Operative Psychological Distress and Functional Outcome after Knee Replacement. ANZ J of Surg. 2010;[E-pub ahead of print] 20/1/2011.

[156] Vissers MM, Bussmann JB, Verhaar JA, Busschbach JJ, Bierma-Zeinstra SM, Reijman M. Psychological factors affecting the outcome of total hip and knee arthroplasty: a systematic review. Semin Arthritis Rheum. 2012 Feb;41(4):576-88.

[157] Rabin R, de Charro F. EQ-5D: a measure of health status from the EuroQol Group. Ann Med. 2001 Jul;33(5):337-43.

[158] Rolfson O, Dahlberg LE, Nilsson JA, Malchau H, Garellick G. Variables determining outcome in total hip replacement surgery. J Bone Joint Surg Br. 2009 Feb;91(2):157-61.

[159] Seligman MEP, Walker, E.F. & Rosenhan, D.L.,. Abnormal psychology, (4th ed.). New York: W.W. Norton & Company, Inc.; 2001.

[160] Quigley L, Nelson AL, Carriere J, Smilek D, Purdon C. The effects of trait and state anxiety on attention to emotional images: An eye-tracking study. Cogn Emot. 2012 May 30.

[161] Montin L, Leino-Kilpi H, Katajisto J, Lepisto J, Kettunen J, Suominen T. Anxiety and health-related quality of life of patients undergoing total hip arthroplasty for osteoarthritis. Chronic Illn. 2007 Sep;3(3):219-27.

[162] Badura-Brzoza K, Zajac P, Brzoza Z, Kasperska-Zajac A, Matysiakiewicz J, Piegza M, et al. Psychological and psychiatric factors related to health-related quality of life after total hip replacement - preliminary report. Eur Psychiatry. 2009 Mar;24(2):119-24.

[163] Brander V, Gondek S, Martin E, Stulberg SD. Pain and depression influence outcome 5 years after knee replacement surgery. Clin Orthop Relat Res. 2007 Nov;464:21-6.

[164] Riddle DL, Wade JB, Jiranek WA, Kong X. Preoperative pain catastrophizing predicts pain outcome after knee arthroplasty. Clin Orthop Relat Res. 2010 Mar;468(3): 798-806.

[165] Chaves JF, Brown JM. Spontaneous cognitive strategies for the control of clinical pain and stress. J Behav Med. 1987 Jun;10(3):263-76.

[166] Sullivan M, Tanzer M, Stanish W, Fallaha M, Keefe FJ, Simmonds M, et al. Psychological determinants of problematic outcomes following Total Knee Arthroplasty. Pain. 2009 May;143(1-2):123-9.

[167] Forsythe ME, Dunbar MJ, Hennigar AW, Sullivan MJ, Gross M. Prospective relation between catastrophizing and residual pain following knee arthroplasty: two-year follow-up. Pain Res Manag. 2008 Jul-Aug;13(4):335-41.

[168] Matthews G, and Ian J. Deary, I.J.,. Personality traits. Cambridge, UK: Cambridge University Press.; 1998.

[169] Fortin PR, Penrod JR, Clarke AE, St-Pierre Y, Joseph L, Belisle P, et al. Timing of total joint replacement affects clinical outcomes among patients with osteoarthritis of the hip or knee. Arthritis Rheum. 2002 Dec;46(12):3327-30.

[170] Fortin PR, Clarke AE, Joseph L, Liang MH, Tanzer M, Ferland D, et al. Outcomes of total hip and knee replacement: preoperative functional status predicts outcomes at six months after surgery. Arthritis Rheum. 1999 Aug;42(8):1722-8.

[171] Merle-Vincent F, Couris CM, Schott AM, Conrozier T, Piperno M, Mathieu P, et al. Factors predicting patient satisfaction 2 years after total knee arthroplasty for osteoarthritis. Joint Bone Spine. 2011 Jul;78(4):383-6.

[172] Valdes AM, Doherty SA, Zhang W, Muir KR, Maciewicz RA, Doherty M. Inverse relationship between preoperative radiographic severity and postoperative pain in patients with osteoarthritis who have undergone total joint arthroplasty. Semin Arthritis Rheum. 2012 Feb;41(4):568-75.

[173] Cushnaghan J, Coggon D, Reading I, Croft P, Byng P, Cox K, et al. Long-term outcome following total hip arthroplasty: a controlled longitudinal study. Arthritis Rheum. 2007 Dec 15;57(8):1375-80.

[174] Croft P, Cooper C, Wickham C, Coggon D. Defining osteoarthritis of the hip for epidemiologic studies. Am J Epidemiol. 1990 Sep;132(3):514-22.

[175] Franklin PD, Li W, Ayers DC. The Chitranjan Ranawat Award: functional outcome after total knee replacement varies with patient attributes. Clin Orthop Relat Res. 2008 Nov; 466(11):2597-604.

Chapter 3

# Preoperative Planning of Total Knee Replacement

A.O. Erdogan, N.S. Gokay and A. Gokce

Additional information is available at the end of the chapter

## 1. Introduction

Total knee replacement (TKR) surgery is the gold standard method in the treatment of end stage knee arthritis with a high success. Relieving pain effectively, restoring range of motion and improving function are the major goals of arthroplasy. Patient satisfaction rates were reported as 90% to 95% after TKR. [1-3] Better clinical results were gained in younger population than the older patients. Unfortunately, primary osteoarthritis is seen mainly in the elderly. However, inflamatory arthritis, trauma, avascular necrosis and hemophilia are some of the secondary causes leading osteoarthritis in younger population.. Nearly 1 million TKR surgeries are performed on earth per year and this number is increasing day by day, with the novel designed surface technologies. Despite the fact that new implant technologies secure better results, a revision procedure may be required in some of the patients. Ofcourse the amount of revision surgeries is also increasing in parallel with primary TKR surgeries. Unfortunately, the clinical result of revision total knee arthroplasty isn't succesfull enough as primary total knee arthroplasty.

Polyethylene (PE) wear, aseptic loosening, instability and infections are counted among the factors leading revision surgery [4,5]. The incidence of PE wear is decreased nowadays by the development of ultra high cross-linked polyethilens (UHMWPE). PE wear is a serious problem leading to aseptic loosening. Malalingment, malrotation and soft tissue imbalance after TKR surgery are the other factors which may cause in aseptic loosening. Instability and problems related with patella are among the other situations in which revision surgery may be requiredIt is very clear that surgical technique of primary TKR is the main risk factor for early failures [6, 7]. Extensive preoperative planning is very important considering aforementioned particulars to achieve accurate prosthetic seating with proper axial alignment. In this chapter, the preoperative planning issues including pre-operative preparations of patient and surgeon will be discussed.

## 2. Pre-operative clinical evaluation

Pre-operative clinical evaluation is very substantial in assessing the current medical status and determining the relative risk profile of the patient. It is very important for the orthopaedic surgeon to understand the basic principles and nuances involved. Preoperative planning initiates with selection of an apropriate candidate for TKR procedure. The patient's expectations and general risk factors plays an import role in this decision. Questioning of the patient's complaints and life quality, assesment of the medical condition and detailed physical examination are the essentials of preoperative clinical evaluation.

## 3. Indication of TKR

Total knee replacement was found to be quite effective in terms of improvement in health-related quality of life dimensions, with the occasional exception of the social dimension. The underlying disease is not a life threatening one. The primary indications for total knee arthroplasty are pain and loss of function. Clinical evaluation of the patient has to be initiated by questioning of the complaints and disabilities.

There must be a significant and disabling pain which is resistant to the medical treatment. Spinal disease, ipsilateral hip pathologies, peripheral vascular disease, meniscal pathologies, and bursitis of the knee should be considered in differential diagnosis. The real source of the knee pain must be displayed.

The patient's quality of life should be questioned and significant reduction might be taken into consideration It should be remembered that the patients, which are less satisfied following TKR, are the ones with mild pre-operative complaints. All conservative treatment modalities should be exhausted before surgery. The frequent indications for TKR surgery are given on table 1.

| |
|---|
| Osteoarthritis |
| Inflammatory arthritis |
| Rheumatoid arthritis |
| Osteochondromatosis |
| Villonodular synovitis |
| Metabolic arthritis |
| Osteonecrosis |
| Gout, pseudogout |
| Posttraumatic arthritis |
| Intraarticular fractures |
| Malaligned ankylosis |
| Failed high tibial osteotomies |

**Table 1.** The major indications for total knee arthroplasty

## 4. Contrendications of TKR

Contraindications must be well known and considered before the surgery decision. Absolute contraindications for total knee arthroplasty include knee sepsis, chronic infection, extansor mechanism dysfunction, severe vascular disease, recurvatum deformity secondary to muscular weakness, presence of well functioning knee arthrodesis. There are also relative and contraversial contraindications. These include medical conditions that preclude safe anesthesia, inadequate soft tissue coverage, morbid obesity, neuropathic arthropathy, and history of osteomyelitis around knee joint. A preoperative condition that can adversly affect the patient's outcome can be considered as a relative contraindication.

## 5. Medical condition of the patient

A comprehensive medical history and physical examination are the cornerstones of the preoperative assessment. Patient's medical comorbidities should be optimized preoperatively. Cardiovascular diseases, cerebrovascular diseases, pulmonary diseases, neurologic conditions, rheumatoid arthritis, uropathy, morbid obesity, haematologic and endocrine diseases are the important situations which may affect the intraoperative and postoperative morbidity and mortality.. Drug history of the patient must be questioned too. Sources of infection such as dental, dermatological, urological or respiratory tract infections must be ruled out. Age alone was not found to be an obstacle for an effective surgery, however age related comorbidities should be considered. Additional risks for infection, previous surgeries should be adressed before surgery. Every patient must have a general medical evaluation including laboratory tests, electrocardiogram and chest graphy. The type of the procedure also may enhance the medical risks. For example, simultaneously performed bilateral TKR may be associated with an increased risk of cardiac, respiratory or neurological complications. Low preoperative mental health has also an influence on outcome after TKR [10].

The detailed physical examination should include the range of motion, ligament status, circulation and skin condition evaluation. Furthermore alignment of lower extremities, patellar instability and gait analysis should to be assessed. Additional knowledge and scientific dissemination of surgery outcomes should help to ensure better management of the patients after total knee arthroplasty and to optimize the procedure [12].

Underlying or predisposing orthopaedic diseases, which may interact the outcome of TKR should be reviewed previously. Examples of such common musculoskeletal conditions are as follows: 1) Nerve entrapments affecting motor functions of lower extremity, 2) Adjacent joint degenerative arthritis 3) Presence of any inflamatory arthritis, which may flare after surgery 4) Any musculoskletal disability affecting postoperative mobility 5) Thromboembolic history or predispositions.

## 6. Radiographic assesment

An apropriate musculoskeletal radiologic study is essential in planning of TKR. The presence of bone defects might be detected and pre-operative decision whether to use a primary or revision implant should be given. Determination of the joint line is also important in determining the flexion/extension space and balance of the ligaments.

Tracking of the quadriceps mechanism and rotational deformites are other important issues for patellar stability, however may not be assessed on direct radiographs especially in deformed knees with fixed valgus position.

Conventional radiographs are usually adequate for initial radiographic evaluation to confirm the diagnosis or assess the severity of the disease. Preoperative radiographic planning for total knee arthroplasty begins by obtaining a high quality standing antero-posterior (AP) and lateral 52-inch casette graphies. Additional views such as Merchant, tunnel, patella sunrise, orthoroentgenogram or advanced imaging modalities such as CT, MRI may be necessary in extraordinary conditions such as congenital dislocation of the patella, post traumatic deformities, severe deformities, tumors and congenital anomalies.

### 6.1. AP view

The AP view should be obtained with the patient in a standing position. The joint space on the weight bearing AP film should be more than 3 mm or within 50% of the joint space of the contralateral knee. Normally, the lateral joint space is wider than the medial space. Articular surfaces of the medial and lateral joint compartments may be best assessed on this view. The presence of associated osteophytes and subcondral bone changes are some of the findings which may be seen on AP graphies.

### 6.2. Lateral view

The lateral aspect of the knee is leaned against the x ray film cassette and flexed 30°. The excessive glide in flexion may be an indicator of posterior cruciate ligament tightness and therefore PCL sacrifiying prosthesis must be considered before the surgery. Patellar height should be assessed on this view using Insall-Salvati ratio. The Insall-Salvati is the ratio of the patellar tendon length (LT) to the length of the patella (LP) (Figure 1). The values above 1,2 is considered as "Patella Alta", while the values belove 0,8 is considered as "Patella İnfera". Suprapatellar and posterior regions must be evaluated in terms of detecting the loose bodies.

Posterior of the knee joint is easily observed on this view and overhanging bone structure or osteophytes should be determined. If left unresected, this overhanging bone can impinge on tibial PE and result with flexion limitation and early wear of the PE.

The lateral view may also allow size selection of the femoral component (Figure 2). Oversizing will create tightness in fexion and increased tension in quadriceps mechanism and undersizing will create looseness in flexion and anterior cortical notching of the femur is also inevitable. Careful preoperative planning with using templates aims to achieve the correct AP dimension for restoring normal kinematics and quadriceps muscle function.

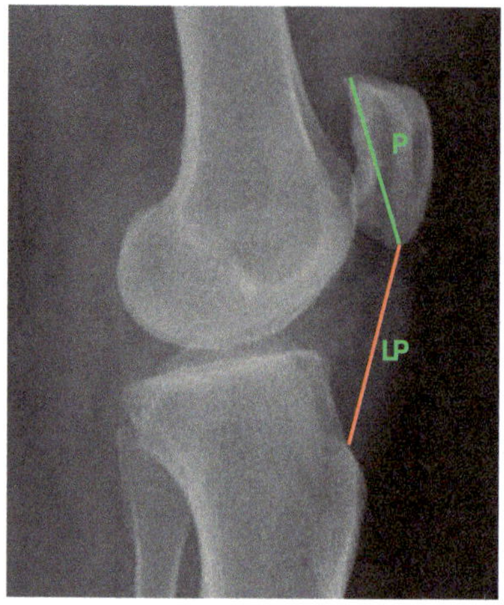


Figure 1. Patella height is assessed via measuring Insall-Salvati ratio (LP/P) on lateral graphies

### 6.3. Standing orthorontgenogram (52-inch casette three joint view)

Standing ap view of the lower extremities from hips to ankles is helpful preoperatively for assessing overall alignment (mechanical axis) of the lower extremity. The knee is normally in 7 degree of valgus alignment on AP view.

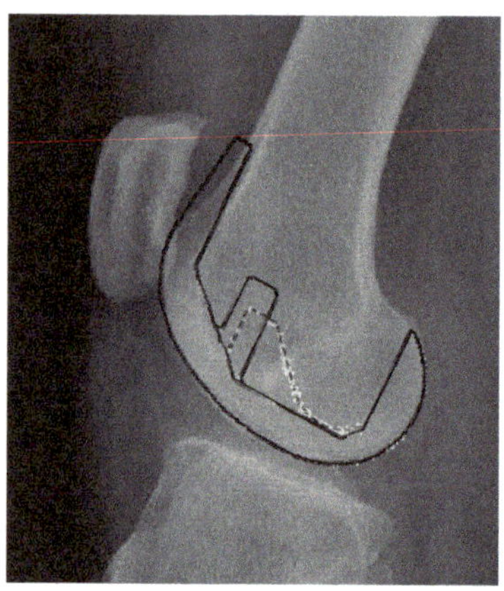

Figure 2. Proper size of the femoral component is assessed via evaluation of the pre-operative lateral radiographs.

The orthorontgenogram allows the surgeon to determine the varus or valgus alignment of the knees, leg length discrepancy and the presence of extraarticular deformities.

It is essential to ensure to take this radiograph in neutral rotation of the legs to obtain the most accurate measurements. It should be confirmed via inspecting the relationship between the tibia and the fibula, distally and proximally.

### 6.4. Merchant view

Merchant view helps to assess the patellofemoral alignment, trochlear grove and articular surfaces. Preoperatively patellar subluxation seen on this view should alert the surgeon for lateral release of the patella during TKR. Merchant view demonstrates both the patellar and trochlear surfaces. Subluxation can be assessed by measuring the congruence angle (Figure 3). Congruence angle demonstrates the relationship of apex of patella with the trochlear grove's bisector. Two lines are drawn to measure the congruence angle. First line is the bisector line of femoral sulcus angle and it establishes a zero reference line. Second line is drawn from the apex of the sulcus angle to the lowest point of the patellar articular ridge.

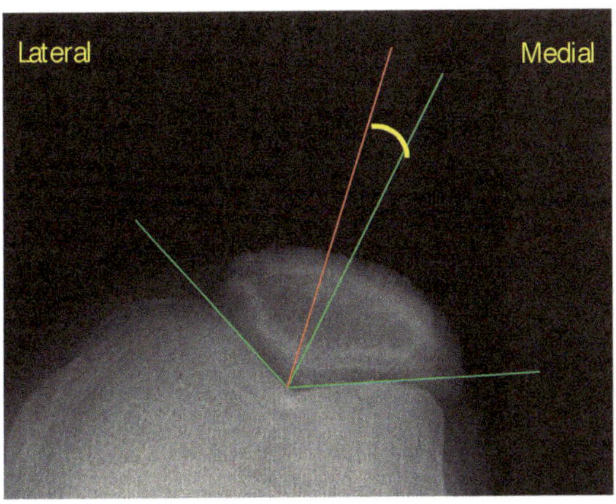


**Figure 3.** The congruence angle (α) lower than 16° to lateral or medial direction is considered as normal.

If congruence angle is lateral to the reference line this means the angle is positive while angles medial to the reference lines are considered as negative. The angles lower than 16 degree are considered as normal.

### 6.5. Tunnel view

Tunnel view shows the posterior aspect of the intercondylar notch and it is useful to evaluate osteocondritis dissecans or intraarticular loose bodies in young patients.

### 6.6. Patella sunrise view

This is called the sunrise view because the patella appears to be rising over the horizon. The sunrise view also helps to identify the patellar malalignment.

## 7. Surgeon's preperation

Preoperative planning is essential component for surgeon in TKR to obtain desired clinical outcome and radiographic result. Correct implant selection with proper size is one of the important stage in preoperative planning. Patient's and surgeon's expectations should be taken into consideration pre-operatively to improve the outcomes and increase the satisfaction after operation [12]. Pre-operative planning of the bone cuts may simplify the surgery. Positioning of the components is very important in acquiring the accurate alignment. Mechanical axis measurement and alignment evaluation on AP and lateral planes may performed on standing X-rays. Also entry points for intramedullary guide pins should be determined for the correct component position.

During the process of planning of TKR, the surgeon aims to obtain the optimal fitting of the implant and the optimal extremity alignment. This is possible for the surgeon by thinking three-dimensionally. The prediction of the surgery pre-operatively should improve the precision of the process and shorten the length of the operation. It should also reduce the complication rate.

## 8. Templating

Most of the knee replacement systems provide a large number of options for treating conditions that are encountered during surgery. The different systems serve the surgeons different sizes of implants in a wide range. Intra-operative determination of the implant sizes was found more accurate than the pre-operative templating. However pre-operative templating is useful in obtaining proper implant positioning. Working with templates is widely accepted approach, which can help determine component sizes, predict amounts of bony resection, and anticipate surgical steps. Acetate templating was found accurate and reliabile [13]. However, with widespread use of digital radiographs the use of digital templating has recently grown due to advances in reducing errors associated with manipulating films and templates (Figure 4).

Combining digital templating with picture archiving and communication system PACS brings advantages include saving health care costs, quick and reproducible planning, remote access, and the ability to keep a permanent digital record of the surgical plan.

Templating should also work in preparing the surgeon to some extreme scenarios which may be encountered during surgery. For example; Standart cruciate retaining or sacrifiying implant systems are usually enough to solve the problem in large majority of cases. Constrained or even more complicated sytems with extension stems or wedges may be necessiated in small number of primary cases (Figure 5). Modular systems should be required due to intraoperative complications such as fractures or ligament tears.

Constrained condylar knee prosthesis (CCK) is commonly used in total knee replacement to overcome the severe ligamentous imbalance problem. CCK may also be preferred if the lateral

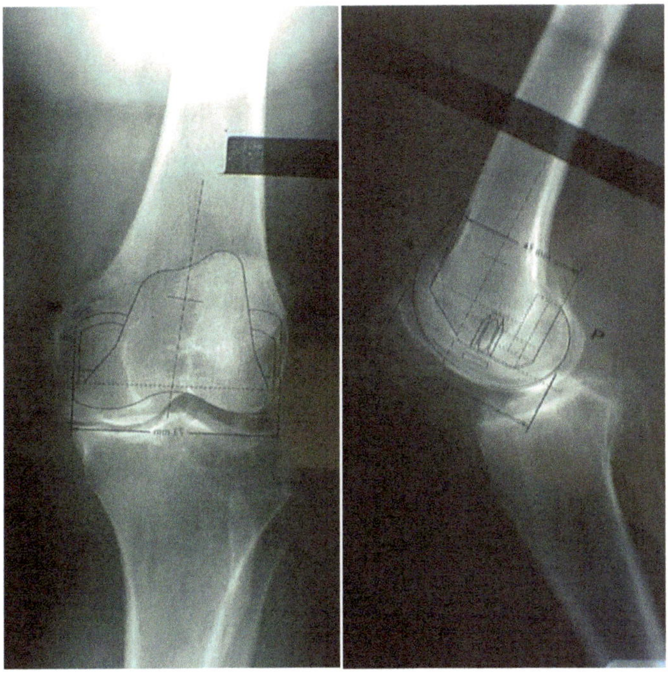

**Figure 4.** Templating

collateral ligament laxity more than 2 mm persists, even after adequate medial soft tissue release in patients with varus deformity of greater than 20°.

Although women have greater functional limitations than men, at the time of the surgery, they recover faster in early post-operative period. Women also have a greater improvement in WOMAC scores than men after primary surgery. Specific anatomic differences are blamed to be responsible for gender-specific differences after TKR. However, there are conflicting data in the literature regarding these gender-specific outcomes [14].

There are also efforts in reducing costs and improving quality of care, which may planned in preoperative period. Template-directed instrumentation was proposed for simplifying the surgical instruments and saving sterilization costs of unnecessary implant trays as saving measurement. In this novel approach, surgical planning combines digital templating with prepared instruments and components used intraoperatively [15].

Computer based navigation should be prefered in complex cases to overcome the heavily distorded anatomy or malalignment. There are also several quite recent technologies, like patient specific surgical cutting guide systems or robotic assisted implantations in cases of surgeon's special interest. Beside the medical aspects surgeons have to deal with cost considerations and even discuss with the patient in preoperative planning period [16].

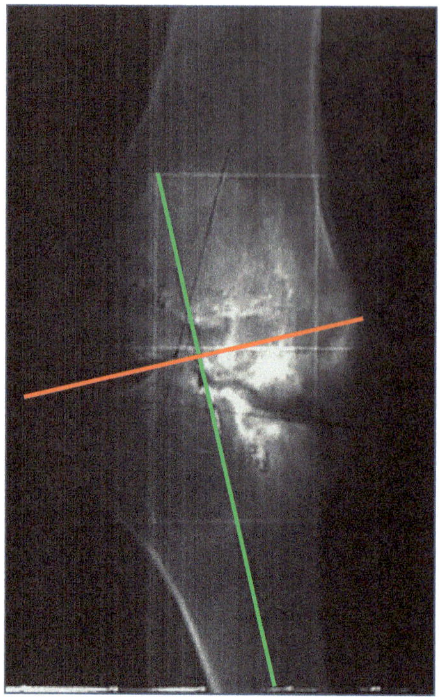

**Figure 5.** Wedge and modular extension stems should be considered in patients which present with a such pre-operative radiograph.

## Author details

A.O. Erdogan, N.S. Gokay and A. Gokce

Namik Kemal University School of Medicine, Department of Orthopaedics and Traumatology, Tekirdag, Turkey

## References

[1] Colizza, W. A, & Insall, J. N. Scuderi GR: The posteriorstabilized knee prosthesis: Assessment of polyethylene damage and osteolysis after a ten-year minimum follow-up. J Bone Joint Surg 77A:(1995)., , 1713-1720.

[2] Emmerson, K. P, & Moran, C. G. Pinder IM: Survivorship analysis of the kinematic stabilizer total knee replacement: A year follow-up. J Bone Joint Surg 78B:441-445, (1996)., 10-14.

[3] Ranawat, C. S, & Luessenhop, C. P. Rodriquez JA: The press-fit condylar modular total knee system: Four to six year results with a posterior-cruciate-substituting design. J Bone Joint Surg 79A:(1997)., 342-348.

[4] Robertsson, O, & Lidgren, L. Annual Report- The Swedish Knee Arthroplasty Register. *Annual Report SKAR* (2008)., 1-37.

[5] Mulhall, K. J, Ghomrawi, H. M, Scully, S, Callaghan, J. J, & Saleh, K. J. Current etiologies and modes of failure in total knee arthroplasty revision. *Clin Orthop Relat Res* (2006)., 446, 45-50.

[6] Manley, M, Ong, K, Lau, E, & Kurtz, S. M. Total Knee Arthroplasty Survivorship in the United States Medicare Population Effect of Hospital and Surgeon Procedure Volume. *J Arthroplasty* (2008).

[7] Schroer, W. C, Calvert, G. T, Diesfeld, P. J, & Reedy, M. E. LeMarr AR. Effects of increased surgical volume on total knee arthroplasty complications. *J Arthroplasty* (2008). Suppl 1):61-67.

[8] Crekarell, J. R, & Guyton, J. L. Arthroplasty of ankle and knee. Canale ST (ed). Campbell's operative orthopaedics. 10th edition, St Louis: Mosby, (2003).

[9] Aydogdu, S. ve ark. Diz artroplastisinde genel ilkeler endikasyonlar. Ege R. Diz sorunları. Ankara, bizim büro basımevi, (1998)., 439-459.

[10] Vissers, M. M, Bussmann, J. B, Verhaar, J. A, Busschbach, J. J, Bierma-zeinstra, S. M, & Reijman, M. Psychological factors affecting the outcome of total hip and knee arthroplasty: a systematic review. Semin Arthritis Rheum. (2012)., 41(4), 576-88.

[11] Ethgen, O, Bruyère, O, Richy, F, Dardennes, C, & Reginster, J. Y. Health-related quality of life in total hip and total knee arthroplasty. A qualitative and systematic review of the literature. J Bone Joint Surg Am. (2004). A(5):963-74., 86.

[12] Ghomrawi, H. M, Mancuso, C. A, Westrich, G. H, & Marx, R. G. Mushlin AI Discordance in TKR Expectations Between Patients and Surgeons; Expectations Discordance Study Group.Clin Orthop Relat Res. (2012). Jul 21.

[13] Peek, A. C, Bloch, B, & Auld, J. How useful is templating for total knee replacement component sizing? Knee. (2012). Aug;doi:j.knee.2011.03.010. Epub 2011 May 10., 19(4), 266-9.

[14] Liebs, T. R, Herzberg, W, Roth-kroeger, A. M, Rüther, W, & Hassenpflug, J. Women recover faster than men after standard knee arthroplasty. Clin Orthop Relat Res. (2011)., 469(10), 2855-65.

[15] Hsu, A. R, Gross, C. E, Bhatia, S, & Levine, B. R. Template-directed Instrumentation in Total Knee Arthroplasty: Cost Savings Analysis. Orthopedics. (2012). Nov 1;35(11):edoi:, 1596-600.

[16] S.David Stulberg Chapter 3 Preoperative Planning and Prosthetic Selectin in book Knee Arthroplasty edited Thomas P. Sculco and Ermanno A. Martucci, New York: Springer Wien; 2002. 250.

Chapter 4

# Special Considerations in Asian Knee Arthroplasty

Hamid Reza Seyyed Hosseinzadeh, Samih Tarabichi,
Ali Sina Shahi, Mehrnoush Hassas Yeganeh,
Usama Hassan Saleh, Gholam Reza Kazemian and
Aidin Masoudi

Additional information is available at the end of the chapter

## 1. Introduction

Human body is a unique correlation between anatomy and physiology. It is mandatory to have adequate knowledge on this issue former to perform any kind of surgery. As in all parts of human body, there are several variations in human knee concerning middle-eastern and Asian ethnicity, which should be considered for performing total knee arthroplasty among these races. These differences involve both in anatomical and physiological features, causing variations in a wide spectrum from metabolic syndromes to morphology of knee components.

During total knee replacement, the accurate bone cutting, adequate balancing of the soft tissues and proper coverage of the resected surface were important factors for achieving a successful outcome. In recent years, many studies have identified shape differences in the knee within the Caucasian population. Total knee replacement is a precise procedure, requiring accurate soft tissue balancing and resection of bone thickness equal to the thickness of the implanted prosthetic component. Proper bone cuts for rotational alignment of the femur and tibia in the axial plane represents the key for a balanced flexion gap and proper patella tracking. Both represent important parameters for high flexion. [1] A properly shaped prosthesis can provide the best coverage and avoid soft tissue impingement. Thus, it becomes important to obtain the anthropometric data to achieve the best stability and longevity for implant. Total knee prostheses based on the accurately morphologic data of knee, gender morphologic difference, and the morphologic correlations between tibia and femur may be expected to give better results.

Differences among males and females have been widely reported, with females having a smaller mediolateral to anteroposterior ratio and more narrow distal femurs and different proximal tibia geometry. [2, 3] However, ethnic differences have not received much focus given that most existing TKA implant designs are based on the Caucasian population. But, many studies have determined that the prostheses designed for Caucasian patients are not suitable for Asian patients. Anatomic differences have been identified between both sex and ethnicity, with Caucasian subjects having a higher tibial torsion angle and lower varus alignment than Japanese.

As mentioned above, accurate sizing and proper placement of prosthetic components plays a major role in the success and long term survival of total knee arthroplasty (TKA). The femoral component sizing is an important determinant for achieving a well-balanced flexion-extension gap in a TKA. Mediolateral sizing of the femoral component is necessary for proper patellofemoral tracking and uniform stress distribution over the resected distal femoral surface; this contributes to the long term stability of the prosthesis. [1] Most of the total knee prostheses currently available have been developed using measurements from Caucasians. Caucasian knees have been shown to be generally larger than Asian knees. [4] It follows that these discrepancies may give rise to implant size mismatch with the resected bony surface of Asian patients. Several studies have found that the femoral aspect ratio (mediolateral [fML]/anteroposterior [fAP]) of the prostheses used in Asia were not suitable for Asian patients. For instance, Ho et al reported that 3 of 5 TKA systems used in China tended to cause mediolateral overhang of the component across the width of the resected femurs of Chinese patients. The authors also found a larger femoral aspect ratio in small knees and a proportionally smaller ratio in large knees, but all the 5 sets of implant systems examined in the study showed little changes in the aspect ratio with AP length. [2]

Iorio et al showed that the Japanese patients had a significantly less postoperative range of motion than white patients. Furthermore, 4.1% Japanese patients required revision after primary posterior cruciate-retaining TKA within an average follow-up of 6.6 years, whereas only 2.6% of their American cohort needed revision within an average follow-up of 9 years. The authors suggested that the racial morphologic differences might be a factor causing the differences in outcome. [5]

Systematic differences have also been observed. ACL laxity among Japanese is higher than Caucasians. [4] It has also been proven that the ACL laxity is significantly different between Malaysians and Caucasians. [6] This could be the result of different life style. The systematic differences are explained further through the chapter.

Some rare complications accompanied by TKA are more common among the ethnicity, such as insufficiency fracture. This could be as a result of having greater rates of risk factors like: osteoporosis, overweight and gross varus deformity. Insufficiency fracture would be presented by no history of trauma, sudden unset pain, knee instability and deformity. The patient surprisingly is unable to walk. Unfortunately it is common to be misdiagnosed as MCL insufficiency.

That's why it is very important to have special consideration while performing total knee arthroplasty among Asian or middle-eastern ethnicity.

These findings on TKA mismatching have led some researchers to suggest that Asia Pacific people should have special designs of TKA prosthesis system.

## 2. Three-dimensional morphology of the knee reveals ethnic differences

In recent years, many studies have identified shape differences in the knee within the Caucasian population. [7, 8, 9] Shape analyses have identified sex differences in the femoral midshaft, distal femur, and patella. [10] Ethnic differences have not received much focus given that most existing TKA implant designs are based on the Caucasian population. Many studies have reported the anatomy and comparison of East Asian populations (Japanese, Chinese, Indian) to existing implant systems. Mahfouz et al in a comprehensive, 3D analysis of the knee morphology identified shape differences in the distal femur and proximal tibia among the ethnic groups. [11]

They found AMs (East Asian Male) had a smaller ML/AP (mediolateral/anteroposterior) ratio than CMs (Caucasian Male) (1.33 ± 0.12 versus 1.4 ± 0.06), contrary to Yue et al. The mean and SD values of the ML for CMs (79 ± 4.6 mm) and CFs (Caucasian Female) (68.6 ± 4.8 mm) were comparable to those published by Yue et al. The normalized ratios and nonlinear shape analysis in this research supported differences between East Asians and Caucasians independent of any scale factor. They also found differences in the ratio between AAF/CF (African American Female/Caucasian Female) and AAM/CM (African American Male/Caucasian Male), with the mean ratio being larger in CMs compared to AAMs and CFs compared to AAFs. [11, 12, 13]

This finding conflicts with Gillespie et al. who reported a larger ML/AP ratio in African Americans than in Caucasians; however, their African American population was from the early 20$^{th}$ century, which could account for differing anatomic features from the current population. [3, 13] The radii of curvature analysis on both the medial and lateral condyles revealed AMs and AFs (American Female) tend to have more curved condyles (ie, smaller radius of curvature) than Caucasians, implying a larger ROM. This finding agrees with Leszko et al. who found an increased ROM of 153° for AF and 151° for AM compared to 146° for CM. [14] Women from all ethnic groups had smaller, narrower knees with a smaller ML/AP ratio.

This study by Mahfouz et al. shows that AAMs and AAFs have larger AP dimensions than their Asian and Caucasian counterparts and AMs and AFs have smaller AP dimensions than CMs and CFs. When compared to CFs with similar AP dimensions, AMs have larger ML dimensions. In analyzing ethnic differences in tibial anatomy, AAMs have larger LAPs (lateral anteroposterior diameter) and smaller MAPs (medial anteroposterior diameter) (Figure 1-B) than CMs, while also having larger ML and AP dimensions than AMs. AMs and AFs have smaller ML and AP dimensions than CMs and CFs. This study also identifies shape differences in the distal femur and proximal tibia between sexes in each ethnic population. Males across all ethnicities have average 9-mm larger ML and 5-mm larger AP dimensions than their female counterparts. AAMs and CFs have shallower patellar grooves than AAFs and CMs. Females have more curved femurs in all ethnicities. Males have larger tibial AP dimensions than females. AAMs and CMs have larger ML dimensions than AAFs and CFs, respectively. Differences in femoral and tibial shapes are also identified in comparing shapes across populations based on differences in ML/AP, AML/PML (anterior mediolateral length/posterior mediolateral length), and MAP/LAP ratios. [11] (Figure 1-A)

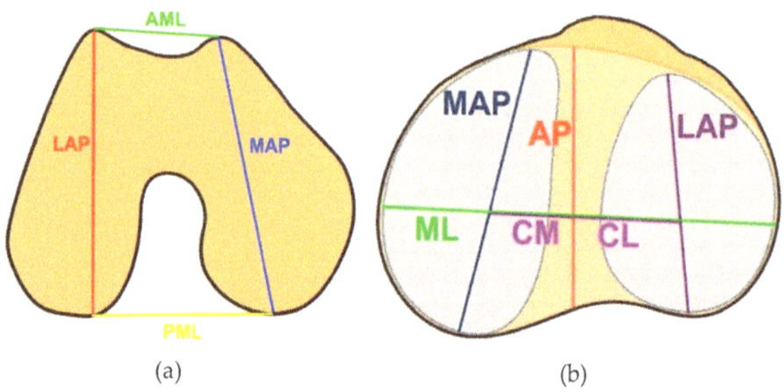


**Figure 1.** A) Diagram illustrating measurements on the distal femur. AML = Anterior mediolateral length, PML = Posterior mediolateral length, LAP = Lateral anteroposterior diameter, MAP = Medial anteroposterior diameter. B) Diagram illustrating measurements on the proximal tibia. ML = Mediolateral width, AP = Anteroposterior length, MAP = Medial anteroposterior length, LAP = Lateral anteroposterior length.

## 3. Normal development of the knee angle

Development of the knee angle from bowlegs (varus) in the infant to knock knees (valgus) in early childhood is a part of normal and physiological development. Several researchers have studied knee angle variation in various parts of the world and many of them have tried to set standards for certain ethnic/social groups. [15, 16, 17]

The TFA has been described as the angle defined by the mechanical axis of the femur intersecting the mechanical axis of the tibia.

There are studies available regarding normal development of the knee angle in whites, Chinese, Nigerians, Koreans, and Turkish children. Saini UC et al. have found that none of the subjects had a varus knee alignment in the more than 3 years age groups. Also, even for the children in the 2 years age group, the mean TFA was positive, indicating a mean valgus alignment in Indian children, even at the age of 2 years. [18] This was contrary to the findings of the largest study carried to date by Cheng et al. in the Chinese population, which showed a mean varus TFA at the age of 2 years. After 3 years, the authors noted a rapid decrease in the mean IMD in the Chinese children, reaching 0 cm at the age of 8 years, with a normal range of ±3 cm. [19] In Turkish children, Arazi et al noted a significantly higher degree of valgus angle than that in previous reports. The maximal mean valgus angle was 9.6° at 7 years of age for boys and 9.8° at 6 years of age for girls. These differences were considered to be racial differences between Turkish children and those of other races. Turkish children aged between 3 and 17 years were found to exhibit up to 11° physiologic valgus. The authors concluded that a measurable varus angle or a valgus higher than 11° during this period should be considered as abnormal. [20] In a study conducted by Heath and Staheli in white children, using clinical measurements of the TFA and the ICD and IMD, children were maximally bow-legged at the age of 6 months and progressed toward approximately neutral knee angles (0.0°) by the age of 18 months. They found the greatest mean knock knee of 8° at the age of 4 years, which was followed by a gradual decrease to a mean of 6° at 11 years of age. Normal children aged 2–11 years had knock knee up to 12° and IMD up to 8 cm. The existence of bowlegs after the age of 2 years was found to be abnormal. [21] Yoo et al. carried out a study on normal healthy Korean children, with full-length anteroposterior view standing radiographs. They found that the overall patterns of the chronological changes in the knee angle were similar to those described previously in western or Asian children, but the knee angle development was delayed, i.e., genu varum before 1 year, neutral at 1.5 years, increasing genu valgum with a maximum value of 7.8° at 4 years, followed by a gradual decrease to approximately 5–6° of genu valgum of the adult level at 7–8 years of age. Although the use of different techniques to estimate the knee angles might be responsible for variations in observations in different studies, it is more likely that these variations are possibly due to the ethnical and racial differences that might exist in different population groups. [22] Arazi et al found the weight of children at a specific age to have a negative correlation with the ICD of the subject. However, this correlation was found to be weak and although statistically significant, it might not be of any clinical significance. The only possible explanation to this might be the relatively thick thighs of the heavier children, which is expected to subjectively decrease the ICD. However, considering the fact that fixed body landmarks on the body should not change even in obese children, this result is hard to explain. [20]

Oginni et al. who measured the knee angles of 2,036 normal Nigerian children up to an age of 12 years. In their study, they found the majority of the knees to be bowed (varus) in the first 6 months. At 21–23 months of age, the distribution of angles became strongly bimodal: about half being varus and half being valgus (knock-kneed). After this, the knee angle was found to be valgus in most of the children. They concluded that the change from varus to valgus in individual infants might be sudden (a few weeks), although the changeover of the whole population appeared smooth and gradual. The authors also concluded that varus knee alignment was uncommon after 2 years in Nigerian children and large knee angles between 2 and 5 years suggested rickets. However, in their study, the children became maximally and uniformly knock-kneed (-7.1° ± 1.4°) between 3 and 3.5 years, with little change thereafter. [23] This is contrary to the findings in Indian children, in whom the maximum valgus has been found to occur at an age of 5–6 years. [18] As the literature shows, there is a wide variation in the normal development of the knee angle, which might be physiological.

### 3.1. Development of tibiofemoral angle in Indian children

Saini et al. observed the highest mean IMD of 4.5 cm in children aged 5 years, with a minimum mean of 1 cm at the age of 9 years. They also found that the maximum mean valgus was seen at the age of 6 years in Indian children. Thereafter, the valgus alignment decreased in Indian children and the mean TFA stabilized to lie between 4 and 5° in most of the children after the age of 10 years. Indian girls overall showed more valgus at the knees than boys and the results were statistically significant, especially at the age of 6 years, when peak valgus was achieved in Indian children. The maximum TFA of 11° was seen in a 6-year-old perfectly healthy girl. They also found a boy with a valgus knee angle of 10.5° at the age of 5 years. [18]

In India, there are statistically significant differences between the mean TFA of boys and girls in the age groups of 3, 5, and 6 years (Table 2). The mean TFA is significantly higher in Indian girls of age groups 3 and 6 years, while Indian boys of age group 5 years showed a significantly higher mean TFA. After the age of 6 years, there are no statistically significant differences between the mean TFA of Indian boys and girls.

Neither height nor body mass of a child at a specific age group have statistically significant correlation with the mean TFA or the ICD or IMD. [18]

| Age in years | Mean TFA of males (±SD) | Mean TFA of females (±SD) |
|---|---|---|
| 2 | 1.0 ± 3.1 | 1.0 ± 3.6 |
| 3 | 1.6 ± 3.6 | 3.4 ± 1.5 |
| 4 | 3.9 ± 1.4 | 4.8 ± 1.3 |
| 5 | 7.5 ± 2.2 | 5.9 ± 1.8 |
| 6 | 7.2 ± 2.6 | 9.0 ± 1.9 |
| 7 | 5.8 ± 1.5 | 6.4 ± 2.0 |
| 8 | 5.7 ± 2.5 | 6.7 ± 1.8 |
| 9 | 5.3 ± 2.2 | 5.9 ± 1.0 |
| 10 | 5.3 ± 2.3 | 5.6 ± 1.9 |
| 11 | 4.58 ± 2.35 | 5.30 ± 2.49 |
| 12 | 4.70 ± 2.15 | 5.16 ± 0.98 |
| 13 | 4.68 ± 1.95 | 5.10 ± 0.87 |
| 14 | 4.56 ± 1.45 | 5.00 ± 0.63 |
| 15 | 4.55 ± 2.13 | 5.00 ± 0.81 |
| Total | 4.61 ± 2.96 | 5.39 ± 2.45 |

**Table 1.** Mean TFA ± SD distribution amongst male and female children at different ages

### 3.2. Development of tibiofemoral angle in Korean children

Yoo JH et al found that in Korean children, knee alignment or aTFA was in varus alignment in infancy, and became neutral at an average age of 1.5 yr. Development into valgus alignment continued until age 4 yr when it peaked at 7.8°. It then decreased slowly to plateau at 5-6° at age 7 to 8 yr, and remained at this level thereafter. This pattern of knee alignment change is similar to that found previously in other ethnic groups, except that the valgus peak occurred later. [22]

### 3.3. Axial alignment of the lower extremity in Chinese adults

Achieving normal axial alignment of the lower extremity is important to surgeons who perform reconstructive surgery of the knee. The normal alignment of the lower extremity in Caucasians has been documented by Moreland et al. with use of radiographs of the lower extremity. [24]

Tang WM et al. showed that the extremities of the Chinese women had a mean of 2.2 ± 2.5 degrees of varus alignment, and those of the Chinese men had a mean of 2.2 ± 2.7 degrees of varus alignment. The knees of Chinese female subjects, therefore, were in more varus alignment than were those in the white female subjects in the study by Hsu et al. [17, 25]

The inferolateral angle (Angle A in figure 2) between the knee joint surface and the mechanical axis of the tibia is an index of knee joint obliquity. If this angle is 90 degrees, the knee-joint surface is perpendicular to the mechanical axis. The knee-joint surface is inclined toward the medial side if this angle is larger than 90 degrees. This angle was a mean (and standard deviation) of 95.4 ± 2.5 degrees (range, 89.0 to 100.0 degrees) in the women and 94.9 ± 2.3 deegrees (range, 90.5 to 102.0 degrees) in the men in this study. The mean medial inclination (Angle B in figure 2) of the knee joint surfaces in Chinese female and male subjects therefore was 5.4 ± 2.5 degrees and 4.9 ± 2.3 degrees, respectively, which is significantly more oblique than the commonly reported 3 degrees. The inferolateral angle in both the right and the left extremity in Chinese male subjects was significantly larger than that in the white subjects in the study by Moreland et al. In the study by Hsu et al., this angle was a mean of 91.0 ± 1.4 degrees in thirty white men (sixty lower extremities) who ranged in age from twenty-five to forty years and a mean of 90.1 ± 1.9 degrees in thirty white women who ranged in age from twenty-five to forty years. [24, 25]

As noted by Insall, one should be cautious in describing what is "normal" because of the substantial individual variations. Currently, designers of most total knee arthroplasty systems recommend placement of the components in such a way that the transverse axis of the artificial knee joint is perpendicular to the mechanical axes of the tibia and the femur. The resulting alignment of the lower extremity, therefore, is in close proximity to the alignment documented by Moreland et al. and Hsu et al. The mechanical axes of the femur and the tibia did not form a straight line in either Chinese males or females. This finding is in contrast to the general consensus that has been described previously. The Chinese females had more varus alignment of the knee than did the white female subjects in the study by Hsu et al. The authors did not find the same difference between the Chinese male subjects and the white male subjects described by Moreland et al. and Hsu et al. Insall and Hungerford et al. described a 3-degree varus alignment of the knee-joint surface with reference to the mechanical axis of the tibia. Although Moreland et al. confirmed this 3-degree varus in white men, the finding was not reproduced in the study by Hsu et al. In this study of Chinese subjects, the surface of the knee joint had a medial inclination with respect to the tibia that was a mean of 5.4 degrees in the women and 4.9 degrees in the men. The values were found to be significantly different from those of the white subjects in the studies of Moreland et al. and Hsu et al. Therefore, if the tibial cut in a total knee arthroplasty is placed perpendicular to the mechanical axis of the tibia, 5 degrees of external rotation of the femoral component instead of the commonly reported 3 degrees might be necessary to produce a rectangular flexion gap in Chinese patients. [24, 25]

Fang et al. showed that femora in Chinese individuals are more bowed. In such patients, a short intramedullary rod entering the femur at the apex of the inter-condylar notch (femoral anatomical axis I) with a 4-degree distal cutting block is more likely to produce a distal femoral cut that is perpendicular to the mechanical axis of the femur. However, the choice of the cutting block should be individualized according to the preoperative planning on weight-bearing radiographs of the whole lower extremity. It is also interesting to note that the designers of some instrumentation systems have recommended use of a distal femoral cutting block with a smaller angle in taller individuals on the basis of the assumption that taller patients have a smaller physiological valgus angle of the femur. [26]

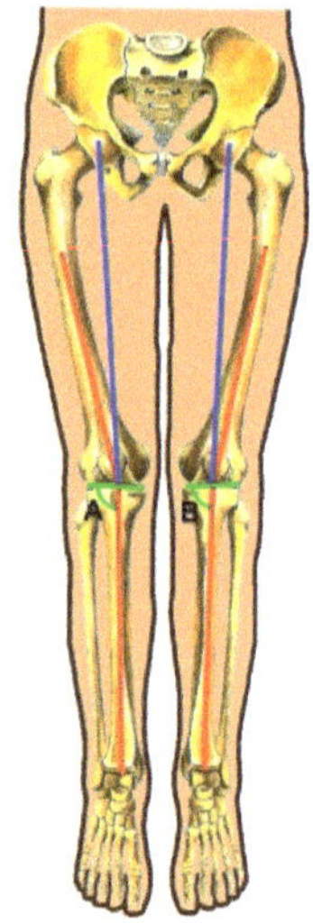


**Figure 2.** Diagram showing the anatomic (red) and mechanical (green) axes of the lower limb and the angles between them.

### 3.4. Axial alignment of the lower extremity in healthy Indian adults

Mullaji et al showed that the mean HKTA angle in healthy indian adults was 1.3° ± 0.8° of varus,mean distal femoral axis-femoral mechanical axis angle was 5.5° ± 0.8°, mean femoral condylarmechanical axis angle was 93.1° ± 1.6°, and mean femoral bow was 0.4° ± 1.2°. [27]

### 3.5. Variances in sagittal femoral shaft bowing

Tang WM et al have confirmed in Chinese patients distal sagittal bowing is a constant and important feature, and it affects the positioning of the femoral component on the sagittal plane. There is a dilemma of implanting the femoral component either according to the anatomy of the distal femur ignoring the bowing, or according the longitudinal axis of the femur on the sagittal plane. On one hand, following the distal anatomy might sufficiently flex the femoral component that it results in an undesirable impingement of the anterior aspect of the polyethylene post on knee extension if posterior-stabilized implants are used and thus become a source of osteolysis-inducing polyethylene particles. However, following the longitudinal axis of the femur might result in an extended femoral component that could compromise the anterior cortex of the distal femur. In Chinese patients who have undergone TKA, distal sagittal bowing of the femur is common but the common pattern is posteromedial osteoarthritis. This apparent inconsistency could be the result of differences in tibial slope and the joint line obliquity in Chinese patients. [28]

## 4. Three dimensional morphometry of the Chinese knees

### 4.1. Proximal tibial morphology

The average tibial mediolateral (tML) and tibial anteroposterior (tAP) measurement for Chinese knees are 73.0±4.6 mm and 48.8±3.4 mm, respectively. Males have larger values for tML and tAP compared with females. The male subject have larger values than female subject in the mediolateral dimension under a given anteroposterior dimension. [29] To evaluate possible differences between the medial and lateral plateau, Bo Cheng et al measured the tMAP and tLAP, and found that the tMAP was larger than the tLAP by an average of 5.6±3.2 mm in males and 5.1±2.2 in females, the CL had larger values than CM (Figure 1, B) by an average of 4.9±2.2 mm in males and 4.3±1.7 mm in females. They also calculated the aspect ratio of the tibia (tML/tAP%). The average aspect ratio of the tibia was 149.7±5.2. (Table 2) The aspect ratio showed a definitely negative correlation with tAP. From the relationship between the aspect ratio (tML/tAP %) and tAP, the authors found that there were large values in the aspect ratio with the smaller tAP, and that males have larger values in the aspect ratio than females having the same values for anteroposterior dimension. Compared with the five tibial components, only one of the prostheses had a declining change in the aspect ratio parallel with the increasing tAP. Even so, but the rate of change did not match that of the Chinese population. [29]

### 4.2. Distal femoral morphology

The femoral mediolateral (fML) and femoral anteroposterior (fAP) measurements are 71.0±3.0 mm and 64.1±2.7 mm, respectively. The male have larger values in fML and fAP compared with female. Comparing the morphological data with similar values for five conventional femoral components currently used in China, Bo Cheng et al found that two of the prostheses had large values in fML dimension with all range of the fAP. This was more evident with reference to female. They found that males have larger values in mediolateral dimension than females under the same value in the anteroposterior dimension. They also found that the fMAP had larger values than fLAP by an average of 0.8±0.3 mm in males and 0.5±0.2 mm in females. The average aspect ratio was 111.1±2.7 (Table 3) and had a negative correlation with the fAP. The femoral aspect ratio was higher for smaller knees and proportionally lower for larger knees. Female subjects had a smaller aspect ratio with the same anteroposterior dimension. Only one of the five femoral components showed a similar negative correlation with the fAP. Even so, the rate of change was not the same as that of the Chinese population. [29]

#### *4.2.1. Morphologic relationships between the tibia and femur*

Bo Cheng et al also analyzed the correlation between the tibial mediolateral (tML) and femoral mediolateral (fML) dimension, and between the tibial mediolateral (tML) and femoral anteroposterior (fAP)measurement. The results showed that the fML and fAP were strongly correlated with the tML. As the tML increasing, the fML and fAP also increased. [29]

| Parameters | Male | Female | Combined |
|---|---|---|---|
| **Tibial mediolateral (tML)** | 76.4±2.8 | 68.8±4.6 | 73.0±4.6 |
| **Tibial middle anteroposterior(tAP)** | 51.3±2.0 | 45.7±1.9 | 48.8±3.4 |
| **Tibial medial anteroposterior (tMAP)** | 53.3±2.5 | 47.5±2.4 | 50.7±2.4 |
| **Tibial lateral anteroposterior (tLAP)** | 47.7±2.7 | 42.4±2.3 | 45.3±2.5 |
| **Medial to central distance (CM)** | 13.2±2.6 | 11.9±2.0 | 12.7±2.1 |
| **Lateral to central distance (CL)** | 18.1±2.4 | 16.2±2.3 | 17.3±2.3 |
| **Aspect ratio (tML/tAP)** | 149.0±5.7 | 150.7±6.1 | 149.7±5.2 |
| **tMAP–tLAP** | 5.6±3.2 | 5.1±2.2 | 5.4±2.8 |

**Table 2.** Average values of the tibia morphology measurement (mm).

| Parameters | Male | Female | Combined |
|---|---|---|---|
| **Femoral anteroposterior (fAP)** | 66.6±2.4 | 61.0±2.7 | 64.1±2.7 |
| **Femoral mediolateral (fML)** | 74.4±2.9 | 66.8±3.1 | 71.0±3.0 |
| **Femoral medial anteroposterior (fMAP)** | 52.6±2.4 | 49.8±3.2 | 51.3±3.3 |
| **Femoral lateral anteroposterior (fLAP)** | 51.8±3.7 | 49.3±4.1 | 50.7±4.0 |
| **Aspect ratio (fML/fAP %)** | 111.7±3.3 | 109.6±3.6 | 111.1±2.7 |
| **fMAP–fLAP** | 0.8±0.3 | 0.5±0.2 | 0.6±0.3 |

**Table 3.** Average values of the femur morphology measurement (mm).

*4.2.2. Utility*

Quantification of the tML and tAP revealed that the female has a smaller tibial surface than the male, and both have smaller values than the Caucasian population. In the tibia of the Chinese population, the morphologic data showed a decreasing aspect ratio (tML/tAP %) as the tAP dimension increased, which is similar in many studies. In contrast, a majority of the implants had a relatively constant aspect ratio. Comparing five major conventional prostheses, it is evident that tML is undersized with the smaller tAP, and overhang with the larger tAP. This is more evident in male knee. In the morphology of the femur, females have a smaller aspect ratio with the same femoral anteroposterior dimension, which suggest that women have generally narrower femora than men when the femoral anteroposterior dimension is adequate. These results suggest that the prostheses which are suitable for Caucasian patients may be larger than ideal for Chinese patients. Bo Cheng et al also found that the femoral condyles in the Chinese population are asymmetric. These results may imply that asymmetric femoral component could prevent soft tissue irritation.

Since the tML is strongly correlated with the fML and fAP, it is important to consider the tibia and femur as a whole. Therefore, the tML and fAP should be considered as the criteria to design gender-specific proper prostheses suitable for most of Chinese population.

### 4.3. Distal rotational alignment of the chinese femur

Yip et al showed a statistically significant difference in Whiteside-epicondylar angle when using the mechanical (2.3°) compared with the anatomic (1.1°) axes in Chinese population. The posterior condylar angle in this study was shown to be 5.1° (for men) and 5.8° (for women). [30] (Figure 3)

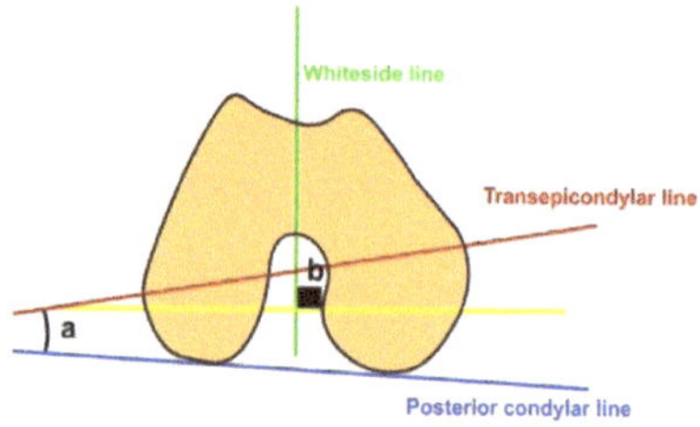


**Figure 3.** The whiteside-epicondylar (a) and Posterior condylar (b) angles.

*4.3.1. The offset of the tibial shaft from the tibial plateau in Chinese people*

Tang et al conducted a study to identify the location of the tibial shaft axis on the tibial plateau with the use of magnetic resonance imaging scans in a Chinese population. All of the measurements were made at three resection levels. The first resection level was just distal to the subchondral bone of the medial tibial plateau, which represented the clinical situation of the level of a bone cut in a proximal tibial segment with mild bone loss. The second resection level was 5mm distal to the subchondral bone of the medial tibial plateau, which represented the level of a bone cut in a proximal tibial segment with moderate bone loss. The third resection level was 10 mm distal to the subchondral bone of the medial tibial plateau, which represented the level of a bone cut in a proximal tibial segment with severe bone loss. They showed that the mean offset (and standard deviation) of the tibial shaft from the tibial plateau was 7.23 ± 2.44 mm (range, 1.62 to 12.26 mm), 6.33 ± 2.26 mm (range, 1.31 to 11.36 mm), and 4.75 ± 2.07 mm (range, 0.46 to 9.36 mm) at the first, second, and third resection levels, respectively. In almost all the knees that were examined, the tibial shaft axis was located anterolateral to the center of the tibial plateau at all resection levels. The anteroposterior and mediolateral offsets and the anteroposterior and mediolateral dimensions of the tibial plateau in the male group were significantly larger than those in the female group at each resection level. [31]

*4.3.2. Utility*

Several studies have revealed that the axis of the tibial shaft is, on the average, located anteromedial to the center of the tibial plateau in the Western population, for whom a medially offset stem seems more suitable. [32-34]

But, these results confirm that the axis of the tibial shaft does not overlap the center of the tibial plateau in Chinese people. Abraham et al. performed total knee arthroplasty in twenty cadaver tibiae and found that the average distance between the center of the tibial diaphysis and the center of the tibial metaphysis was 4.1 mm at the resection level of the fibular head. In view of the findings of Abraham et al. [35] as well as this study, it would appear that an offset stem would be more suitable for Chinese patients who need a long-stemmed tibial component. These authors also noted that there was a large variation in the offset of the tibial shaft from the tibial plateau, ranging from0.46 to 12.26 mm, so it would be desirable to have a wide range of offset stems available—for example, from 0 to 16 mm, in 2-mm or 4-mm increments. [35]

In a study on Iranian normal adult knees, we assessed the tibial plateau shift angle (TPSA) in order to assess our hypothesis that the proximal tibia of Iranian knee is not the same as the western knees. Our TPSA findings demonstrate that tibial plateau was not symmetrical and the Cp passes medial to Cs. This shows that the tibial plateaus in Iranian knees have a medial offset in regard to tibial shaft. So we consider that the center of the tibial plateau should not be used as a landmark of the tibial component.

Yoo et al. studied the placement of the tibial stem in close relation to the medial tibial cortex when using total knee replacements (TKRs) with medially-offset tibial stems in Korean patients. They found that the midline of the tibial stem was located medial to the tibial shaft axis in 79.7% of knees. In 6.5% of knees there was radiological contact between the tibial stem or cement mantle and the medial tibial cortex. This study has shown that the medially-offset stem in the tibial component may not be a good option for knees undergoing replacement Korean patients. (Figure 4) These researches show that some tibial base-plates specifically designed for Caucasians may not be suitable for Asian people and it remains a necessity to design a special tibial base-plate for these ethnic groups. [36] (Figure 5)

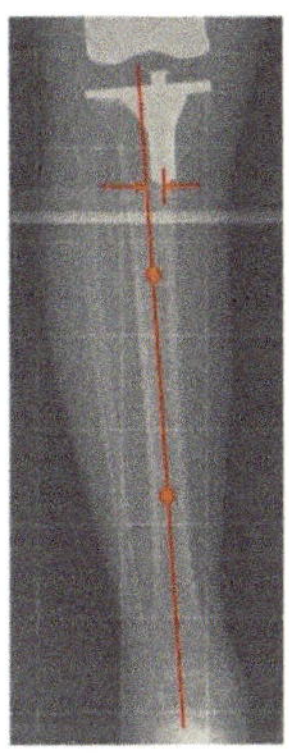

**Figure 4.** Anteroposterior postoperative radiograph showing the distance between the tip of the stem and the tibial shaft axis (between arrows)

### 4.4. Posterior slope of tibial plateau in Chinese

Kapandji found that the tibial plateau was inclined posteriorly for 5 ° to 6 ° with the horizontal and called this *retroversion* in the sagittal plane of the tibia. Insall and Kelly quoted that the posterior slope was approximately 10 ° with respect to the shaft of the tibia in western population. [38] Chiu et al. studied the posterior tibial slope in Chinese population. On visual inspection, they found that the posterior slope of the medial tibial plateau was 14.8 °

(SD, 4.2°; range, 5°-25°), and that of the lateral tibial plateau was 11.8 ° (SD, 3.8°; range, 4°-23°). The association between the posterior slopes of the medial and lateral tibial plateau was not strong.

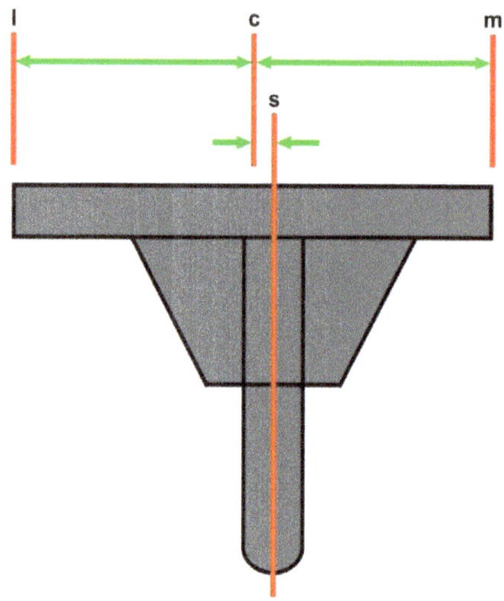


**Figure 5.** Diagram showing a right tibial component with a medially-offset stem. The tip of the stem (s) is located medial to the center of the tibial tray (c) which is equidistant from the medial (m) and lateral (l) borders of the tibial component. The distance between c and s corresponds to the amount of medial offset.

The difference between the posterior slopes of the medial and lateral tibial plateau was statistically significant. On radiographic assessment, they showed that the posterior slope was 14.7 ° (SD, 3.7°; range, 5°-22 °) with the extramedullary alignment line and 11.5 ° (SD, 3.6°; range, 2°-18.5 °) with the intramedullary alignment line. The association between the posterior slopes with the 2 alignment lines was strong. The difference between the posterior slopes with the 2 alignment lines was statistically significant. The posterior slope of the medial tibial plateau on visual inspection showed stronger correlation to the posterior slopes determined by radiographs. The posterior slope of the lateral tibial plateau on visual inspection had weaker correlation to the posterior slopes with the intramedullary alignment line and extramedullary alignment line in the radiographs. [38]

### 4.5. Ethnical differences of knee anthropometry

#### *4.5.1. Between Chinese and white men and women*

Recent anthropometric studies have suggested that current design of total knee arthroplasty (TKA) does not cater to racial anthropometric differences. Most of the commercially available TKA prostheses are designed according to the anthropometric data of white knees, which has been suspected as the cause of the component mismatch in Asian people. Several studies have compared the morphology of Asian knees to that of TKA prostheses currently used in Asia and found that the femoral aspect ratio (mediolateral [fML]/anteroposterior [fAP]) of these prostheses were not suitable for Asian patients. Iorio et al showed that the Japanese patients had a significantly less postoperative range of motion than white patients. Furthermore, 4.1% Japanese patients required revision after primary posterior cruciate-retaining TKA within an average follow-up of 6.6 years, whereas only 2.6% of their American cohort needed revision within an average follow-up of 9 years. The authors suggested that the racial morphologic differences might be a factor causing the differences in outcome. [5]

Yue B et al showed that the fML dimension of Chinese females (72.8 ± 2.6 mm; range, 70.0-79.1 mm) was significantly smaller than that of white females (76.4 ± 4.0 mm; range, 70.3-82 mm) (P =.002). The fAP dimension was 58.8 ± 2.5 mm (range, 53.2-63 mm) for Chinese females and 59.7 ± 2.6 mm (range, 54.6-64.1 mm) for white females. The difference in fAP dimension was not statistically significant. A statistically significant difference was noted between the fML/fAP ratios of Chinese females (1.24 ± 0.04; range, 1.17-1.32) and white females (1.28 ± 0.06; range, 1.16-1.39). The morphological data showed a progressive decline in the fML/fAP ratio with increasing fAP dimension for both races. However, there was a distinct offset between the fML/fAP ratio of Chinese and white females, indicating that the Chinese females had a smaller fML/fAP ratio than white females for the same fAP dimension.(Table 5) Measurements of tibia showed that the tibial size of Chinese females was generally smaller than that of white females. However, the tibial aspect ratio did not show any significant difference between Chinese (1.78 ± 0.1; range, 1.56-1.96) and white females (1.76 ± 0.08; range, 1.58-1.89). The medial/lateral posterior tibial slopes showed no difference between the 2 groups. The average medial slope was 5.4° ± 2.3° (range, 1.4°-10.1°) for Chinese females and 6.5° ± 2.9° (range, 0.6°-10.7°) for white females. The average lateral slope was 4.8° ± 2.8° (range, 0.3°-10.6°) for Chinese females and 5.8° ± 2.7° (range, 0.8°-10.4°) for white females. Chinese males had an average fML dimension of 82.6 ± 3.6 mm (range, 72.6-87.1 mm), which was significantly smaller than that of white males (86.0 ± 5.6 mm; range, 74.9-100.2 mm). The fAP size averaged 65.0 ± 2.8 mm (range, 59.4-70.3 mm) for Chinese males and 67.5 ± 3.6 mm (range, 62.4-75.3 mm) for white males. The difference was statistically significant between fAP size of Chinese and white males. The femoral aspect ratio (fML/fAP) of Chinese males averaged 1.27 ± 0.03 (range, 1.22-1.33) and white males 1.28 ± 0.07 (range, 1.12-1.37), and there was no statistically significant difference. The tibial dimension of Chinese males was generally smaller than that of white males. A significant difference was noted for the tibial aspect ratio, with Chinese males averaging 1.82 ± 0.07 (range, 1.70-1.95) and white males averaging 1.75 ± 0.11 (range, 1.58-1.87). The morphological data showed a progressive decline in the tibial aspect ratio with increasing average tAP dimension for both races. The lines representing change in tibial aspect ratio with increasing average tAP dimension for Chinese and white males were nearly coincident. Therefore, the differences in tibial aspect ratios between the 2 groups may be caused by the average tAP dimensions of Chinese males that were generally smaller than those of white males. The medial/lateral plateau posterior slope showed no significant difference between the 2 groups.

The average medial slope was 6.0° ± 2.5° (range, 2.7°- 12.0°) for Chinese males and 5.1° ± 3.3° (range, −3.0° to 11.1°) for white males. The average lateral slope was 5.2° ± 3.6° (range, −1.8° to 14.0°) for Chinese males and 5.6° ± 2.7° (range, 2.5°-15.1°) for white males. [39] (Table 5)

| | fML (mm) | fAP (mm) | fML/fAP |
|---|---|---|---|
| **Chinese female** | 72.8 ± 2.6 (70.0-79.1) | 58.8 ± 2.5 (53.2-63) | 1.24 ± 0.04 (1.17-1.32) |
| **White female** | 76.4 ± 4.0 (70.3-82) | 59.7 ± 2.6 (54.6-64.1) | 1.28 ± 0.06 (1.16-1.39) |
| **Chinese male** | 82.6 ± 3.6 (72.6-87.1) | 65.0 ± 2.8 (59.4-70.3) | 1.27 ± 0.03 (1.22-1.33) |
| **White male** | 86.0 ± 5.6 (74.9-100.2) | 67.5 ± 3.6 (62.4-75.3) | 1.28 ± 0.07 (1.12-1.37) |

**Table 4.** Femoral Measurements Categorized by Race and Sex.

| | Tibial Plateau Dimensions | | | | | Posterior Tibial Slope (deg) | | |
|---|---|---|---|---|---|---|---|---|
| | MPAP (mm) | LPAP (mm) | Average AP (mm) | tML (mm) | tML/Avg. tAP | MPPS | LPPS | Average Posterior Slope |
| Chinese female | 41.5 ± 3.0 (37.6-48.6) | 33.2 ± 3.2 (28.7-40.2) | 37.3 ± 2.8 (34.5-44.1) | 66.2 ± 2.1 (63.1-69.5) | 1.78 ± 0.10 (1.56-1.96) | 5.4 ± 2.3 (1.4-10.1) | 4.8 ± 2.8 (0.3-10.6) | 5.1 ± 2.3 (1.4-9.9) |
| White female | 43.4 ± 1.9 (39.2-46.5) | 35.2 ± 3.8 (26.5-40.0) | 39.3 ± 2.6 (34.1-43.3) | 69.0 ± 4.2 (61.3-74.4) | 1.76 ± 0.08 (1.58-1.89) | 6.5 ± 2.9 (0.6-10.7) | 5.8 ± 2.7 (0.8-10.4) | 6.1 ± 2.5 (0.7-9.8) |
| Chinese male | 46.1 ± 2.4 (42.0-49.5) | 36.8 ± 2.1 (34.1-40.7) | 41.5 ± 2.1 (38.0-45.1) | 75.2 ± 3.6 (67.6-81.5) | 1.82 ± 0.07 (1.70-1.95) | 6.0 ± 2.5 (2.7-12.0) | 5.2 ± 3.6 (-1.8-14.0) | 5.6 ± 2.8 (0.4-11.9) |
| White male | 49.3 ± 3.1 (42.5-53.5) | 40.7 ± 2.9 (35.6-48.4) | 45.0 ± 2.8 (39.9-50.2) | 78.7 ± 5.4 (67.1-89.1) | 1.75 ± 0.11 (1.58-1.97) | 5.1 ± 3.3 (-3.0-11.1) | 5.6 ± 2.7 (2.5-15.1) | 5.3 ± 2.5 (0.8-12.7) |

**Table 5.** Tibial Measurements Categorized by Race and Sex

The present study showed that the dimensions of Chinese knees were generally smaller than white knees. In addition, Chinese females had a significantly narrower distal femur than white females, whereas Chinese males had a wider proximal tibia than their white counterparts. These results proved the hypothesis that there is a distinct difference in size and shape between the Chinese and white knees. [39] Harvey et al also showed that there are more valgus alignment of the distal femur in Chinese. [40]

A proper design of femoral aspect ratio of femoral TKA components is critical to obtain an ideal coverage of the resected bone surface. It must be noted that the differences in average values of femoral aspect ratio between Chinese and white females cannot be explained by differences in knee size alone, and this may point to a distinct variation in femoral shape between the 2 races. Given this, it is possible that the components designed based on white knee data may produce a mediolateral component overhang in Chinese females. [41]

The geometry of tibial plateau has a direct influence on the biomechanics of tibiofemoral joint and is considered as an important factor in TKA design and implantation. [9, 42]

The study by Yue et al. showed that Chinese subjects generally had a smaller size of proximal tibia than white subjects in both sexes. Interestingly, the tibial aspect ratio of Chinese males was significantly larger than that of white males (1.82 ± 0.07 vs 1.75 ± 0.11). However, the present study also found a larger tibial aspect ratio in small knees and a proportionally smaller ratio in large knees. Therefore, the differences of the tibial aspect ratios between the 2 groups may be caused by the average tAP dimensions of Chinese males that were generally smaller than those of white males. This study showed that there was no difference in medial/lateral posterior slope between Chinese and white subjects in either sex. [39]

#### *4.5.2. Anthropometry of the Japanese proximal tibia*

Uehara et al, in a comparative study between CT and intraoperative measurements of tibial dimensions, showed that the average ML length on the CT scan was significantly larger (74.3 ± 6.6 mm [mean ± SD]) compared with the intraoperative measurement (71.4 ± 5.0 mm). In contrast, the average AP length on the CT scan was significantly smaller (48.3 ± 5.4 mm) compared with the intraoperative measurement (50.3 ± 3.6 mm). [43]

#### *4.5.3. Variations between Japanese and Caucasian populations in the healthy young adult knee joint*

Hovinga et al showed that there was a significant difference in alignment between Caucasian and Japanese groups. The mechanical alignment in Caucasians was slightly varus (0.55 ± 0.338, 57%varus), while78% of Japanese subjects exhibited a varus alignment (1.64 ± 0.438). A significant difference also existed between male and female subjects, with women exhibiting a higher percentage of valgus alignment (50%) than men (36%). The average torsion angle was 37.58 for all subjects. Tibial torsion measurements showed significant differences with ethnicity; Caucasians demonstrated a higher torsion angle than Japanese. No difference based on gender was observed. The tibial width for all subjects was 74.1 ± 0.77 mm. The lateral width was 39.4 ± 0.52 mm, while the medial width was 34.6 ± 0.42 mm. Medial and lateral widths were greater in males than in females, but no ethnic differences were found. The laxity measurement for Caucasian females was 6.4 ± 0.36 mm, and for males was 4.9 ± 0.35 mm. For Japanese females, the laxity was 8.1 ± 0.65 mm, and for males 6.9 ± 0.56 mm. Significant differences were found for both gender and ethnicity. [4]

Based on this study, a higher varus alignment, lower tibial torsion, and higher ACL laxity were found in Japanese compared to Caucasian populations. Males demonstrated a higher varus alignment, larger tibial width, and lower ACL laxity compared to females. [4]

Tamari et al performed a clinical study aimed to investigate whether or not there were ethnic, gender, and age-related differences in FTA and torsion of the lower limb among healthy Japanese and Australian Caucasian populations. They found that the Japanese had significantly greater FTA than the Australian Caucasians. Moreover, there was gender difference in this variable, that is, the female subjects had significantly smaller FTA than the males. The femoral antetorsion was significantly smaller in middle and older age groups compared to the younger age group in the Japanese subjects. Femoral antetorsion of the Japanese was significantly greater than that of the Australian subjects. Further, the females had greater femoral antetorsion than the male subjects. They also found that the tibiofibular torsion was significantly larger in the younger and middle age groups compared to the older age group of the females, whereas there were no significant age-related differences in the male subjects. But, there was no ethnic difference in tibiofibular torsion. Tibiofibular torsion of the females was significantly smaller than that of the male subjects. [7]

#### *4.5.4. Morphometry of the Korean proximal tibia*

Kwak et al assessed the morphometry of the proximal tibia of Korean ethnicity. Their results are as follows. (Table 6)

##### *4.5.4.1. ML and AP dimensions*

The average mediolateral (ML) and middle anteroposterior (AP) dimensions for the Korean population were 73.5±5.6 mm and 47.3±3.8 mm, respectively. The males were found to have larger values for the AP and ML dimensions when compared to the females. Comparison of the AP and ML dimensions to the height of the person showed a statistically significant, positive correlation with the height of the person. [44]

##### *4.5.4.2. Medial and lateral anteroposterior dimensions of the tibial condyle*

The medial tibial plateau is larger than the lateral tibial plateau anteroposteriorly by an average of 3.9±2.9 mm in the males and 3.7±2.7 mm in the females. This result favors the need for asymmetry in the tibial component for the Korean population.

Accordingly, the gross size of the proximal tibia (ML and AP) in the females was found to be smaller than that in the males. Both the AP and ML lengths were found to be smaller than the Caucasian population. This research shows that the ML dimension is more strongly correlated to the height of the person when compared to the AP dimension. They also found that the MAP was located closer to the centre of the tibial plateau (C) as compared to the LAP, which further confirmed the asymmetry of the proximal tibia. [44]

This study revealed a higher aspect ratio for the smaller AP dimensions of the proximal tibia and a lower aspect ratio for the larger AP dimensions of the proximal tibia. In other words, this means that with every increase in the AP dimension of the proximal tibia, the shape of the anticipated tibial component becomes less oval (mediolaterally) for use in the Korean population. In the Japanese study, the aspect ratio in women varied from 138 to 142.86, however, they found that as the ML dimensions increased the aspect ratio increased. In contrast, to the pattern of the study population, the majority of the symmetric conventional implants showed a relatively constant aspect ratio or an increase in the aspect ratio (NexGen) with the increase of the AP dimension of the proximal cut. Thus, a tibial component that would be suitable for the Korean population would be one whose aspect ratio decreased with increase in the anteroposterior dimension. [44]

*4.5.5. Anthropometric measurements of knee joints in Thai population*

Chaichankul et al assessed the knee morphology in Thai population and found that the femoral aspect ratio and the tibial aspect ratio were significantly different between males and females. This study also demonstrated that when the tibial AP dimension increased, there was a decreasing tibial AP/ML aspect ratio, while most implants had a relatively constant aspect ratio. [45] (Table 7 and 8)

| Parameter | Male | Female | Combined |
|---|---|---|---|
| Mediolateral length (ML) | 76.1±4.0 | 67.64±3.12 | 71.9±5.6 |
| Middle anteroposterior length (AP) | 48.2±3.3 | 43.2±2.3 | 45.7±3.8 |
| Medial anteroposterior (MAP) | 48.5±3.7 | 43.5±2.9 | 45.9±4.2 |
| Lateral anteroposterior (LAP) | 44.6±3.2 | 39.8±2.5 | 42.2±3.7 |
| Medial to centre distance (CM) | 14.4±5.1 | 12.9±3.5 | 13.7±4.4 |
| Lateral to centre distance (CL) | 19.7±3.5 | 15.9±5.6 | 17.8±5.1 |
| Aspect ratio | 158 | 156 | 157 |
| Height (cm) | 165.9±4.8 | 156.4±5.0 | 161.2±6.8 |
| MAP–LAP difference | 3.9±2.9 | 3.7±2.7 | 3.8±2.8 |

**Table 6.** Average values (in mm) of the measured data from the cadavers

| Parameters | Total | Male | Female |
|---|---|---|---|
| | Mean±SD (range) | Mean±SD (range) | Mean±SD (range) |
| Resected AP length (mm) | 45.43±4.5 (35–56.9) | 48.55±3.73 (40–56.9) | 43.32±3.69 (35–55) |
| Resected ML width (mm) | 64.06±6.31 (52–78.9) | 70.15±3.87 (61.4–78.9) | 59.91±3.75 (52–76.3) |
| Aspect ratio (ML width/AP length)×100 | 141±12 (111–177) | 145±11 (124–177) | 139±12 (111–177) |

**Table 7.** The distal femoral condyle dimensions.

| Parameters | Total | Male | Female |
|---|---|---|---|
| | Mean±SD (range) | Mean±SD (range) | Mean±SD (range) |
| Resected AP length (mm) | 46.04±4.4 (37.6–56.6) | 50.15±3.09 (44–56.6) | 43.23±2.57 (37.6–52) |
| Resected ML width (mm) | 68.8±5.8 (57.8–86) | 74.44±3.44 (65.6–86) | 64.95±3.45 (57.8–78.6) |
| Aspect ratio (ML width/AP length)×100 | 67±3 (59–77) | 67±3 (61–75) | 67±3 (59–77) |

**Table 8.** The proximal tibial dimensions.

### *4.5.6. Anthropometric measurements of the Indian population*

Vaidya et al examined the anthropometric characteristics of Indian normal knees by CT scan and dry bone measurement. They found that the mean anteroposterior diameter of the femur in men was 61.09 mm and in women was 55.58 mm. Most men (27 of 38) had a range of anteroposterior diameter between 55 and 65 mm, whereas most women (40 of 48) had a range between 49 and 59 mm. In the cadaveric study, the mean anteroposterior diameter was 55.26 mm, and most (19 of 25) had a range between 52 and 60 mm. [46]

Assuming the lowest cut-off value of the anteroposterior diameter of the lower end of the femur in the study population to be 55 mm (55 mm being the smallest size of commercially available prosthetic femoral component), it was observed that a statistically significant number of Indian population (approximately 40%) had measurements lower than this value. This percentage was more significant in women (60.4%), in whom the mean anteroposterior diameter was 52.01 mm, than in men. The clinical implication of this statistical analysis is that there is a substantial number of Indians in whom the problem of component oversizing is likely to occur. [46]

### *4.5.7. Morphology of proximal tibia in Iranian*

#### *4.5.7.1. Lateral offset of tibial shaft in relation to tibial plateau*

In a study on Iranian normal adult knees, we assessed the tibial plateau shift angle (TPSA) in order to assess our hypothesis that the proximal tibia of Iranian knee is not the same as the western knees. TPSA is the angle formed between central line (Cs)of the tibial shaft and the mechanical axis of the tibia which goes through the central point (Cp) of the tibial articular surface and the center of ankle. Our results are shown in Table 9.

| | Our study | | | Japanese | | | Americans | | | France |
|---|---|---|---|---|---|---|---|---|---|---|
| **Parameter** | **Mean** | **SD** | **Range** | **Mean** | **SD** | **Range** | **Mean** | **SD** | **Range** | **Mean** |
| **TA** | 93.8 | 1.54 | 90.3-98 | 97.2 | 3.8 | 89-106 | 93 | 1.6 | 90-96.5 | 93 |
| **TPSA** | 2.11 | 3.64 | -3.4-7.4 | 2.21 | 1.5 | -3.0-7.0 | - | - | - | - |

**Table 9.** Representation of the amount of tibial shaft offset in Iranian and its comparison with other studies.

Our TPSA findings demonstrate that tibial plateau was not symmetrical and the Cp passes medial to Cs. This shows that the tibial plateaus in Iranian knees have a medial offset in regard to tibial shaft. So we consider that the center of the tibial plateau should not be used as a landmark of the tibial component.

#### *4.5.7.2. Posterior tibial slope*

We assessed the tibial slope in normal adults in Iran. The mean slope angle was 9.4±1.8 degrees. We found no statistical relationship between age and gender and posterior tibial slope. The normal posterior tibial slope angle in this Iranian population was different from other ethnic groups (Table 10). It may be necessary to consider these differences in designing tibial components for knee arthroplasty. [47]

| Study | Ethnic group | Number | Range of slope (degrees) | Mean ± (SD) |
|---|---|---|---|---|
| **Moore et al (1974)** | American | 50 | 7 – 22 | 14 ± 3.7 |
| **Jiang et al (1994)** | Thai | 50 | 0 – 20 | 10 ± 4 |
| **Matsuda et al (1999)** | Japanese | 30 | 5 – 15.5 | 10.7 |
| **Chiou et al (2000)** | Chinese | 25 | 5 – 22 | 14.7 ± 3.7 |
| **Our study (2009)** | Iranian | 108 | 2 – 18 | 9.4 ± 1.8 |

**Table 10.** Comparison of posterior tibial slope between Iranians and other ethnic groups

## 5. Patella

Patella-related problems are among the issues of concern during and after TKA. Information regarding anthropometric patellar dimensions can play an important role during the design of patellar prostheses and the development of surgical techniques. [48] Thickness, height/width ratio, and relative position of the median ridge all have implications relating to the selection of patellar components, patellofemoral contact stress, and patellar tracking in the trochlear groove. [49]

Patellar thickness is a challenging consideration during patellar resurfacing for TKA. A thin patella can reduce patellofemoral contact force but also poses the potential risk of stress fracture and anteroposterior instability. Increasing patellar thickness might be expected to increase effective quadriceps moment arm at low flexion angles of the knee but potentially reduces range of motion and predisposes to patellar subluxation. It commonly is assumed that it is desirable for a resurfaced patella to be equal to its original thickness, and a bony patellar thickness of at least 15 mm should be maintained. However, it is not uncommon to find, intraoperatively, the patella is too thin to simultaneously satisfy these criteria. Three surgical options should be considered with a thin patella: (1) leave the patella unresurfaced; (2) restore the original patellar thickness by removing bone to account for the thickness of the prosthesis, while accepting thin residual bone; and (3) leave residual bone of adequate thickness, while accepting an increase in overall patellar thickness. To solve this problem, the only versatile option is to use a specifically designed patellar prosthesis with less thickness. [9, 50]

Patellar height/width ratios and the position of the median patellar ridge have clinical implications for TKA with patellar resurfacing. Because the mediolateral width of a patella typically is larger than its height, a dome-shaped patella component chosen by the height does not cover the entire resected surface of the patella. It has been recommended the patella be placed at the medial margin of a resected patella to help patellofemoral tracking by decreasing the Q angle. In addition, the position of the median ridge is another factor to consider when selecting the size of a patellar component. The median ridge can act as a fulcrum for patellofemoral tracking and thus can influence restoration of normal kinematics after TKA with patellar resurfacing. If an orthopaedic surgeon attempts to restore the original position of the median ridge, he or she may have to select a smaller component, which reduces patellofemoral articulation contact area. [9]

The only article in the literature that we could find on this subject was by Kyun Kim et al. They performed an anthropometric assessment of patella on Korean knees (Figure 6) and its comparison to the western knees. They found that Koreans had thinner and smaller patellae than Westerners. The mean central ridge thickness was 21.2 mm in women and 23.1 mm in men, whereas corresponding reported mean thicknesses in Western patients are 21.8 to 22.5 mm and 23.9 to 26.1 mm. In Koreans, mean heights and widths were 33.1 mm and 41.0 mm in women and 36.2 mm and 45.6 mm in men, whereas corresponding values in Western patients are 35.0 mm and 42.7 mm in women and 39.4 mm and 49.5 mm in men. However, despite these differences in thicknesses, widths, and heights, the width/height ratios and ridge positions were similar in Koreans and Westerners. [50] (Table 11)

Some studies have advocated reestablishment of original thickness and adequate residual bony thickness as key surgical guidelines. However, in Korean patients, these two guidelines often cannot be satisfied. In such cases, the surgeon is forced to choose between restoring the original thickness while accepting a low residual bony thickness and retaining sufficient residual bony thickness while accepting an increased overall thickness. But if Koreans can have a specifically designed patellar prosthesis with less thickness, this problem will be better resolved. [51]

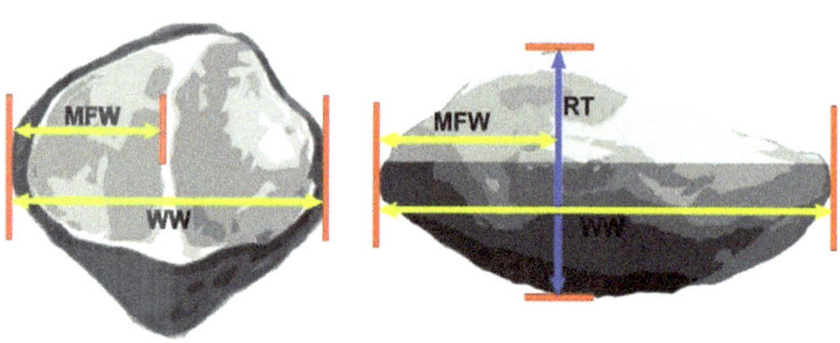


**Figure 6.** The schematic drawings show anthropometric dimensions before bone resection, including medial facet width (MFW), whole patella width (WW), and thickness at the median ridge (RT).

| Study | Thickness at central ridge (mm) | Ridge position | Mediolateral width (mm) | Superoinferior height (mm) | Width/height Ratio | Residual bony thickness after bone resection (mm) | Overall thickness after implantation (mm) |
|---|---|---|---|---|---|---|---|
| **This study** | | | | | | | |
| **Female (n = 713)** | 21.2 (17–26) | 0.45 (0.23–0.67) | 41.0 (25–51) | 33.1 (23–43) | 1.24 (0.72–1.78) | 12.5 (10–15) | 21.2 (17–25) |
| **Male (n = 39)** | 23.1 (20–26) | 0.44 (0.23–0.52) | 45.6 (36–52) | 36.2 (31–52) | 1.27 (0.81–1.50) | 13.5 (12–16) | 22.7 (20–26) |
| **Baldwin and House (2005)** | | | | | | | |
| **Female (n = 57)** | 21.8 (18–27) | 0.43 | 42.7 (32–50) | 35.0 (28–43) | 1.22 (1.06–1.56) | | |
| **Male (n = 35)** | 23.9 (20–30) | 0.42 | 49.5 (44–64) | 39.4 (34–45) | 1.26 (1.05–1.51) | | |
| **Chmell et al.(1996)** | | | | | | | |
| **Female (n = 123)** | 22.6 (17.5–28) | | | | | | |
| **Male (n = 75)** | 26.1 (20–33) | | | | | | |
| **Hitt et al.(2003)** | | | | | | | |
| **Female (n = 209)** | 22.5 | | | | | | |
| **Male (n = 128)** | 25.3 | | | | | | |

**Table 11.** Comparisons of the anthropometric dimensions of the patellae of Korean and Western patients (based on published values)

## 6. Is ethnicity influencing in vivo normal knee kinematics?

Current TKA reduces pain, restores mobility, and provides satisfactory longevity. Surgery is sometimes refused in non-Western cultures due to the anticipated limited postoperative ROM. [52]

Therefore, improvements to facilitate deep flexion activities are required in the present TKA designs to be accepted by Asian people. To make design changes, it is important to understand which factors influence deep flexion capabilities. Since Asian populations can achieve more flexion than Caucasians (156.9°, 157.3°, 159.6°, 160°, 162° or even 165° for Asian populations and 143.8°, 145° for Caucasian), ethnicity might reveal certain factors leading to higher knee flexion. [53 - 55]

Physiologic and anatomic characteristics can vary considerably between individuals. Research data originating from different regions of the world suggest ROM may be a function of ethnicity or a lifestyle. Caucasians can flex to about 140°, while in societies where daily activities require full kneeling or squatting as in Japan, India, or the Middle East, subjects achieve up to 165°, providing an energy-saving flexed posture. Saudi Arabian men flex their knees, on average, to 159.6°, 15° more than Scandinavians. Muslims maintain the flexion of 157.3° in their prayer position. [54, 55]

Leszko et al. assessed the knee kinematics in Asian and Caucasian population. They found that Caucasian women achieved similar maximum flexion as the Japanese women and Japanese men. These three groups also outnumbered the Caucasian males capable of achieving knee flexion greater than 150°. Consequently, the average maximum flexion was lower for Caucasian men than for Caucasian women or Japanese men. These differences were also apparent when comparing the flexion ROM; the highest was attained by Japanese women, followed by Japanese men, Caucasian women, and Caucasian men. The maximum axial rotation was lower for Caucasian men compared to Caucasian women. Caucasian women and both Japanese groups achieved similar average maximum axial rotation. The absolute range of axial rotation revealed a similar trend; it was lower for Caucasian men than for the three other groups, and there was no difference among the three other groups. When compared at each flexion increment, the femur rotated externally with increasing flexion, in a similar pattern for all four groups. [9]

However, in deep flexion, Caucasian men had the least amount of external rotation. For all groups, the femur was slightly abducted at the beginning of the activity but adducted with increasing knee flexion. Above 120° of flexion, the femur remained about 4° adducted for Caucasian women and both Japanese groups, while for Caucasian men, the adduction reduced and the femur became slightly abducted at 150° of flexion. The lateral tibio-femoral contact point translated posteriorly in virtually the same pattern for all four groups and there was no difference at any flexion increment or in the absolute range of translation between any of the groups. The AP translation of the medial tibio-femoral contact point was also similar for all groups, except at maximum flexion where it was more posterior for Caucasian men than for Caucasian women. Similarly, the AP translation of the lateral femoral flexion facet center was similar between the groups at any flexion as was the medial femoral flexion facet center translation at each flexion increment. However, the posterior translation of the femoral flexion facet center from full extension to maximum flexion was higher for Caucasian men than for any other group. The medial and lateral condyles moved in different modes. The lateral condyle was spinning and rolling posteriorly throughout the ROM. However, the medial condyle counter-translated in the early flexion and then was spinning until 120°. Above 120°, the motion changed to more of a rolling type for both condyles, which may justify the use of the term "posterior femoral rollback." There were no differences in the type of motion of the lateral condyle between the analyzed groups at any flexion increment. However, above 120° of flexion, the medial condyle revealed more rolling for Caucasian men compared to Caucasian women and both Japanese groups. [9]

This study suggested higher axial rotation is not related to the lateral condyle, as its motion was almost identical for all three groups (the lateral femoral condyle was spinning and rolling in the same manner for all four groups). The differences were observed on the medial condyle.

From full extension to maximum flexion, for Caucasian men, the medial tibio-femoral contact point and flexion facet center translated more posteriorly than for any other group. The medial condyle was also rolling more for the Caucasian men than for any other group above 120°. In fact, for the three other groups, the medial condyle remained more stationary, spinning close to the center of the tibial plateau, possibly allowing the lateral condyle to pivot about it and to rotate more externally. The ability to achieve more external rotation may also be related to ACL laxity, as it was higher for Japanese than for Caucasians. [9]

## 7. Conclusion

Almost all prosthetic implants have been designed and manufactured to accommodate the knee anatomy of Western Caucasians, and there is some doubt about the application of these systems to Asians, as the size of Asians differs from that of Caucasians. Moreover, even if the smallest size from each Western prosthesis company is used, it may be too big for some Asian subjects.

However, all the problems with matching a conventional knee prosthesis with Asian knees is not the mere size. It is important not to consider Asian knees as a smaller western Caucasian knees. As we reviewed in above paragraphs, there are many differences in various anatomic parameters between Asian and Caucasian knees. In Chinese, Korean and Iranian knees, it has been shown that the tibial anatomic axis does not pass through the same point of plateau as the western Caucasian knees. It is a noteworthy point to consider while marking the tibial entry point, otherwise, in Asian knees, the tibial component would be inserted in varus or the tibial medial cortex would be fractured.

Besides, the relationship between these parameters in Asian knees are far different from western Caucasian knees. As it was described in multiple studies in Chinese, Japanese, Korean and Indian population, the mediolateral diameter of the distal femur is smaller than their counterpart in western population with the same AP diameter. There is also a more important aspect of difference between these two groups of knees, which is great disparity among changes in these parameters. In other words, in contrast to western Caucasian knees, there are some parameters in the Asian knees which decrease upon increasing the other parameters and the size of the knee. As it has been shown in Chinese knees, the femoral aspect ratio was higher for smaller knees and proportionally lower for larger knees and female subjects had a smaller aspect ratio with the same anteroposterior dimension. On the tibial side, the aspect ratio (tML/tAP %) showed a definitely negative correlation with tAP, which means that there were large values in the aspect ratio with the smaller tAP, and that males have larger values in the aspect ratio than females having the same values for anteroposterior dimension. Although, there are some prostheses that consider this negative correlation between tibial aspect ratio and tAP, however, the rate of change did not match that of the Asian population.

There is also a huge number of differences in the angular parameters between Asian and western Caucasian knees. Distal femoral coronal angle, posterior femoral condylar angle, proximal tibial varus angle and posterior tibial slope have all been shown to be different in Asian from western Caucasian knees. It means that standard considerations while preparing and cutting distal femur and proximal tibia may not be appropriate for Asian knees, otherwise, soft tissue tension, ligament balancing and ROM of the joint may be disturbed.

Patellar dimensions are also different between these two ethnic groups, so although specific considerations in patellar resurfacing techniques for Asians are necessary, a specifically designed patellar prosthesis with less thickness is imperative to accommodate thinner patella of Asian ethnicity.

Aside from technical considerations for Asian knees which of course must be different from western knees, there seems to be necessary to have some specifically designed knee prostheses for Asian population. These prostheses must take into account not only the differences in size, but also the variations in aspect ratios in size parameters and their specific changes with changes in other parameters. Another consideration in Asian knee prostheses is their need for more flexion than their western counterparts. For achieving deep flexion after TKA, prosthesis design, although not as important as the technical consideration, is an significant point.

## 8. Summary

As you've read through the chapter it is clear that knees are different in different ethnic population.

These differences vary in a wide spectrum. For example, three-dimensional morphology of the Knee represents that the shape of the distal femur and proximal tibia is different among the ethnic groups. The normalized ratios and nonlinear shape analysis of the studies supported differences between East Asians and Caucasians independent of any scale factor.

There is a strong correlation between the femoral mediolateral (fML) and femoral anteroposterior (fAP) dimensions with the tibial mediolateral (tML) measurements, and as the latter increases, there is an increase in the formers.

Quantification of the tML and tAP (tibial anteroposterior) revealed that among Chinese population females have a smaller tibial surface than males, and both have smaller values than the Caucasian population. The morphologic data of the tibia showed a decreasing aspect ratio (tML/tAP %) as the tAP dimension increased, which is similar in many studies. In contrast, a majority of the implants had a relatively constant aspect ratio. Comparing five major conventional prostheses, it is evident that tML is undersized with the smaller tAP, and overhang with the larger tAP. This is more evident in male knees. In the morphology of the femur, females have a smaller aspect ratio with the same femoral anteroposterior dimension, which suggest that women have generally narrower femora than men when the femoral anteroposterior dimension is adequate. These results suggest that the prostheses which are suitable for Caucasian patients may be larger than ideal for Chinese patients. Since the tML is strongly correlated with the fML and fAP, it is important to consider the tibia and femur as a whole. Therefore, the tML and fAP should be considered as the criteria to design gender-specific proper prostheses suitable for most of Chinese population.

Dimensions of Chinese knees were generally smaller than white knees. In addition, Chinese females had a significantly narrower distal femur than white females, whereas Chinese males had a wider proximal tibia than their white counterparts. These prove the hypothesis that there is a distinct difference in size and shape between the Chinese and white knees. Another point is that the femoral condyles are asymmetric among Chinese population.

Anatomical differences could be observed even during childhood developments. Arazi et al found a negative correlation between the weight of children at a specific age with the ICD of the subject. However, this correlation was found to be weak and although statistically significant, it might not be of any clinical significance. The only possible explanation to this might be the relatively thick thighs of the heavier children, which is expected to subjectively decrease the ICD. Literature shows that there is a wide variation in the normal development of the knee angle, which might be physiological.

Axial alignment of the lower extremity has also seemed to be different among different races. Achieving normal axial alignment of the lower extremity is important to surgeons who perform reconstructive surgery of the knee.

In the study by Tang et al, the extremities of Chinese women had a mean of 2.2 ± 2.5 degrees of varus alignment, demonstrating that the knees of Chinese female is in more varus alignment than those in the white females.

Several studies have revealed that the axis of the tibial shaft is, on the average, located anteromedial to the center of the tibial plateau in the Western population, for whom a medially offset stem seems more suitable. But, some studies confirm that the axis of the tibial shaft does not overlap the center of the tibial plateau in Chinese people. It seems that an offset stem would be more suitable for Chinese patients who need a long-stemmed tibial component. Among Asian population, there is a large variation in the offset of the tibial shaft from the tibial plateau, ranging from 0.46 to 12.26 mm.

In a study on Iranian normal adult knees, we assessed the tibial plateau shift angle (TPSA) in order to assess our hypothesis that the proximal tibia of Iranian knee is not the same as the western knees. Our TPSA findings demonstrate that tibial plateau was not symmetrical and the central point (Cp) passes medial to central shaft line (Cs). This shows that the tibial plateaus in Iranian knees have a medial offset in regard to tibial shaft. So we suggest that the center of the tibial plateau should not be used as a landmark of the tibial component. Therefore, some tibial base-plates specifically designed for Caucasians may not be suitable for Asian people and it remains a necessity to design a special tibial base-plate for these ethnic groups.

Some variances have also been observed in sagittal femoral shaft bowing. In Chinese patients distal sagittal bowing is a constant and important feature, and it affects the positioning of the femoral component on the sagittal plane. There is a dilemma of implanting the femoral component either according to the anatomy of the distal femur ignoring the bowing, or according the longitudinal axis of the femur on the sagittal plane. On one hand, following the distal anatomy might sufficiently flex the femoral component that it results in an undesirable impingement of the anterior aspect of the polyethylene post on knee extension if posterior-stabilized implants are used and thus become a source of osteolysis-inducing polyethylene particles. However, following the longitudinal axis of the femur might result in an extended femoral component that could compromise the anterior cortex of the distal femur. In Chinese patients who have undergone TKA, distal sagittal bowing of the femur is common but the common pattern is posteromedial osteoarthritis. This apparent inconsistency could be the result of differences in tibial slope and the joint line obliquity in Chinese patients.

The posterior tibial slope has also a unique feature in Asians. Kapandji found that the tibial plateau was inclined posteriorly for 5 ° to 6 ° according to the horizontal plane and called this *retroversion* in the sagittal plane of the tibia. We assessed the tibial slope in normal adults in Iran. The mean slope angle was 9.4±1.8 degrees. We found no statistical relationship between age and gender and posterior tibial slope. The normal posterior tibial slope angle in this Iranian population was different from other ethnic groups. It may be necessary to consider these differences in designing tibial components for knee arthroplasty.

**Special considerations in total knee arthroplasty for Asians:** Recent anthropometric studies have suggested that current design of total knee arthroplasty (TKA) does not cater to racial anthropometric differences. Most of the commercially available TKA prostheses are designed according to the anthropometric data of white knees, which has been suspected as the cause of the component mismatch in Asian people. Several studies have compared the morphology of Asian knees to that of TKA prostheses currently used in Asia and found that the femoral aspect ratio (medio-lateral [fML]/antero-posterior [fAP]) of these prostheses were not suitable for Asian patients.

Patella-related problems are among the issues of concern during and after TKA. Information regarding anthropometric patellar dimensions can play an important role during the design of patellar prostheses and the development of surgical techniques. Thickness, height/width ratio, and relative position of the median ridge all have implications relating to the selection of patellar components, patella-femoral contact stress, and patellar tracking in the trochlear groove. The only article in the literature that we could find on this subject was by Kyun Kim et al. They found that Koreans had thinner and smaller patellae than Westerners. Patellar thickness is a challenging consideration during patellar resurfacing for TKA. A thin patella can reduce patella-femoral contact force but also poses the potential risk of stress fracture and anteroposterior instability. It commonly is assumed that it is desirable for a resurfaced patella to be equal to its original thickness, and a bony patellar thickness of at least 15 mm should be maintained. However, it is not uncommon to find, intra-operatively, the patella is too thin to simultaneously satisfy these criteria. To solve this problem, the only versatile option is to use exclusively designed patellar prosthesis with less thickness.

Yet the importance of these issues is more distinguished when one considers the geographical variation in the epidemiology of osteoarthritis, which has been well documented. The ratio of knee osteoarthritis to hip osteoarthritis is 9:1 for Chinese individuals in Hong Kong,

3:1 for white individuals in the United States, and 1:2 for Swedish individuals. The racial differences in the axial alignment of the lower extremity may contribute to the variation in this ratio. The authors suspect that the larger knee-joint-obliquity angle in Chinese individuals may contribute to the higher ratio of knee osteoarthritis to hip osteoarthritis among Chinese adults.

One should be cautious in describing what is "normal" because of the substantial individual variations. Currently, designers of most total knee arthroplasty systems recommend placement of the components in such a way that the transverse axis of the artificial knee joint is perpendicular to the mechanical axes of the tibia and the femur. The resulting alignment of the lower extremity, therefore, is in close proximity to the alignment documented by Moreland et al. and Hsu et al. The mechanical axes of the femur and the tibia did not form a straight line in either Chinese males or females. This finding is in contrast to the general consensus that has been described previously.

And ultimately, the answer to this question: "Are in vivo normal knee kinematics influenced by ethnicity?" is, **YES**.

## Author details

Hamid Reza Seyyed Hosseinzadeh[1*], Samih Tarabichi[2], Ali Sina Shahi[1], Mehrnoush Hassas Yeganeh[1], Usama Hassan Saleh[2], Gholam Reza Kazemian[1] and Aidin Masoudi[1]

*Address all correspondence to: hhosseinzadehmd@yahoo.com

1 Shahid Beheshti Unversity of Medical Sciences, Tehran, Iran

2 American Hospital, Dubai, United Arab Emirates

## References

[1] Hofmann S, et al. Bone Cuts and Implant Positioning to Achieve High Flexion. Techniques in Knee Surgery, 2011; 10(2): 77-86.

[2] Bellemans J et al. Both Morphotype and Gender Influence the Shape of the Knee in Patients Undergoing TKA. Clin Orthop Relat Res (2010) 468:29–36

[3] Gillespie RJ, et al. Gender differences in the anatomy of the distal femur. J Bone Joint Surg Br. 201;93(3):357-63.

[4] Hovinga KR, et al. (2009). Anatomic variations between Japanese and Caucasian populations in the healthy young adult knee joint. J Orthop Res. 2009;27(9):1191-6.

[5] Iorio R, et al. Primary posterior cruciate-retaining total knee arthroplasty: a comparison of American and Japanese cohorts. J Surg Orthop Adv. 2007 Winter;16(4):164-70.

[6] Kamarul T, et al. Normal Anterior Cruciate ligament Laxity in the Malaysian Population. J Malaysian Orthopaedic. 2007; Vol 1: No 2.

[7] Tamari K, et al. Ethnic-, Gender-, and Age-Related Differences in Femorotibial Angle, Femoral Antetorsion, and Tibiofibular Torsion. Clinical Anatomy 19:59–67 (2006)

[8] Henry D, et al. Restoration of Femoral Anatomy in TKA With Unisex and Gender-specific Components. Clin Orthop Relat Res (2008) 466:2711–2716

[9] Hitt K, et al. Anthropometric Measurements of the Human Knee: Correlation to the Sizing of Current Knee Arthroplasty Systems. J Bone Joint Surg Am. 85-A; Supplement 4: 2003

[10] Conley S, et al. The Female Knee: Anatomic Variations. J Am Acad Orthop Surg 2007;15 (suppl 1):S31-S36

[11] Mahfouz M, et al. Three-dimensional morphology of the knee reveals ethnic differences. Clin Orthop Relat Res. 2012;470(1):172-85.

[12] Nelson AE, et al. Static knee alignment measurements among Caucasians and African-Americans: The Johnston County Osteoarthritis Project. J Rheumatol 2009;36(9): 1987–1990

[13] Yue B, et al. Gender differences in the knees of Chinese population. Knee Surg Sports Traumatol Arthrosc. 2011;19(1):80-8.

[14] Leszko F, et al. Comparison of in vivo patellofemoral kinematics for subjects having high-flexion total knee arthroplasty implant with patients having normal knees. J Arthroplasty. 2010;25(3):398-404.

[15] Espandar R, et al. Angular Deformities of the Lower Limb in Children. Asian Journal of Sports Medicine, 2010;Vol 1 (No 1): 46-53

[16] Sabharwal S, Zhao C. The Hip-Knee-Ankle Angle in Children: Reference Values Based on a Full-Length Standing Radiograph. J Bone Joint Surg Am. 2009;91:2461-8

[17] Tang WM, Zhu YH, Chiu KY. Axial alignment of the lower extremity in Chinese adults. J Bone Joint Surg Am. 2000; 82-A(11):1603-8.

[18] Saini UC, et al. Normal development of the knee angle in healthy Indian children: a clinical study of 215 children. J Child Orthop. 2010;4(6):579-86.

[19] Cheng N, Shi QY. Rehabilitation exercises after single total knee replacement: a report of 38 cases. Zhongguo Gu Shang. 2010; 23(3): 220-1.(Abstract)

[20] Arazi M, et al. Normal development of the tibiofemoral angle in children: a clinical study of 590 normal subjects from 3 to 17 years of age. J Pediatr Orthop. 2001; 21(2): 264-7.

[21] Heath CH, Staheli LT. Normal limits of knee angle in white children—genu varum and genu valgum. J Pediatr Orthop. 1993; 13(2): 259-62.

[22] Yoo JH, et al. Development of tibiofemoral angle in Korean children. J Korean Med Sci. 2008; 23(4): 714-7.

[23] Oginni LM, et al. Knee angles and rickets in nigerian children. J Pediatr Orthop. 2004; 24(4): 403-7.

[24] Moreland JR, et al. Radiographic analysis of the axial alignment of the lower extremity. J Bone Joint Surg Am. 1987; 69(5): 745-9.

[25] Hsu RW, et al. Normal axial alignment of the lower extremity and load-bearing distribution at the knee. Clin Orthop Relat Res. 1990; (255): 215-27.

[26] Fang Y, et al. The biomechanical study of rotating-arm self-locking intramedullary nails in comminuted femoral shaft fractures. Sheng Wu Yi Xue Gong Cheng Xue Za Zhi. 2006 Oct;23(5):1041-4.(Abstract)

[27] Mullaji AB, et al. Distal femoral rotational axes in Indian knees. J Orthop Surg (Hong Kong). 2009; 17(2): 166-9.

[28] Tang WM, et al. Sagittal bowing of the distal femur in Chinese patients who require total knee arthroplasty. J Orthop Res. 2005; 23(1): 41-5.

[29] Cheng FB, et al. Three dimensional morphometry of the knee to design the total knee arthroplasty for Chinese population. Knee. 2009; 16(5): 341-7..

[30] Yip DK, et al. Distal rotational alignment of the Chinese femur and its relevance in total knee arthroplasty. J Arthroplasty 2004; 19: 613.

[31] Tang Q, et al. The offset of the tibial shaft from the tibial plateau in Chinese people. J Bone Joint Surg Am. 2010. 18; 92(10): 1981-7.

[32] Hicks CA, et al. The anatomy of the tibial intramedullary canal. Clin Orthop Relat Res. 1995; 321: 111-16.

[33] Westrich GH, et al. Resection specimen analysis of proximal tibial anatomy based on 100 total knee arthroplasty specimens. J Arthroplasty. 1995; 10: 47-51.

[34] Wevers HW, et al. Improved fit by asymmetric tibial prosthesis for total knee arthroplasty. Med Eng Phys. 1994;16: 297-300.

[35] Abraham R, et al. An anatomical study of tibial metaphyseal/diaphyseal mismatch during revision total knee arthroplasty. J Arthroplasty. 2007 Feb; 22(2): 241-4.

[36] Yoo JH, et al. The relationship of the medially-offset stem of the tibial component to the medial tibial cortex in total knee replacements in Korean patients,. J Bone Joint Surg [Br] 2008; 90-B: 31-6

[37] Kapandji IA. The knee ligaments as determinants of trochleo-condylar profile. Med Biol Illus. 1967; 17(1): 26-32.(Abstract)

[38] Chiu KY, et al. Posterior slope of tibial plateau in Chinese. J Arthroplasty. 2000; 15(2): 224-7.

[39] Yue B, et al. Differences of Knee Anthropometry Between Chinese and White Men and Women. J Arthroplasty. 2011; Vol. 26: No. 1

[40] Harvey WF, et al. Knee alignment differences between Chinese and Caucasian subjects without osteoarthritis. Ann Rheum Dis. 2008; 67(11): 1524-8.

[41] Hosaka K, et al. Asian-Specific total knee system: 5-14 year follow-up study. Musculoskeletal Disorders 2011, 12:251

[42] Hashemi J, et al. The Geometry of the Tibial Plateau and Its Influence on the Biomechanics of the Tibiofemoral Joint. J Bone Joint Surg Am. 2008; 90-A: 12.

[43] Uehara K, et al. Anthropometry of the proximal tibia to design a total knee prosthesis for the Japanese population. J Arthroplasty. 2002; 17(8): 1028-32.

[44] Kwak DS, et al. Morphometry of the proximal tibia to design the tibial component of total knee arthroplasty for the Korean population. Knee. 2007; 14(4): 295-300.

[45] Chaichankul C, et al. Anthropometric measurements of knee joints in Thai population: correlation to the sizing of current knee prostheses. Knee. 2011; 18(1): 5-10.

[46] Vaidya SV,et al. Anthropometric measurements to design total knee prostheses for the Indian population. J Arthroplasty. 2000; 15(1): 79-85.

[47] Hosseinzadeh HR, et al. Measurment of Posterior Tibial Slope. Iranian Journal of Orthopaedic Surgery Vol 9, No 2, Spring 2010:121-5

[48] Hsu HC, et al. Influence of patellar thickness on patellar tracking and patellofemoral contact characteristics after total knee arthroplasty. J Arthroplasty. 1996; 11: 69–80.

[49] Baldwin JL, House CK. Anatomic dimensions of the patella measured during total knee arthroplasty. J Arthroplasty. 2005; 20: 250–257.

[50] Kim TK, et al. Clinical implications of anthropometric patellar dimensions for TKA in Asians. Clin Orthop Relat Res. 2009; 467(4): 1007-14.

[51] Koh JS, et al. Influence of patellar thickness on results of total knee arthroplasty: does a residual bony patellar thickness of 12 mm lead to poorer clinical outcome and increased complication rates? J Arthroplasty. 2002; 17: 56–61.

[52] Noble PC, et al. Does total knee replacement restore normal knee function? Clin Orthop Relat Res. 2005; 431: 157–165.

[53] Hemmerich A, et al. Hip, knee, and ankle kinematics of high range of motion activities of daily living, J Orthop Res. 2006; 24: 770–781.

[54] Freeman MA, Pinskerova V. The movement of the knee studied by magnetic resonance imaging. Clin Orthop Relat Res. 2003; 410: 35–43.

[55] Freeman MA, Pinskerova V. The movement of the normal tibiofemoral joint. J Biomech. 2005; 38: 197–208.

Section 2

# Surgical Techniques and Technologies

Chapter 5

# The Acrylic Bone Cement in Arthroplasty

Hamid Reza Seyyed Hosseinzadeh,
Mohammad Emami, Farivarabdollahzadeh Lahiji,
Ali Sina Shahi, Aidin Masoudi and Sina Emami

Additional information is available at the end of the chapter

## 1. Introduction

### 1.1. The genesis and evolution of acrylic bone cement

#### *1.1.1. History*

Otto Röhm is known as the developer of polymethylmethacrylate (PMMA) in 1901. Industrial-size chemical synthesis of MMA was achieved in the 1920s in the laboratories of Rohm and Haas, and the first biomedical applications of PMMA was the fabrication of dentures. In the 1930s it was discovered that the mixing of MMA monomer and benzoyl peroxide initiator with prepolymerized PMMA powder resulted in the formation of a dough-like material which could slowly harden into a glassy polymer. This two-component polymer (cement) was initially used to close cranial defects. Because of the transparency, strength, and stability of polymethylmethacrylate, the commercial production of cast sheets of it in the early 1930s led to its utilization as a denture base and prosthetic material. Originally pieces of the material were molded under heat and pressure.[1, 2, 3] In 1935, an injection molding technique was introduced by ICI for dentures in which the melted PMMA was injected into dried plaster molds under hydraulic pressure. These techniques proved to be too cumbersome. In 1936, as was mentioned above, it was discovered that mixing of methyl methacrylate monomer with the ground polymer produced a dough that could be shaped in plaster molds and could be polymerized into a solid mass by using benzoyl peroxide as a polymerization initiator. In the next few years, it was found that improved molding characteristics could be obtained using a powder that was a mixture of ground and spherical (bead) polymer particles.[1, 2]

The discovery of the dough molding technique led to the near universal use of these acrylic resins for dentures and prostheses for cranioplasties in the 1940s.[4] In 1943, German chemists discovered that if a tertiary amine such as dimethyl-pare-toluidine was added along with the benzoyl peroxide, the dough could be polymerized at room temperature. Based on this development, Kulzer and Degussa companies refined a dough-like, workable form of PMMA in 1943. Their developments led to the introduction of cold-cured PMMA, which hardens at room temperature. In the 1940s, with the advent of acrylic femoral hemiarthroplasties by Jean and Robert Judet, PMMA attracted interest in the field of orthopaedics. Kiaer and Haboush separately reported using PMMA to affix femoral implants in the early 1950s. The success with and the popularity of PMMA in orthopaedics is attributable to Sir John Charnley, whose work was affected by his exposure to the field of dentistry (because his father was a dentist) and his inherent interest in biomaterials. Charnley's early clinical accomplishments established a foundation for the continued use of PMMA in orthopaedics. Charnley had a long experience in producing his own instruments and gadgets. Charnley was interested in the work on thin sectioning of bones and rocks embedded in cast acrylic resin. He also performed a research into Judet prostheses and acrylic joints cast in alginate molds. He performed some arthroplasties with acrylic bone cement and reported the preliminary results of six cases in the British Journal of Bone and Joint Surgery in 1960. It is important to appreciate that this advance was not simply the use of acrylic cement but rather a conscious recognition of its ability to fill completely the medullary canal and adapt to the bone interface, so facilitating stress transfer, minimizing local stresses, and thereby stabilizing and anchoring the prosthesis. It was a new technique and provided the basis for the development of Charnley's concept of low friction arthroplasty during the next decade.[1, 2]

For over 40 years, poly(methylmethacrylate) (PMMA)-based bone cement, commonly known as acrylic bone cement, has been used for fixation of total joint replacement prostheses to periprosthetic bone. Today, most acrylic bone cements on the market consist of two components: a liquid and a powder one, which are mixed in the operating room until they become dough-like and are then applied to the bone prior to insertion of the component of the joint replacement prosthesis. The primary function of cements is to fix the joint replacement prosthesis to the periprosthetic bone tissue.[5] The basic component of acrylic bone cements is methylmethacrylate (MMA), which is an ester of methacrylic acid. In 1951, Kaier and Jansen in Copenhagen were the first to use PMMA bone cement for the fixation of acrylic cups to the subchondral bone of the femoral head. In 1953, Haboush used bone cement as a seating material for femoral head replacements without inserting it into the medullary canal. In 1958, Sir John Charnley used acrylic bone cement to fix femoral prostheses in the femur, as is done in modern-day joint arthroplasty these days. Charnley used a self-curing PMMA cement called Nu-Life, which was a pink-colored denture repair material. These early total hip replacements had a high incidence of failure, and it was not because of the cement or stems but because of the use of polytetrafluoroethylene (PTFE) acetabular cups. In 1966, CMW began to supply the first sterilized bone cement, formulated specifically for fixation of total joint replacement prostheses.[5] Nowadays, uncemented total hip replacement prostheses designs have largely been introduced in the orthopedic market, but acrylic cements continue to be one of the best primary methods of fixation of joint replacement prostheses, especially for knee replacement prostheses. In addition, injectable formulations of acrylic bone cements have been used for applications in vertebroplasty.

Several factors such as their chemical composition, viscosity, porosity, radiopacifiers and antibiotic additives, mixing methods, sterilization, temperature during handling, mechanical properties, and biocompatibility, affect the clinical performance of bone cements.

## 2. Composition and chemistry

The methylmethacrylate monomer consists of two carbon atoms that are covalently bound, with one of the carbon atoms covalently bonded to two hydrogen atoms and the other attached via a covalent bond to a methyl and acrylic group. Polymerization of MMA monomer produces PMMA, which is a polymer or a macromolecule. Hardened acrylic bone cement consists of linear, uncross-linked PMMA macromolecules of various lengths ranging from a few tens of thousands to a few million grams per mole. Acrylic bone cements comprise two components, often supplied in a 2:1 ratio: (a) a powder component, usually in a 40 g package, and (b) a liquid component, in a 20 mL ampoule.[2, 6](Table 1) There are several reasons for using a two-component bone cement instead of simply polymerizing pure MMA monomer:

The polymerization of MMA monomer is too slow and can take several hours or days, depending on the type and amount of reaction initiator used.

Pure MMA monomer has a very low viscosity and can easily diffuse into the blood stream, which can lead to cardiorespiratory and vascular complications.

The heat of polymerization can easily increase the temperature of the cement to over 100°C (boiling point for MMA = 100.3°C), which could lead to boiling of the volatile MMA monomer. The use of less amount of monomer and the presence of prepolymerized PMMA beads in the powder decreases the number of polymerization reaction and hence, the amount of released heat and assists in heat dissipation, decreasing the overall temperature.

After polymerization of pure MMA into PMMA, there would be a volumetric shrinkage of 21% due to differences in the density of the MMA monomer and the PMMA polymer. This amount of shrinkage is unacceptable and would lead to a large gap at the cement-bone and cement-prosthesis interface, compromising the fixation of the prosthesis.

The powder is the variable part in composition of bone cements among different brands, which contributes to differences in properties. (Figure 1) The powder component primarily consists of prepolymerized PMMA beads of 10 to 150 μm diameter, contributing to 83% to 99% of the powder. The prepolymerized beads of different bone cements include copolymers of MMA with styrene, methyl acrylate, or butyl methacrylate comonomers. The remaining components include a radiopacifier, either barium sulfate ($BaSO_4$) or zirconium dioxide ($ZrO_2$) (8% to 15% by weight), as well as an initiator, benzoyl peroxide (0.75% to 2.6%). The MMA monomer can self-polymerize under exposure to heat and light, but, this reaction is very slow. Therefore, dibenzoyl peroxide (BPO) reaction initiator in powder form is included in the powder component. Other variations include the initiator tri-n-butylborane and accelerator 2,5-dimethylhexane- 2,5-hydroperoxide(in Bonemite, chlorophyll dye and ethanol and ascorbic acid. The initiator, radiopacifier, and antibiotic powders all consist of particles of approximately 1 μm in diameter. [7]

| Constituent | Role |
|---|---|
| **Powder components** | |
| Polymer | Polymethylmethacrylate |
| Co-polymer (e.g. MA-MMA) | Alter physical properties of the cement |
| Barium sulphate or Zirconium dioxide | Radio-opacifiers |
| Antibiotics* | Antimicrobial prophylaxis |
| Dye (e.g. chlorophyll) | Distinguish cement from bone |
| **Liquid components** | |
| Monomer | Methylmethacrylate monomer |
| N,N-dimethyl-p-toluidine (DMPT) | Initiates cold curing of polymer |
| Benzoyl peroxide | Reacts with DMPT to catalyze polymerization |
| Hydroquinone | Stabilizer preventing premature polymerization |
| Dye (e.g. chlorophyll) | Distinguish cement from bone |

*Plain bone cements do not contain antibiotics

**Table 1.** Commercial constituents of bone cement

The monomer, a colorless liquid with a characteristic odor, is packaged in ampules. The liquid components remain relatively constant among commercially available cements. 97% to 99% of this liquid consists of methylmethacrylate. N,N-dimethyl-para-toluidine (DMPT) makes up 0.4% to 2.8% by weight and acts as an accelerator to speed up the polymerization and setting of the cement. Since MMA can spontaneously polymerize during storage, addition of trace amounts of a stabilizer, usually hydroquinone (15 to 75 ppm), stabilizes and prevents premature polymerization of monomers.

MMA polymerizes by the mechanism of free radical polymerization, which consists of three steps: initiation, propagation, and termination. The initiation step involves decomposition of BPO monomer into radicals at room temperature.[7] (Figure 2)

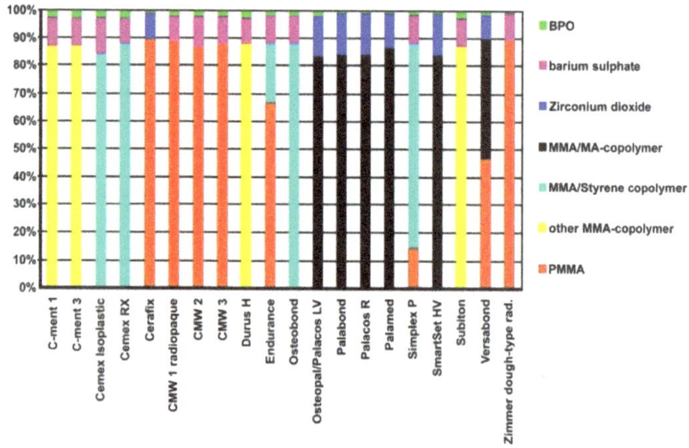


**Figure 1.** The composition of the powder of several PMMA bone cements on the market.

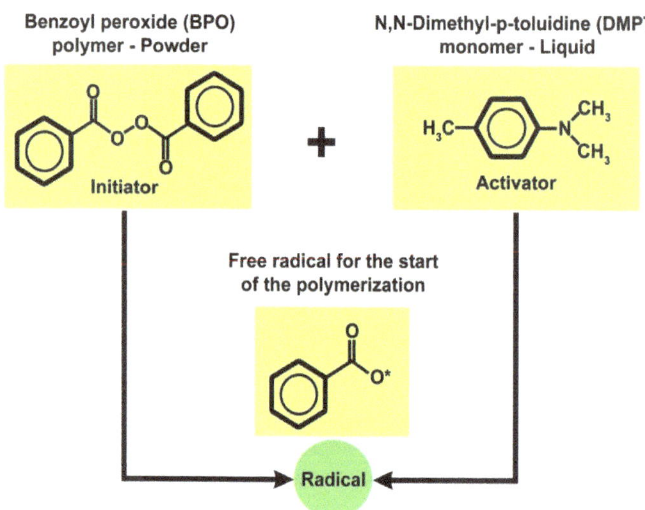


**Figure 2.** The initiation of the polymerization of MMA: BPO from the powder and DMPT from the liquid react to form radicals, starting the curing of bone cements.

Upon mixing of the two components, the DMPT in the liquid component decomposes BPO into a benzoyl radical and a benzoate anion as follows:

$$(C_6H_5COO)_2 + CH_3C_6H_4N(CH_3)_2 \longrightarrow C_6H_5COO^* + C_6H_5COO^- + CH_3C_6H_4N(CH_3)_2^{+} \longrightarrow CH_3C_6H_4NCH_3CH_2^{*} + H^{+} \quad (1)$$

where BPO = $(C_6H_5COO)_2$, DMPT= $CH_3C_6H_4N(CH_3)_2$, benzoyl radical = $C_6H_5COO^*$, and benzoate anion = $C_6H_5COO$-.

The second step of the free radical polymerization is chain propagation in which the benzoyl radical reacts with the MMA monomer as follows:

$$C_6H_5COO^* + CH_2{=}CCH_3COOCH_3 \longrightarrow C_6H_5COO\text{-}CH_2\text{-}CCH_3COOCH_3 + CH_2{=}CCH_3COOCH_3 \longrightarrow C_6H_5COO\text{-}CH_2CCH_3COOCH_3\text{-}CH_2CCH_3COOCH_3 \quad (2)$$

The free radical attacks one of the double bonds of the MMA monomer. One electron of the double bond pairs up with the electron of the free radical to form a bond between the oxygen of the benzoyl free radical and one of the carbon atoms of the MMA monomer while the second electron of the double bond shifts to the other carbon atom, which then turns into a free radical. This free radical then attacks another MMA monomer and the chain propagates until a PMMA of relatively high molecular weight, on the order of 100,000 to 1,000,000 g/mol, is achieved. Finally, chain termination can be achieved by chain coupling as follows:

$$\text{-}CH_2CXCH_3^* + {}^*CXCH_3CH_2\text{-} \longrightarrow \text{-}CH_2CXCH_3\text{-}CXCH_3CH_2\text{-} \quad (3)$$

or, to a lesser extent, by disproportionation via transfer of a hydrogen atom as follows:

$$\text{-}CH_2CXCH_3^* + {}^*CXCH_3CH_2\text{-} \longrightarrow \text{-}CH_2C_XCH_2 + CXH{=}CH\text{-} \quad (4)$$

where X refers to the substituent $COOCH_3$.

The glass transition temperature of PMMA is about 105°C, but the glass transition temperature of hardened PMMA-based bone cement can be lower due to plasticization effects of residual monomer and water. With proceeding of polymerization, the growing polymer chains slowly turn into a hard, glassy material, and it becomes difficult for the monomer to diffuse through the hardened PMMA matrix to continue chain propagation. [8]

The hardened acrylic bone cement consists primarily of linear, uncross-linked PMMA macromolecules of various lengths, but their length (or molecular weight) can vary widely. The molecular weight of the hardened cement depends on several factors, such as (a) the molecular weight of the monomer used (usually MMA), (b) the molecular weight of the prepolymerized beads, (c) the ratio of the initiator and the accelerator, (d) the presence of stabilizers, (e) the ambient temperature during polymerization, and (f) the sterilization method.[7, 8]

# 3. Properties

## 3.1. Heat production during polymerization

Combining powder and liquid monomer initiates an exothermic reaction. In vitro, the peak temperatures reach 113°C. In vivo temperatures are reported to be between 40° and 56°C. Methylmethacrylate monomer, the basic building block of PMMA, contains carbon-carbon double bonds, which react with the free radical produced by the activator and initiator. The monomer free radical interacts with other monomer molecules, creating a growing polymer chain. During the polymerization, the powder changes to a workable dough. [7]

This reaction releases 52 KJ/mole of monomer, equating to heat production of 1.4 to $1.7 \times 10^8$ $J/m^3$ of cement. The production of heat by the curing cement has been studied *in vitro* and *in vivo* and modeled using finite element analysis. *In vitro* studies have shown that the thicker cement mantles, the higher ambient temperatures and the greater ratio of monomer to polymer the more heat is produced. Recorded temperatures range between 70°C and 120°C. Collagen denatures with prolonged exposure to temperatures in excess of 56°C, and the risk of causing thermal damage to bone has been emphasized by several authors. However, *in vivo* studies have recorded lower peaks of temperature. In 1977, Reckling and Dillon measured the temperature at the bone cement interface in 20 THRs. The maximum temperature was 48°C.[9] The reasons for the lower in vivo temperature are:

1. The thin layer of the bone cement
2. Blood circulation
3. The large surface area of the interface
4. Poor thermal conductivity of the cement
5. Heat dissipation to the prosthesis and to the vital tissue.

So, the temperature increase greater than the coagulation temperature of proteins is avoided.

Harving, Soballe and Bunger recorded temperatures above 56°C but only for two to three minutes. Even though, such temperatures may sometimes be reached, animal studies have shown no adverse effects. Nevertheless, concerns regarding thermal and chemical injury persisted.[3]

## 3.2. Curing of a bone cement

By mixing the powder and liquid, two different processes are started. First, the polymer powder takes up the monomer liquid, forming a more or less viscous fluid or a dough. This phenomenon is because of the swelling and dissolution processes of monomer and polymer powder. Swelling and dissolution processes are physical processes and they are important for the working characteristics of a bone cement. Second, a chemical process is initiated, which is responsible for the final hardening of the bone cement. The initiator BPO from the polymer powder and the activator DMPT from the liquid interact to produce free radicals in the so-called "initiation reaction". These radicals are able to start the polymerization of MMA by adding to the polymerizable double-bond of the monomer molecule. This results in a growing polymer chain that builds up macromolecules. Because of the high number of radicals generated, many rapidly growing polymer chains are formed and, therefore, there is a fast conversion of MMA to PMMA. If two growing polymer chains meet, the chains are terminated by combining both, resulting in an unreactive polymer molecule. The polymerization of MMA is an exothermic reaction, resulting in a temperature increase in the curing bone cement.[7] This temperature maximum can be influenced by:

1. The chemical composition of the cement
2. By the powder to liquid ratio
3. By the radiopacifier.

### 3.3. Volume shrinkage

Because a polymerization means a conversion of a large number of monomer molecules to a much smaller number of polymer molecules, there is a volume shrinkage during curing of the bone cement. The reason for this shrinkage is the decreasing molecular distance between free monomer molecules before the polymerization and the molecular distance of the molecules bonded in the polymer chain. The volume shrinkage of pure MMA is approximately 21%. By using prepolymerized powder, the content of MMA in commercially available bone cements is reduced to approximately one third of the whole mass. The theoretic volume shrinkage of bone cements is therefore approximately 6%–7%. The real shrinkage is lower, however, because of the air inclusions in the cement dough. So, the real volume shrinkage of hand-mixed bone cement thus might be lower than the shrinkage of vacuum-mixed bone cement, because vacuum-mixed cement has hardly any air inclusions. Because acrylic bone cement absorbs water, its volume shrinkage is compensated by the expansion caused by the water-uptake.[8]

## 4. Processing and handling of bone cement

The handling characteristics and setting times of acrylic cements are of great importance for orthopedic surgeons. The handling of bone cements can be described by four different phases with their corresponding viscosities:

1. The mixing phase (up to 1 minute) is the period during which the powder and the liquid are homogenized thoroughly. The powder and the liquid can be mixed manually by using a bowl and a spatula or by a special mixing system, applying vacuum to avoid the formation of voids.
2. The waiting phase (up to several minutes, according to the type of cement and the handling temperature) is the period to reach a non-sticky state of the cement.

3. The working phase (2–4 minutes, according to the type of cement and the handling temperature) is the period during which the surgeon can inject the cement and insert the prosthesis. The viscosity of the cement has to be high enough to withstand the bleeding pressure. Blood pervasion of the cement results in a reduction of the strength of the cement. A late application at a too high viscosity level may result in poor interfaces between the prosthesis, the cement, and the bone.

4. The hardening phase (1–2 minutes) is the period of the final setting process and the development of the polymerization heat.

The effect of the temperature on the length of the phases is clearly visible. The information given by the temperature versus time curves of different cements is not always comparable, because manufacturers use different determination methods resulting in variant lengths of the working phases. This disagreement is caused by the lack of a universal detection method. A wide experience and knowledge by the surgeon is therefore helpful to find the optimal range of time to inject the cement and to fix the prosthesis. The method described in ISO 5833 and ASTM F 451 to determine a viscosity-like parameter is the intrusion test. This is not really a test method for the determination of the true viscosity. To perform this test, the mixed cement is placed in a plastic mold and is loaded with a force of 49 N for 1 minute. The depth of the intrusion of the cement into four drill holes is measured. This method is only available for high viscosity bone cements. In the standard ASTM F 451, there is another extrusion viscosity test described with a capillary rheometer for low viscosity bone cements. [7]

In the Standards, there are two further time parameters defined: the doughing time and the setting time. The doughing time end by the beginning of the working phase and it is determined by recording from the start time of mixing until the mixture is able to separate cleanly from a gloved finger. The second time parameter is the setting time, which is defined as the time to reach a temperature midway between ambient and maximum. The end of setting time marks the final hardening of the bone cement. [8]

During the waiting period swelling of the beads occurs and allows the polymerization to proceed, leading to an increase in viscosity. At this stage, the cement turns into a sticky dough. The working period begins when the cement is no longer sticky but of sufficiently low viscosity to permit the surgeon to easily apply the cement into the prepared place. During this period, the chain propagation continues, along with an increase in viscosity. The viscosity of the cement must be carefully assessed before inserting the cement because with a very low viscosity the cement would not be able to withstand the bleeding pressure. This would result in blood lamination in the cement, which can weaken the cement. The heat produced during this period, results in thermal expansion of the cement. On the other hand, there is a volumetric shrinkage of the cement as the MMA monomer converts into the denser PMMA polymer.

The final stage is the hardening period, when the polymerization terminates and leads to a hardened cement. The temperature of the cement continues to elevate during this period and then slowly decreases to body temperatures. During this period, the cement undergos volumetric shrinkage along with thermal shrinkage as the cement cools down to body tem- 9
perature. While the manufacturer can determine the hardening period length using in vitro

measurements at a controlled temperature and humidity in a laboratory environment, it is difficult to predict the hardening period in vivo, with accuracy due to variations in the ambient environment in the operating room, the body temperature, and thickness of the cement mantle, all of which can alter the setting times of the cement. Several factors, such as the type of mixing method used, the viscosity of the cement, the precooling of the monomer and/or powder, the preheating of the powder component, and the preheating of the prosthesis, can also significantly alter the times of some of the handling phases. Thus it is important for the surgeon to know each of the factors that can alter the duration of each phase. [7]

### 4.1. Viscosity and handling properties

The dynamic viscosity (η) of fluids is denoted by shear stress (F)/shear rate (S) [$\eta = F/S$]. Fluids are designated as Newtonian if shear stress is linearly related to shear rate. Cement in its liquid phase of curing behaves as a non-Newtonian fluid with viscosity decreasing as shear rate is increased. This is called pseudoplastic or shear thinning behaviour. However, the viscosity of all cements increases during polymerisation as the polymer chains lengthen.[10]

The mixed cement begins as a viscous liquid, then turns into a viscoelastic material, and finally hardens into a predominantly elastic solid. Thus, it is important to monitor both the dynamic viscosity as well as the viscoelastic parameters, such as storage modulus (G'), loss modulus (G"), and tanδ (their ratio). A high storage modulus indicates that the material is more solid-like whereas a high loss modulus shows that the material is more viscous.[7]

The viscosity of bone cements at the dough stage is determined mainly by the chemical composition and the powder to monomer ratio. These aspects should never be modified in the operating theater to modify the viscosity. There are some methods to modify the viscosity without changing other characteristics of the cement, however. One of them is the prechilling of the cement. The velocity of the reaction, and with it the viscosity, depends on the temperature. Prechilling of cements, especially of high viscosity cements, has been introduced with the introduction of mixing systems to make mixing of cement in these systems more convenient and to improve the quality of the mixture, especially with respect to porosity. [8]

Another method for applying this change is preheating the cement, to accelerate the polymerization and thus, reducing the operation time. But it has been shown that by this heat application to the cement powder, various characteristics of the cement itself or the cemented construct are either enhanced, degraded, or marginally affected, which depends on the structure of the cement powder and its stability against the heat. Specifically, these properties are significantly decreased when the principal constituent in the powder has a low resistance to degradation by the preheat temperature (as is the case of the PMMA polymer in Cemex XL and CMW 1 cements) but are not when the resistance is high (as in the case of a mixture of PMMA + MMA styrene copolymer in Surgical Simplex P cement).[11]

Manufacturers can also change the viscosity of cement by changing the molecular weight, by using co-polymers, and by varying the methods of sterilization. In addition, the curing process itself can be controlled by altering the proportions of the initiator (Toluidine) and the monomer, and this can change the working properties.

The cement must be liquid enough during the working phase to be forced through a delivery device and then flow under pressure to penetrate the interstices of cancellous bone, achieving micro-interlock. Bone cements are usually divided into three categories: high, medium and low viscosity:

*Low.* These have a long waiting phase of three minutes, also known as a sticky phase. The viscosity rapidly increases during the working phase and the hardening phase is one to two minutes long.

*Medium.* There is a long waiting phase of three minutes, but during the working phase, the viscosity only increases slowly. Hardening takes between one minute 30 seconds, and two minutes 30 seconds.

*High.* A short waiting/sticky phase is followed by a long working phase. The viscosity remains constant until the end of the working phase. The hardening phase lasts between one minute 30 seconds and two minutes. High viscosity cements are therefore forgiving for the surgeon and are in predominant use in orthopaedics. [3]

However, the rates of curing are very sensitive to environmental factors. Low ambient temperatures during storing and mixing, and high humidity both prolong setting time. Typical representatives of high viscosity cements are Palacos R (Biomet Inc.; Warsaw/USA; Schering-Plough; Heist-op-den-Berg/Belgium; Heraeus Kulzer; Wehrheim/Germany), Palamed (Biomet Merck; Ried/Switzerland; Heraeus Kulzer), CMW 1 (DePuy; Blackpool/England), Simplex P (Stryker; Limerick/Ireland), and Cemfix 1 (Teknimed; Vic en Bigorre/France), whereas Osteopal (Biomet Merck; Heraeus Kulzer), Palacos LV (Schering-Plough; Heraeus Kulzer), Osteobond (Zimmer; Warsaw/USA), Versabond (Smith & Nephew; Memphis/USA), Cemfix 3 (Teknimed), Sulcem 3 (Zimmer; Baar/Switzerland), and CMW 3 (DePuy) are examples of low viscosity cements. [7]

The high viscosity during mixing might be a disadvantage, because this supports the entrapping of air. The viscosity is the most important handling property for the surgeon and determines the working properties of the cement.

### 4.2. Residual monomer and monomer release

Radical polymerization of the MMA in bone cement generally does not proceed to completion, because the mobility of remaining monomer molecules is inhibited at high conversion rates. There will remain, therefore, some residual monomer. Directly after curing, the content of residual monomer is approximately 2%–6%. In the following 3 weeks this content decreases to approximately 0.5%. The main part (approximately 80%) of the total residual monomer is post-polymerized slowly. A smaller part of the residual monomer is released from the cement and metabolized to carbon dioxide and water in the citric acid cycle.(Figure 3) In earlier times, released MMA was considered the main reason for perioperative respiration and circulation upset. However, these effects are definitely the result of the increase in the intramedullary pressure and fat embolism. They are not caused by the residual monomer. [7]

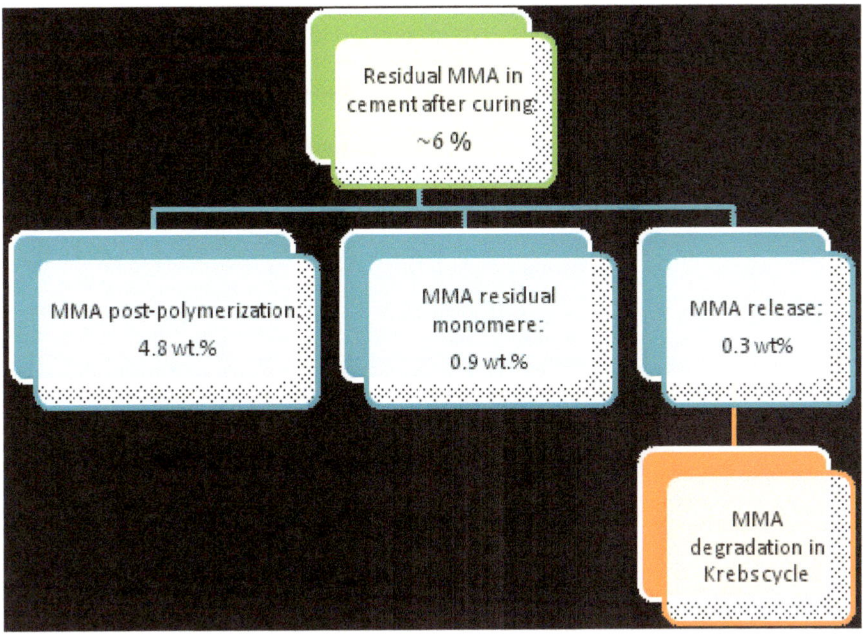


**Figure 3.** Residual monomer in acrylic bone cement: post-polymerization and release with subsequent degradation.

### 4.3. Radiopacity

After a total joint replacement, if the cement does not have a distinct opacity, the surgeon cannot monitor the healing process clearly. This is the reason why radiopaque materials are added to bone cements, so the hardened cement is radiopaque. Barium sulfate or zirconium dioxide is used as opacifiers in all available bone cements.(Figure 4) The radiopacifier does not contribute to the polymer chain. It is dispersed uniformly in the polymer powder and in the resulting solid bone cement. Animal experiments and in vivo studies with different cell cultures showed more osteolytic changes by using barium sulfate than by using zirconium dioxide. Despite the low solubility of barium sulfate, toxic barium ions can be released. On the other hand, the abrasive properties of zirconium dioxide seem to be a disadvantage. All bone cements examined contain 8.0%–15.0% opacifier within the polymer. Zirconium dioxide provides higher opacity to bone cements compared to barium sulfate. Bone cements with more than 15.0% zirconium dioxide in the polymer have the most distinct opacity.[2, 3, 7]

### 4.4. Molecular weight and sterilization

The molecular weight of the polymer powder particles is affected strongly by the sterilization procedure used. Sterilization by $\gamma$-irradiation or $\beta$-irradiation significantly lowers the molecular weight, whereas sterilization by ethylene oxide has no influence on the molecular weight of the polymer. The molecular weight influences the swelling properties and the mechanical properties of the bone cement; therefore, low molecular weights have a few disadvantages. Sterilization by ethylene oxide is the preferred method for bone cements, because there is no change in material properties during sterilization. [12]

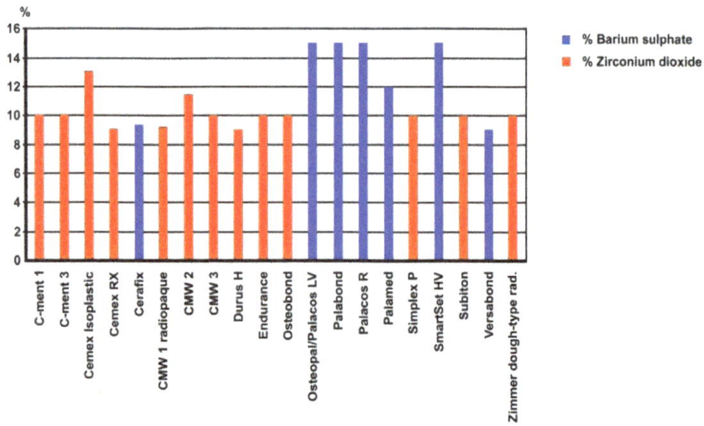


**Figure 4.** Content of radiopaquer in the powder of several acrylic bone cements; two radiopaquer agents are used in commercial products: Barium sulfate and Zirconium dioxide.

## 5. Cement morphology

The composition of hardened cement consists of prepolymerized beads of PMMA or their copolymers fused with the polymerized MMA monomer, in addition to radiopacifiers and additives, such as powders of antibiotics, as well as pores or voids and residual initiator. These parts of a cement composition act as flaws. These flaws can be due to: (a) air dissolved within the powder particles; (b) air entrapment during mixing of powder and liquid monomer; (c) incomplete fusion of prepolymerized PMMA beads with the setting MMA; (d) evaporation of the volatile monomer due to the heat of reaction during setting; (e) air entrapment during transfer of the dough to the gun; and (f) air entrapment during introduction of cement into the medullary canal. The major problem associated with the presence of flaws is that when a critical flaw size is achieved, the flaws act as sites of stress concentration, leading to weakening of the cement. But if the critical flaw size is not reached, they act as crack blunting part of the cement upon its fracture. In other words, the cracks deviate from their path when they encounter flaws in their path associated with pores and radiopacifier particles. The Griffith crack criterion assumes that there exists a critical flaw size unique to each material above which its fracture strength is compromised. For PMMA, the critical flaw size is 70 μm. Thus, if the pores are smaller than the critical flaw size for PMMA, the porosity will not compromise the fracture strength of bone cement. It is generally well known that hardened bone cement contain macropores (pore diameter greater than 1 mm) and micropores (pore diameter 0.01-1.0 mm). Based on the Griffith theory, elimination of the macropores would be more important than elimination of the micropores, especially the pores much smaller than 70 μm in diameter. The most common method of eliminating pores is to use centrifugation and vacuum mixing methods. Another source of flaws that can be potential sites of high stress concentration is radiopacifier powder particles. A radiopacifier powder, usually barium sulfate or zirconium oxide, consists of particles with a broad range of sizes, from approximately 0.2 to 2 μm in diameter. Zirconium oxide is a harder material than barium sulfate. Thus, if there is loosening, there could be concerns with regards to third body abrasive wear in the bearing surface of the joint replacement. Barium sulfate is generally insoluble, but there are concerns about toxicity of barium ions. Poor spread of radiopacifier particles in the region between the prepolymerized cement beads can affect both crack initiation and crack propagation, especially if they are larger than the critical flaw size for PMMA. The radiopacifier particles do not bond with PMMA and instead reside within pores, which are larger than these particles due to cement shrinkage. [13, 8]

## 6. Mixing techniques and its effect on porosity

Mixing techniques are of great importance in determining the content and size of flaws that can affect the cement toughness. Historically, three methods of mixing of cement have been employed: (a) hand mixing in air; (b) hand mixing followed by centrifugation; and (c) hand mixing in an evacuated mixing device, commonly known as "vacuum mixing." [8, 14]

Hand mixing involves mixing of the liquid and powder components in an open bowl using a spatula at a speed of 1 to 2 Hz for a period of duration of approximately 2 minutes. The hand-mixing method can introduce a porosity of 7% or higher. It is confirmed that excessive mixing can lead to increased porosity. By decreasing the number of beats and waiting for a short duration after wetting the powder component with the monomer the porosity of cement can be reduced to approximately 5%. Centrifugation was later introduced as a method to eliminate pores. In this method, the liquid and powder components are initially hand mixed and then placed in a tube and subjected to centrifugation at a speed of 2300 to 4000 rpm for a duration of 0.5 to 3 minutes. With this method the total porosity decreases to 1% or less, which is significantly lower than the porosity observed in hand mixing. It is obvious that for centrifugation to be effective, the viscosity of the cement must be relatively low, allowing the air bubbles to flow to the surface of the cement under the centrifugal force. One way to assist centrifugation is to chill the MMA monomer prior to mixing. One potential disadvantage of the centrifugation mixing technique is that it can lead to an inhomogeneous distribution of radiopacifier particles in the centrifuged cement, due to the difference in density of radiopacifier particles and PMMA and MMA monomer. The third type of mixing technique is vacuum mixing, in which the two components of bone cements are placed in a mixing bowl and are mixed after subjecting the bowl to vacuum conditions. The vacuum-mixing devices have proven to substantially decrease porosity in cements to less than 1% and consequently to increase their fatigue properties. Another major reason for using vacuum mixing is that MMA monomer is contained within the mixing bowl, which limits exposure to its vapors. Toxicology information obtained from materials safety data sheets (MSDSs) show that MMA monomer is harmful if inhaled, swallowed, or absorbed through the skin. [8, 14]

It must be noted that this reduction in the porosity of cement mantle with vacuum-mixing, is not always the case. Messick et al found that vacuum-mixed cement does not result in overall lower porosity of the cement, but the distribution of porosity may be different when compared with that of hand-mixed cement.(Figure 5) It has also been demonstrated that very high vacuum levels can be associated with the presence of cracks in the cement.[15]

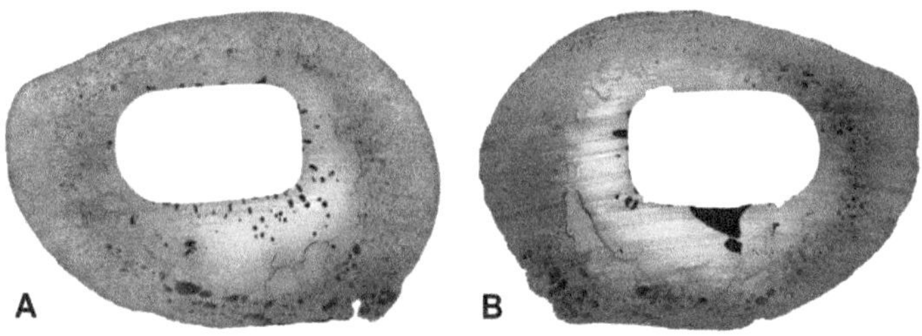


**Figure 5.** Representative sections illustrating the distribution of porosity for A) hand- and B) vacuum-mixed cement.

## 7. Mechanical and physical properties

### 7.1. Static mechanical properties (Table 2)

The main function of acrylic bone cement is the stable fixation of endoprostheses. The cement must endure considerable stresses, thus, sufficient strength is one of the most important demands to achieve a stable fixation and to guarantee long-term stability of the implant. The cement layer has the effect of an elastic buffer between prosthesis and bone. Because of its close adaptation to bone and its viscoelastic properties, it can reduce the stress concentrations at the interface with the bone. In the end, transferring load from the prosthesis to the bone as efficiently as possible also is decisive for the long-term stability of the implant. The mechanism of loading is especially complex for hip arthroplasty; therefore, it is difficult to define what sufficient strength actually means. The total load affecting bone cement is a mixture of compressive loading combined with bending, tension, shear, and torsion. It has been extremely difficult to simulate this complex situation in the laboratory. Two mechanical tests have been introduced into ISO 5833, the relevant standard for testing acrylic bone cements. These tests are the compression and the four-point bending test for the determination of the compressive strength, the bending strength and the bending modulus (modulus of elasticity or Young's modulus), respectively. The standard ASTM F 451 includes the compression test only. Generally there are two different fundamental measuring principles to determine mechanical properties of bone cements: applying static (also called quasistatic) stresses and dynamic stresses. Static tests are destructive tests with a uniaxial single loading, increasing until failure, in contrast to dynamic tests that involve a cyclic loading.[16]

The compression test according to the standards ISO 5833 and ASTM F 451 is a static method in which the compressive strength is defined as the maximum stress that a material can withstand before failure in compression. The test is executed with a universal testing machine equipped to record load versus crosshead displacement. The minimum requirement for the compressive strength is 70 MPa according to the standards. All commercial antibiotic and plain bone cements meet this requirement. Between both cement types, no significant differences in compressive strength are observable.[10]

The second mechanical test according to ISO 5833 is the four-point bending test, also performed with a universal testing machine. According to ISO 5833 the minimum requirement for the bending strength is 50 MPa and for the bending modulus it is 1800 MPa, respectively. Again, all commercial cements clearly fulfill the requirements. The addition of antibiotics reduces the bending strength, but the differences between antibiotic and plain cement are not always statistically significant. The bending modulus represents the ratio of stress to corresponding strain of the material within the elastic range characterizing the relative stiffness of the material. Stiff materials have a high modulus, eg, glass and ceramics; ductile materials like rubber have a low modulus. Within the elastic range the stress and strain are directly proportional following Hooke's Law, and if the load is released, the material regains its initial dimensions. The elastic range is limited by a stress limit, the so-called "proportional limit" at which the physical properties of the material actually change and the material might not recover its initial shape after releasing load. As already mentioned the cement acts as a mechanical buffer. For this purpose the modulus of elasticity of bone cement has to be lower than the moduli of the metallic prosthesis and the bone. The modulus must not decrease to below a minimum value, however; therefore, a lower limit for the modulus is established in ISO 5833. The modulus varies with temperature, which means the higher the temperature, the lower the modulus. Testing bone cement at 23°C is not a really convenient way to get meaningful results for the application in the human body. The mechanical performance of bone cements is influenced by various parameters, such as composition of the cement, porosity, and preparation of the cement. The addition of radiopacifier and antibiotics to a bone cement slightly decreases the mechanical strength. These additives are necessary to get radiograph opacity and antibiotic protection of the implant, which are important attributes of bone cements. Despite these additives, the resulting cements easily meet the requirements. [16,17]

Although bone cement has a high compressive strength, it is susceptible to fracture that might result from tensile loading. Tensile tests therefore are performed according to ISO 527-1 or ASTM D 638. These standards describe a static test method applicable for all polymer materials. The uniaxial tensile test is executed with flat tapered specimens. The ultimate tensile strength is defined as the maximum stress that a material can withstand before failure in tension. The tensile strength is approximately 50 –60 MPa and there are no significant differences between the tested materials. Again, the addition of antibiotics seems to reduce the tensile strength, but the differences between antibiotic and plain cement are not statistically significant. [18]

The compressive strength of bone cement is higher than the flexural strength and that is higher than the tensile strength. This descending order is found in all polymer materials. That means tensile loading may be a higher risk factor for failure than compressive loading. In vivo, simple tensile loading, however, does not play an important part in reality; complex combinations of different loading types are more relevant. From a physical point of view, bending is a mixture of compressive and tensile loading; therefore, the bending test actually is a realistic test. [17]

One further static test applied with bone cements is the shear strength test according to ASTM D732. This mechanical parameter is important because debonding of the stem–cement interface has been implicated in the initiation of failure of cemented femoral stems. The interface static shear strength is influenced by surface roughness, cement type, and porosity. Surface finish has the greatest effect on the interface strength. Increasing the surface roughness increases the interface shear strength. Increasing the surface roughness to greater than a certain value, however, has no additional affect. Cement type and porosity have a minor influence on the static interface strength. [19]

Furthermore, there are methods to determine fracture properties, such as fracture toughness (ASTM E399 and ISO 13,586) and impact strength (ISO 179/ISO 180/DIN 53,435). There is a correlation between the two methods. For a given specimen configuration, g-irradiation produced a statistically significant decrease in fracture toughness because of the concomitant depreciation in molecular weight. Impact strength is a measure of the energy required to cause a material to fracture when struck by a sudden blow. The addition of radiopacifier and antibiotics together with pores in the cement might have a negative effect on the impact strength. [20]

### 7.2. Water uptake and glass transition

When considering the mechanical tests described previously, one fact should be taken into account: most of the tests are executed with dry specimens at room temperature. The cement has to perform its task in the human body, however, in contact with body fluid and at a temperature of 37°C. Mechanical properties of polymers vary relative to their temperature and water uptake. The absorption of water results in a lower modulus of elasticity and in a less stiff material. The decreasing stiffness may even be advantageous for fracture resistance and long-term stability of the implant. The water uptake of commercial bone cements is approximately 1%–2% for plain bone cements and slightly higher for antibiotic bone cements. There is high initial water uptake during the first days of incubation at 37°C. The bone cements are completely water-saturated 4–8 weeks after incubation. The glass transition temperature is a physical parameter defining the softening range of a material. Softening means a transition from a hard and rigid glassy state with a high modulus to a soft rubbery state with a low modulus by heating the polymer. If the material for anchoring endoprosthesis is in the rubbery state, there would be a high risk for subsidence of the femoral stem and no stable fixation of the implant would be possible. Bone cements therefore can be used only for fixation of endoprostheses at temperatures less than their glass transition temperature in the glassy state. The glass transition temperatures of acrylic bone cements in a dry state range from 80°–100°C. These are high temperatures compared with the temperature of the human body. The water absorption of the cement, however, results in a reduction in glass transition temperature of approximately 20°–30°C after 8 weeks of incubation in water. The glass transition temperatures of water-saturated bone cements are approximately 60°–70°C. The addition of antibiotics does not lower the glass transition significantly. Considering the pronounced difference between the glass transition temperature and the temperature of the human body, the risk for sinking of the implant caused by creep seems to be very low.[16]

| Property | Value range (MPa) |
|---|---|
| Ultimate tensile strength | 36 to 47 |
| Ultimate compressive strength | 80 to 94 |
| Bending strength (4 point configuration) | 67 to 72 |
| Shear strength | 50 to 69 |
| Mean fracture toughness ($K_{Ic}$)** | 1.52 to 2.02 (MPa$\sqrt{m}$) |

*Simplex P, Palacos R, CMW1

**$K_{Ic}$, mean fracture toughness of brittle materials

**Table 2.** Mechanical properties of three cement brands*

### 7.3. Creep behavior

Polymers such as PMMA bone cements exhibit a combination of elastic and viscous behavior called viscoelasticity. When a polymer is subjected to a constant load, the resulting deformation can be divided into two parts: the immediate elastic deformation and the time-dependent, continuous deformation. The immediate elastic deformation happens instantaneously by applying load. It is a recoverable deformation essentially independent of time. Following this rapid deformation there is a delayed continuous deformation resulting from stress. One part of this deformation is recoverable in time after releasing load. This part is called delayed elastic deformation or primary creep. The second part of this continuous deformation is a non-recoverable permanent deformation called secondary creep.[21]

Different test methods are described in the standard ASTM D 2990 to measure creep. The specimen is loaded by tensile, compressive, or flexural stress. In each method the change in length of the specimen is measured and divided by the original length for the calculation of creep. All plastic materials including acrylic bone cement creep to a certain extent. The degree of creep depends on several factors, such as composition of the material, temperature, load, and load duration. Delayed injection time of acrylic bone cement increased creep compared with bone cement prepared according to standard injection procedures. Creep therefore depends not only on the material properties, but also on the cement handling by the surgeon.[22] It has been proposed that creep of acrylic bone cement may contribute to loosening of cemented total joint replacements. The long-term prosthetic subsidence rates caused by creep of acrylic cement, however, are small. On the other hand, cement creep relaxes cement stresses and creates a more favorable stress distribution at the interfaces. [3, 16]

### 7.4. Fatigue behavior

To ensure survival of the cement in the human body, the bone cement must be able to withstand the varying loads it endures. The fatigue properties of the cement thus are of particular significance, and they may determine when a correctly used cement will fail or not. Many studies have dealt with this topic, measuring fatigue properties in different ways. Today three different standard testing procedures are used to characterize the fatigue behavior:

- Four-point bending arrangement recommended by ISO 5833 standard
- Uniaxial pure tensile test with flat tapered specimens according to ISO 527
- Uniaxial compression–tension test with cylindrical tapered specimens according to ASTM F2118
- The first method is equivalent to the bending test method according to ISO 5833.

### 7.5. Fatigue testing

Fatigue testing is a dynamic test and is executed with a sinusoidal cyclic loading under stress control. The tests are continued until failure or until run-out. The run-out limit is a predetermined number of cycles at which the testing on a specimen is stopped, eg, 5 million or 10 million cycles. The second method is equivalent to tensile testing according to ISO 527. Again, the test run is performed with a sinusoidal cyclic loading under stress control until failure or until run-out. The third method is according to ASTM F2118. The specimens are subjected to fully reversed compressive and tensile loading in a sinusoidal cyclic manner. Again, the tests are continued until failure or until the run-out limit is reached. Most fatigue tests run at a specified frequency, eg, 5 Hz, in buffered saline solutions at 37°C.[16]

For tension–compression, the preliminary results exhibit a steeper decrease that might be caused by a possibly stronger deterioration from the additional compressive loading. The materials behave in a similar way under bending and uniaxial tension. The simplest test configuration is the standardized four-point bending test according to ISO 5833. Additionally the preparation of the specimens for the tension–compression is much more complex than the preparation of specimens for the bending test. For these two reasons the four-point bending is the preferred method for fatigue testing. The environmental conditions in which these experiments are conducted have a considerable influence on the fatigue life. Bone cements have different fatigue behavior if tested dry or in aqueous solution. The tests in air at room temperature result in a stress-number of cycles-curve (S-N-curve) of considerably higher slope. To simulate the body environment, tests should be performed in an appropriate liquid, such as simulated body fluid or Ringer's solution. The results of tests in air at laboratory temperature should be rated carefully.

Furthermore, the sterilization process of the polymer powder has an influence on fatigue behavior of acrylic bone cements. Sterilization by $\gamma$-irradiation or b-irradiation significantly lowers the molecular weight of the polymer powder and the resulting cured bone cement, whereas sterilization by ethylene oxide has no influence on the molecular weight of the polymer. Bone cement with high molecular weight has a better fatigue performance than a cement with low molecular weight.[17]

Porosity is a major cause of reduced fatigue life of bone cement. Pores or other inclusions serve to concentrate stress in the material and often initiate fatigue cracks within the bone cement. These cracks ultimately lead to failure. The sources of porosity are air initially surrounding the powder, which is trapped during wetting of the powder, air trapping in the cement during mixing, and air trapping in the cement during transfer from mixing container to application device. Hand-mixed bone cement in an open bowl has a significantly higher number of pores than bone cement mixed in a vacuum mixing system. Modern cement mixing systems reduce cement porosity and enhance cement strength by eliminating the chances of air entrapment in the cement.[23]

## 8. Antibiotics

Buchholz and Engelbrecht were the first to add gentamicin antibiotic to a bone cement.[3] Initially the antibiotic was added by hand, and subsequently during manufacture, making antibiotic-loaded acrylic cement widely available as part of antimicrobial prophylaxis in primary arthroplasty. It was shown later, that oxacillin, cefazolin, and gentamicin are all stable in PMMA bone cement and were released in active form. The largest release of antibiotics occurred in the first 24 hours, but high bactericidal concentrations of the antibiotics were measured in the periprosthetic bone for up to 21 days after implantation. A small amount of antibiotic elution is observed even after 5 years. Bone cement without any antibiotics had no bacteriostatic effect on *Staphylococcus aureus, Escherichia coli,* and *Pseudomonas aeruginosa* organisms. [24]

Bone cements can function as a matrix for the local application of antibiotics. Because of the high local concentration of an antibiotic in the surroundings of the implant, the use of bone cements has great advantages compared with a systemic antibiotic therapy. The artificial implant is especially sensitive to bacterial contamination on its surface, because the microorganisms may proliferate there almost unhampered by the immune defense of the body. As the bacteria rapidly generate a protective mucus layer and go to an inactive state with low sensitivity to antibiotics, a local antibiotic treatment is important. The pharmacokinetics of the antibiotic release from the matrix is of clinical importance. The local antibiotic concentrations reached must be clearly greater than the minimal inhibitory concentration and the minimal bactericidal concentration for the organisms. Not all antibiotics are suitable for use in bone cements. To avoid the development of resistant strains, a high initial level with a subsequent controlled release for days or weeks is important. The following bacteriologic and physical and chemical factors should be considered in the choice of an antibiotic:

1. Broad antibacterial spectra, including gram-positive and gram-negative organisms
2. Good bactericidal effect in low concentrations
3. Low incidence of primary resistant germs
4. Low rate of development of resistances
5. Low protein bonding
6. Low allergic potential
7. Little effect on bone cement mechanics
8. Chemical and thermal stability
9. Good solubility in water
10. Good release from bone cement

Based on these requirements and release tests, gentamicin has become the favorite antibiotic for bone cements since the early 1970s. Gentamicin is the most common additive because it has, amongst other features, a good spectrum of concentration-dependent bactericidal activity, thermal stability and high water solubility. [7]

Antibiotics are added in the form of powder, which is unable to diffuse through a hard, glassy polymer. So the mechanism of elution of the antibiotics is believed to be closely related to water-absorbing properties of the cement with respect to time and distance from the surface of the cement. The diffusion rate of the antibiotics depends on several factors, such as the chemical composition of the cement, the surface area at the cement-bone interface, and cement handling. For example, Palacos cement containing prepolymerized beads of P(MMA-co-MA) were shown to elute gentamicin at more rapidly than Simplex containing prepolymerized beads of P(MMA-co-S). In addition, vacuum mixing, which decreases the porosity in bone cement, can also alter the kinetics of the elution of antibiotics and was shown to decrease their rate of elution by 50%.[25]

Penner et al investigated the release of vancomycin and tobramycin from bone cement separately or combined in nonvacuum preparations. They observed that the combined use of the 2 antibiotics led to an increased elution of both from cement. Baleani et al also showed that the presence of meropenem broadened the antibacterial spectrum and enhanced the elution of vancomycin from cement. [26]

Since powder gentamicin is a costly antibiotic and is not available for hand-mixing with bone cement in operating rooms, many researchers have tried to add liquid gentamicin to bone cements. The liquid gentamicin, a much less costly antibiotic (1/20 the price of tobramycin) with a broad antimicrobial spectrum, is widely available throughout the world, but there is always a fear of deteriorating the mechanical properties of the bone cement by adding liquid gentamicin. Hsieh PH et al investigated the use of liquid gentamicin, alone and in combination with vancomycin, incorporated into acrylic bone cement as a potential treatment of complex orthopedic infections. They assessed the cement specimens loaded with

480 mg of liquid gentamicin, 4 g of powdered vancomycin, or both antibiotics for elution characteristics, bioactivity, compressive strength, and porosity. Vancomycin elution was enhanced by 146% with the addition of gentamicin liquid, and gentamicin elution was enhanced by 45% when combined with vancomycin. Bioassay confirmed the bactericidal activity of the released antibiotics. Adding liquid gentamicin increased porosity, whereas adding vancomycin did not. Compressive strength decreased by 13%, 37%, and 45% in specimens containing vancomycin, liquid gentamicin, and both antibiotics, respectively.(Table 3) Despite inferior mechanical properties, the temporary nature of cement beads and spacers makes the liquid gentamicin–vancomycin mixture a potentially more cost-effective regimen in bone cement to treat musculoskeletal infections. [27]

| | Vancomycin | Gentamicin | Both antibiotics |
|---|---|---|---|
| Porosity* (%) | 5.8 ± 2.6 | 16.8 ± 1.9 | 22.4 ± 3.4 |
| Compressive strength (MPa) | 79.69 ± 6.2 | 57.99 ± 1.5 | 50.32 ± 4.9 |

*Porosity as a percentage of the total area.

**Table 3.** Porosity and ultimate compressive strength of the specimens

Other antibiotics with suitable spectra against orthopaedic infecting organisms, such as cefazolin, ciprofloxacin, linezolid, levofloxacin and rifampin, have been tested according to their elution and bactericidal activities and have been shown that all these antibiotics may be suitable for incorporation into polymethylmethacrylate for management of orthopaedic infections.[28] (Table 4)

But it worth noting that all antibiotics are not suitable for adding to bone cements. Goss et al have shown that amphotericin B does not elute from polymethylmethacrylate bone cement. However, addition of this antifungal increases the mechanical strength by forming covalent crosslinks in the PMMA matrix, imparting better mechanical properties. [29]

Antibiotics premixed into the cement by the manufacturer can be advantageous since the addition of antibiotic powder manually can lead to agglomeration and a decrease in the mechanical strength of the cement. Antibiotics are added to cement in the powdered form since it was demonstrated that the addition of liquid antibiotics resulted in a decrease in mechanical strength due to interference with the early stages of polymerization of the MMA monomer. The amount of antibiotic powder required for a therapeutic level of elution is approximately 0.5 to 2 g in a standard 40-g package of prepolymerized PMMA powder. Note that antibiotic powder, like radiopacifiers and pores, also results in defects or flaws in bone cement. The flexural strength of antibiotic-containing cement was shown to be lower than that of cement without antibiotics, and the toughness of antibiotic-containing cement decreased further with excessive amounts of antibiotics. A likely reason for this is that excess amounts of undissolved antibiotics agglomerate into aggregates exceeding the critical flaw size for PMMA. However, doses of 2 g of well-dispersed antibiotic powder may not have any adverse effect on the mechanical properties of bone cement if the size of the inclusions remains below the critical flaw size for PMMA.

| Antimicrobial | Amount (%) | AUC (μg/mL/h) | Peak concentration (μg/mL) | Time no longer detectable (h) | Percent in the bead before elution |
|---|---|---|---|---|---|
| Cefazolin | 2.5 | 18 ± 3 | 15 ± 2 | 2 ± 0 | 56 ± 2 |
| | 7.5 | 162 ± 33 | 62 ± 23 | 10 ± 1 | 42 ± 4 |
| | 15 | 792 ± 47 | 147 ± 22 | 26 ± 1 | 54 ± 5 |
| Ciprofloxacin | 2.5 | 23 ± 5 | 5 ± 0 | 45 ± 3 | 36 ± 3 |
| | 7.5 | 112 ± 3 | 15 ± 1 | 45 ± 5 | 36 ± 7 |
| | 15 | 307 ± 10 | 54 ± 3 | 48 ± 0 | 31 ± 3 |
| Gatifloxacin | 2.5 | 157 ± 34 | 15 ± 2 | 48 ± 0 | 45 ± 2 |
| | 7.5 | 190 ± 65 | 19 ± 1 | 48 ± 0 | 47 ± 4 |
| | 15 | 499 ± 51 | 51 ± 3 | 48 ± 0 | 50 ± 3 |
| Levofloxacin | 2.5 | 33 ± 4 | 7 ± 1 | 48 ± 0 | 28 ± 3 |
| | 7.5 | 123 ± 7 | 26 ± 3 | 48 ± 0 | 23 ± 3 |
| | 15 | 291 ± 59 | 52 ± 10 | 48 ± 0 | 24 ± 3 |
| Linezolid | 2.5 | Not detected | <5 | 0 ± 0 | 96 ± 5 |
| | 7.5 | 213 ± 53 | 43 ± 4 | 12 ± 4 | 88 ±4 |
| | 15 | 224 ± 155 | 64 ± 47 | 22 ± 2 | 84 ± 4 |
| Rifampin | 2.5 | 5 ± 2 | 4 ± 1 | 2 ± 1 | 21 ± 1 |
| | 7.5 | 147 ± 15 | 15 ± 2 | 37 ± 1 | 27 ± 4 |
| | 15 | 409 ± 46 | 31 ± 11 | 48 ± 0 | 24 ±1 |

AUC: area under the curve

**Table 4.** Parameters of release from PMMA for studied antimicrobials

### 8.1. Costs of antibiotic-loaded bone cement

Currently the increased acquisition cost of commercially available antibiotic-loaded bone-cement products is considerable. Compared with the cost of plain bone-cement products, the cost of equivalent antibiotic-loaded bone-cement products is increased anywhere from $284 to $349 (United States dollars) per 40-g packet. If the historical 11% usage of antibiotic-loaded bone cement increased to 50% of the estimated 500,000 primary total joint arthroplasties performed annually in the United States, and if two packets of cement (at a $300 increased cost per packet) were used for each joint replacement, the increase in overall health-care costs would be $117,000,000 for the 195,000 additional cases. This estimated increased health-care cost must be balanced with the potential cost savings associated with a realized reduction in the rate of infection associated with routine use of antibiotic-loaded bone cement for prophylaxis in primary total joint replacement. At an approximately $50,000 cost for the treatment of an infection at the site of a total joint replacement, there would have to be 2340 fewer infected patients among the additional 195,000 patients for the routine use of antibiotic-loaded bone cement to be fiscally neutral. With a rather high estimated infection rate of 1.5%, a deep postoperative infection could be expected to develop in 2925 of 195,000 patients. In other words, the rate of deep periprosthetic infection would need to be reduced from this 1.5% to 0.3% to recover the costs associated with the routine use of commercially available low-dose antibiotic-loaded bone cement in primary total joint arthroplasty. Moreover, while the estimated costs for the treatment of an infection at the site of a total joint arthroplasty do not account for morbidity and mortality associated with the treatment required, the increased costs associated with the treatment of more drug-resistant organisms are unknown. [30]

### 8.2. Choice of antibiotic in antibiotic-loaded bone cement used prophylactically

The aminoglycoside antibiotics were originally selected for use in antibiotic-loaded bone cement because of their broad bacterial coverage and their low allergy profile. Because the level of gentamicin or tobramycin in the joint is often ten times greater than safe blood levels, the efficacy of those drugs is excellent unless the organism has a specific resistance to them. Gentamicin and tobramycin are also the only antibiotics currently available in commercially premixed low-dose antibiotic-loaded bone-cement preparations. As mentioned above, however, low doses of other types of antibiotics, including several of the cephalosporins, have been hand-mixed into bone-cement preparations, and those preparations have had good success in prophylactic applications. Allergic reactions have not been reported, to our knowledge, but it is prudent for the surgeon to consider the individual patient's allergy history before selecting the antibiotic for antibiotic-loaded bone cement. There has been considerable research on the primary bacterial contaminants in total joint surgery.

Al-Maiyah et al. took 627 blood-agar impressions of the gloved hands of surgical personnel during the performance of fifty total hip arthroplasties in England. Bacteria grew on culture of fifty-seven impressions (9%); 69% were coagulase-negative staphylococci, 12% were Micrococcus, 9% were diphtheroids, and 6% were *Staphylococcus aureus*. Of the coagulase-negative staphylococci, only 52% were sensitive to cefuroxime. In contrast, Ridgeway et al. found *Staphylococcus aureus* in 50% of the surgical site infections (both superficial and deep) in their multiple-hospital study in England. More than half of the *Staphylococcus aureus* isolates were methicillin-resistant. Thus, it appears that staphylococcal species are the primary bacteria toward which antibiotic-loaded bone cement would be directed. The currently available commercial gentamicin or tobramycin-loaded bone cements provide sufficient elution concentrations to be bactericidal even against methicillin-resistant organisms. Vancomycin may also be added to bone cement, but it has a lower efficacy than gentamicin or tobramycin at these concentrations. The use of vancomycin should be considered in revisions following primary arthroplasties in which gentamicin or tobramycin-loaded bone cement had been used because of the prevalence of gentamicin resistance in association with such revisions. Cephalosporins may also be considered for antibiotic-loaded bone cement that is to be used prophylactically but may not be effective against methicillin-resistant organisms.[30]

## 9. Adverse effects of bone cement

### 9.1. Cardiopulmonary complications

Cardiopulmonary complications associated with PMMA have been reported in conjunction with hip arthroplasty and VA. Prior studies have postulated that PMMA-associated hypoxia, hypotension, and death may occur as a result of the toxic effects of monomer or anaphylaxis. Other literature indicates that the application of PMMA may lead to embolization of marrow debris and neurogenic reflex, thus adversely affecting cardiopulmonary function. Pulmonary infarction and death have been reported as a result of embolization of PMMA that was injected in liquid state following VA. [2]

### 9.2. Hypersensitivity to components of methylmethacrylate, especially benzoyl peroxide

A small but significant proportion of cemented total knee arthroplasties develop early aseptic loosening. Polyethylene debris is unlikely to be the cause in the small subgroup that experiences early loosening. Allergy to polymethylmethacrylate bone cement or its constituents has been reported in dentistry, dermatology, and joint arthroplasty. Although allergy to polymethylmethacrylate bone cement or its constituents is unusual, the possibility of a systemic inflammatory response and consequent pain and loosening must be considered. Benzoyl peroxide is an essential component of bone cement. Direct evidence for allergic reactions to benzoyl peroxide has been reported in dental and dermatological literature. The currently accepted model for this delayed hypersensitivity is that a hapten such as benzoyl peroxide conjugates with a body protein, which creates a neoantigen capable of stimulating an immune response. This hypersensitivity places the patient at risk of developing insidious pain, a systemic inflammatory response, and possibly aseptic loosening. After revision to uncemented femoral and tibial components, the patient's symptoms vastly improved.[31]

### 9.3. Presence of components of methylmethacrylate in serum and breast milk

Singh et al. reported dose-related teratogenic and fetal toxic effects of methacrylic acid administered via the intraperitoneal route in rats. McLaughlin et al. exposed pregnant mice to very high vapor concentrations of methacrylic acid of 1330 parts per million for two consecutive hours, twice daily. The mice demonstrated no evidence of fetal toxicity or teratogenic effects; in fact, there was a slight increase in fetal weight with methacrylic acid exposure. The only published study that has addressed methacrylic acid exposure during lactation involved a patient undergoing arthroplasty, not operating room personnel who were exposed to methacrylic acid vapors. In that study, Hersh et al. found undetectable levels of polymethylmethacrylate in breast milk that was collected thirty-six hours after hybrid total hip arthroplasty in a twenty-nine-year-old woman who was five months postpartum. Linehan et al. showed undetectable levels of methacrylic acid (at the 0.5-part-per-million level) in the serum and breast milk of two lactating surgeons who had been exposed to typical operating room conditions without the use of personal exhaust systems. [32]

## 10. Composite bone cements

PMMA-based bone cement has a high modulus but low toughness compared with ductile polymers. In order to address the lack of fracture toughness and fatigue strength, many investigators who have developed new composite PMMA cements use the concept of fiber reinforcement and incorporate a low-volume fraction of chopped fibers of approximately 1% to 2%.[33] Several types of fibers, such as fibers made of carbon, polyethylene terephthalate, oriented PMMA, ultra high molecular weight polyethylene, titanium, aramid, Kevlar, graphite, steel, and zirconia fibers with and without acrylic coating have been used to reinforce PMMA-based bone cement.[33-6] While these composites have displayed improved fatigue failure properties, biocompatibility concerns and complications of processing have prevented their implementation in the manufacture of PMMA bone cement.

## Author details

Hamid Reza Seyyed Hosseinzadeh, Mohammad Emami, Farivarabdollahzadeh Lahiji, Ali Sina Shahi, Aidin Masoudi and Sina Emami

Akhtar Orthopaedic Hospital, Shahid Beheshti University of Medical Sciences, Iran

## References

[1] Dennis, C., et al. (2005). The genesis and evolution of acrylic bone cement Orthop Clin N Am , 36(2005), 1-10.

[2] Todd, J., et al. (2010). DO Polymethylmethacrylate: Properties and Contemporary Uses in Orthopaedics, J Am Acad Orthop Surg 2010; , 18, 297-305.

[3] Webb, J. C. J., et al. (2007). The role of polymethylmethacrylate bone cement in modern orthopaedic surgery J Bone Joint Surg [Br] 2007;B:851-7., 89.

[4] Kuehn KD, et al. Acrylic bone cements: Composition and properties. Orthop Clin North Am (2005). , 36, 17-28.

[5] Charnley, J., et al. (1964). The bonding of prostheses to bone by cement. J Bone Joint Surg Br 1964; , 46, 518-529.

[6] Webb JC, et al. (2007). The role of polymethylmethacrylate bone cement in modern orthopaedic surgery. J Bone Joint Surg Br 2007; , 89, 851-857.

[7] Klaus-Dieter, K., et al. (2005). Acrylic bone cements: composition and properties Orthop Clin N Am , 36(2005), 17-28.

[8] Anuj Bellare, et al. (2007). orthopaedic bone cement, the adult hip, second edition, 2007, LWW, , 144-155.

[9] Reckling FW, et al. (1977). The bone- cement interface temperature during total joint replacement. J Bone Joint Surg 1977;59A: , 80-2.

[10] Lewis, G., et al. (1997). Properties of acrylic bone cement: state of the art review. J Biomed Mater Res 1997; , 38, 155-82.

[11] Gladius Lewis, et al. (2007). Preheating Acrylic Bone Cement Powder Is Not Recommended for All Brands. *The Journal of Arthroplasty*, 22(3).

[12] Lewis, G., et al. (1998). Effect of sterilization method on properties of Palacos R acrylic bone cement. *Biomaterials*, 117 EOF-24 EOF.

[13] Bridgens, J., et al. (2008). Stockley Orthopaedic bone cement DO WE KNOW WHAT WE ARE USING? J Bone Joint Surg [Br] 2008;B:643-7., 90.

[14] Macaulay, W., et al. (2002). Differences in bone-cement porosity by vacuum mixing, centrifugation, and hand mixing. J Arthroplasty 2002; , 17, 569-75.

[15] Messik, K. J., et al. (2007). Vacuum-mixing cement does not decrease overall porosity in cemented femoral stems. J Bone Joint Surg [Br]2007;B:1115-21., 89.

[16] Klaus-Dieter Kuehn, et al. (2005). Acrylic bone cements: mechanical and physical properties Orthop Clin N Am , 36(2005), 29-39.

[17] Demian HW, et al. (1998). Regulatory perspective on characterization and testing of orthopedic bone cements. *Biomaterials*, 19, 1607-18.

[18] Harper EJ, et al. (2000). Tensile characteristics of ten commercial acrylic bone cements. J Biomed Mater Res 2000; , 53(5), 605-16.

[19] Wang JS, et al. (2003). Factors affecting the static shear strength of the prosthetic stem-bone cement interface. J Mater Sci Mater Med 2003; , 14, 55-61.

[20] Lewis, G., et al. (2000). Correlation between impact strength and fracture toughness of PMMA-based bone cements. *Biomaterials*, 21(8), 775-81.

[21] Verdonschot, N., et al. (2000). Creep properties of three low temperature-curing bone cements: a preclinical assessment. J Biomed Mater Res 2000; , 53, 498-504.

[22] Lee AJ, et al. (2002). Factors affecting the mechanical and viscoelastic properties of acrylic bone cement. J Mater Sci Mater Med 2002; , 13, 723-33.

[23] Lewis, G., et al. (1999). Effect of two variables on the fatigue performance of acrylic bone cement: mixing method and viscosity. Biomed Mater Eng 1999; , 9, 197-207.

[24] Armstrong, M., et al. (2002). Antibiotic elution from bone cement: a study of common cement-antibiotic combinations. *Hip International*, 12, 23-7.

[25] Perry AC, et al. (2002). Antimicrobial release kinetics from polymethylmethacrylate in a novel continuous flow chamber. Clin Orthop Relat Res. 2002; , 403, 49-53.

[26] Baleani, M., et al. (2008). Biological and biomechanical effects of vancomycin and meropenem in acrylic bone cement. J Arthroplasty. 2008 Dec; Epub 2008 Apr 14., 23(8), 1232-8.

[27] Hsieh PH, et al. (2009). Liquid gentamicin and vancomycin in bone cement: a potentially more cost-effective regimen. J Arthroplasty. 2009 Jan; Epub 2008 Feb 14., 24(1), 125-30.

[28] Anguita-Alonso, P., et al. (2006). Comparative study of antimicrobial release kinetics from polymethylmethacrylate. Clin Orthop Relat Res. 2006 Apr; , 445, 239-44.

[29] Goss, B., et al. (2007). Elution and mechanical properties of antifungal bone cement. J Arthroplasty. 2007 Sep; Epub 2007 Jul 25., 22(6), 902-8.

[30] Jiranek WA, Hanssen AD, Greenwald AS. ((2006). )Antibiotic-loaded bone cement for infection prophylaxis in total joint replacement. J Bone Joint Surg Am. 2006 Nov; Review., 88(11), 2487-500.

[31] Edwards SA, et al. (2007). Hypersensitivity to benzoyl peroxide in a cemented total knee arthroplasty: cement allergy. J Arthroplasty. 2007 Dec; Epub 2007 Jan 18., 22(8), 1226-8.

[32] Linehan CM, et al. (2006). Serum and breast milk levels of methylmethacrylate following surgeon exposure during arthroplasty. J Bone Joint Surg Am. 2006 Sep; , 88(9), 1957-61.

[33] Kotha, S., et al. (2009). Reinforcement of bone cement using zirconia fibers with and without acrylic coating. J Biomed Mater Res A. 2009 Mar 15; , 88(4), 898-906.

[34] Kotha SP, et al. (2006). Improved mechanical properties of acrylic bone cement with short titanium fiber reinforcement. J Mater Sci Mater Med. 2006 Aug; , 17(8), 743-8.

[35] Kotha SP, et al. (2006). Improved mechanical properties of acrylic bone cement with short titanium fiber reinforcement. J Mater Sci Mater Med. 2006 Aug; , 17(8), 743-8.

[36] May-Pat, A., et al. (2011). Flores-Gallardo SG. Comparative study on the mechanical and fracture properties of acrylic bone cements prepared with monomers containing amine groups. J Mech Behav Biomed Mater. 2012 Feb; Epub 2011 Nov 17., 6, 95-105.

Chapter 6

# Short-Stem Hip Arthroplasty

Kálmán Tóth and Gellért Sohár

Additional information is available at the end of the chapter

## 1. Introduction

Total hip arthroplasty has become a remarkably successful operation for treating osteoarthritis in the last half century. The increased need for better quality of life has led the operation to be extended to younger patients. However, long term results showed a rise in the number of revision surgeries. The longer life expectancy of the patient population led to the demand for multiple revision surgeries for the same patient. In revision surgery numerous technical difficulties are encountered because of bone loss due to the loosening. In addition, these solutions are exceptionally expensive. The search for alternatives led to the modification of the primary components. Improvements have introduced changes to achieve more proximal load transfer to the femur in order to reduce proximal stress shielding and thus preserve bone stock for potential revision surgery. As hip resurfacing declines in popularity, it is likely that there will be a corresponding increase in the number of short stem femoral components in use. Metaphyseal stems combine the advantages of straight stem implant design and hip resurfacing.

The aim of this chapter is to outline the recent developments in short (metaphyseal) stem arthroplasty.

## 2. Concise review of the pertinent literature

### 2.1. Rationale

Short metaphyseal femoral stems have been developed in order to improve the results of the standard non-cemented stems. Different designs of short stems are available, with differences in operative technique and published outcomes [Mai et al., 2010; McElroy et al., 2011]. The new generation short-stem hip implants are designed to encourage physiological-like loading to minimize stress-strain shielding and therefore implant loosening in the long term.

Traditionally, femoral stems are tapered, anatomical, or cylindrical. The classic tapered stem has rectangular cross-section, 4 corners and 4 flat surfaces that are compressed into the proximal femur. The second, equally popular design consists of anatomically shaped stems designed to match the shape of the proximal femur. The third design, with its different philosophy of fixation, consists of cylindrical, straight, nontapered, and extensively coated stems achieving distal fixation at the isthmus by means of a "scratch fit" between the fully roughened porous surface of the implant and the slightly smaller, underreamed femoral canal [Mai et al., 2010].

Proximal loading short stems have been designed to improve the results of the traditional non-cemented stems. [d'Imporzano & Pierannunzii, 2006; Renkawitz et al., 2008]. In a study by Westphal et al. the migration and cyclic motion were compared between a new short-stemmed hip prosthesis (Proxima™) and two clinically successful shaft prostheses in order to estimate the primary stability of the new stem [Westphal et al., 2006b]. Initially the short stem migrated more than the shaft prostheses. When cortical contact was achieved or the cancellous bone was compacted sufficient stability was acquired. Therefore, correct positioning and good bone quality are important factors for the short stem. Bony ingrowth is more favorable with the short stem because of the lowered cyclic motion after implantation. The effects of stress shielding are reduced by more physiological loading of the femur because of the new stem's lower bending stiffness [Westphal et al., 2006b].

The following advantages have been reported:

1. bone stock and soft tissue (m. gluteus medius et minimus insertation) preservation, in the greater trochanteric and sub-trochanteric regions, at the time of implantation for future revisions [Khanuja et al., 2011; Morrey, 1989] Fig. 1,

2. decreased stress shielding, caused by metaphyseal bone resorption and diaphyseal cortical hypertrophy [Pipino, 2000],

3. stress concentration at the tip of a distal fixation traditional component causes thigh pain, with the short stem this is eliminated [Khanuja et al., 2011; Mai et al., 2010],

4. the iliotibial band's tension band effect provides compression forces both medially and laterally in the proximal femur. [Leali et al., 2002] Fig. 2, lateral cortex provides a strong support as a second compression column [d'Imporzano & Pierannunzii, 2006]

5. transfers load to the metaphysis from a superior to an inferior direction in a physiological manner [Leali et al., 2002; Walker et al., 1999],

6. the method of implantation eases minimally invasive approaches [McElroy et al., 2011] Fig. 1,

7. wide range of indication (over surface arthroplasty risk index grade 3), all types of bone stock with normal femoral morphology are acceptable [Kim et al., 2011],

8. revision surgery becomes easier because of minimally invasive approach, less soft tissue damage, and the intact bone stock below the lesser trochanter [d'Imporzano & Pierannunzii, 2006].

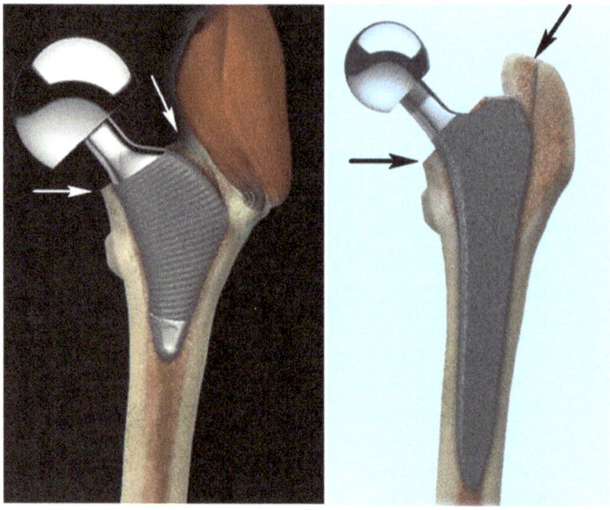

**Figure 1.** More bone stock and soft tissue preservation (arrows) in the greater trochanteric and sub-trochanteric regions at the time of implantation. Revision surgery becomes easier because of minimally invasive approach and less tissue damage.

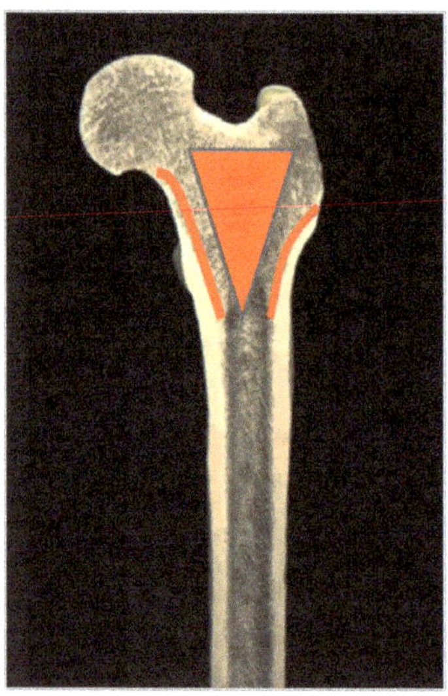

**Figure 2.** The lateral flare geometry of short stem femoral components loads the proximal wider metaphyseal lateral and medial cortices of the femur. This additional contact area creates a wider base for support and provides a more physiologic load distribution in the proximal femur.

The design and geometry of the implant impacts its ability to transfer loads to the femur [Westphal et al., 2006a]. The lateral flare geometry of short stem femoral components loads the proximal femur more evenly [Walker et al., 1999]. The lateral flare component is stabilized by resting upon the lateral column of cortical bone. This additional contact area creates a wider base for support and provides a more physiologic load distribution in the proximal femur [Leali et al., 2002; Dabirrahmani et al., 2010]. Therefore, femoral components that engage the metaphysis and load the femur both medially and laterally are more stable [Leali et al., 2002]. The stem does not need to be 'press-fitted' into the femur or driven distally. The stem rests upon the proximal wider metaphyseal lateral and medial cortices of the femur [Leali et al., 2002; Walker et al., 1999].

## 2.2. Outcomes of different short stems

There are no long-term clinical studies available to prove the benefits of these short-stem implants so far. Owing to this lack of clinical data, numerical simulation may be used as a predictor of longer term behaviour. This finite element study predicted both the primary and long-term stability of a short-stem implant. The primary implant stability was evaluated in terms of interface micromotion. This study found primary stability to fall within the critical threshold for osseointegration to occur. Longer term stability was evaluated using a strain-adaptive bone remodelling algorithm to predict the long-term behaviour of the bone in terms of bone mineral density (BMD) changes. No BMD loss was observed in the classical Gruen zones 1 and 7 and bone remodelling patterns were comparable with hip resurfacing results in the literature [Dabirrahmani et al., 2010]

In previous reports on short stems, the HHS values showed an increase of 56 points for the Mayo® stem [Hube et al., 2004] and 33 points for the CUT® stem [Thomas et al., 2004] after a minimum follow-up period of three-months after operation. Our results showed an increase of 39 points with the Proxima™ stem [Tóth et al., 2010]. At a minimum follow-up time of 12 months, an increase in the HHS of 51 [Ender et al., 2007] and 34 points [Thomas et al., 2004] with the CUT® stem, 51 with both the Proxima™ [Ghera & Pavan, 2009] and the Mayo® stem [Morrey, 1989] have been reported. In a similar study [Tóth et al., 2010], we noted a 50 points increase in the HHS with the Proxima™ stem one year post operatively, which is comparable with previous reports.

Some studies reported a vertical or horizontal (varus) migration of short stems requiring a subsequent revision [Ender et al., 2007; Morrey, 1989; Thomas et al., 2004], others described significant radiolucent lines or progressive proximal femoral osteolysis around the short stems without a need for revision [Gilbert et al., 2009; Goebel & Schulz, 2009]. In our reported study [Tóth et al., 2010], no horizontal or vertical migration was found at follow-up at that time, not even with the under-sized and varus positioned stem (Fig. 3). The patient cohort is continuously followed both by radiological and clinical examination. After average follow-up of 4.5 years still no horizontal nor vertical migration was seen.

Thigh pain is a common complaint following traditional non-cemented hip arthroplasty. Among the Proxima™ hip cases evaluated by Tóth et al [Tóth et al., 2010], none of the patients reported any thigh pain even after 4.5 years. Ghera and Pavan reported similar findings with Proxima™ stems [Ghera & Pavan, 2009]. Hube et al also did not find any thigh pain following THA with the Mayo® stem [Hube et al., 2004]. Other studies reported severe thigh pain following short stem implantation (Mayo®, CUT®), requiring revision [Ender et al., 2007; Gilbert et al., 2009; Thomas et al., 2004].

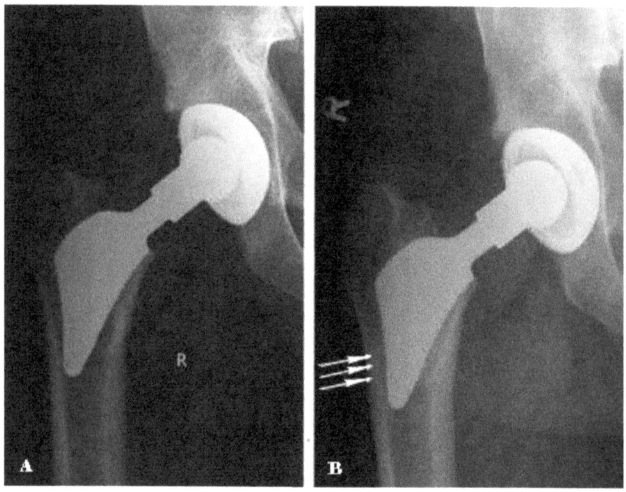


**Figure 3.** Undersized Proxima™ short-stem in severe varus position (a) immediate postoperative radiograph (b) radiograph 4 year post-op. Even though the long neck is biomechanically disadvantageous, after 4 years the position of the stem is the same. Strengthening of the trabecular structure against the lateral aspect of the stem (arrows) is stimulated by proximal loading (Wolf's law).

Survival of the implanted short stems are summarized in Table 1.

| Type | Author | Follow-up | Survival |
|---|---|---|---|
| May® Conservative Stem (Zimmer) | Morrey et al, 2000 | 5 and 10 years | 98.2% |
| CFP™ | Gill et al, 2010 | 3 years | 97% |
| CFP™ | Pons, 2010 | 3,1 years | 100% |
| Cut® (ESKA) | Steens et al, 2010 | 6.6 years | 98% |
| Metha™ | Synder et al, 2009 | 1 year | 100% |
| Metha™ | Floerkemeier et al, 2012 | 2.75 years | 96% |
| Proxima™ (DePuy) | Santori et al, 2010 | 8 years | 100% |
| Proxima™ (DePuy) | Tóth et al, 2010 | 2.1 years | 100% |
| Proxima™ (DePuy) | Kim et al, 2012 | 4.1 years | 100% |
| Proxima™ (DePuy) | Ghera et al, 2009 | 1.7 years | 100% |
| SPS™ | Sariali et al 2012 | 10 years | 100% |
| TaperLoc® Microplasty™ | Molli et al 2012 | 1.8 years | 99.7% |

**Table 1.** Reported survival of different short stems

## 3. Authors' own experience

### 3.1. Materials and methods

At the Orthopedic Department of the University of Szeged, implantation of the short-stemmed Proxima™ (DePuy; Leeds, UK) began in September 2006. Proxima™ was chosen of all the short stemmed designs on the market because the 36 stem options provide broader variety for the anatomical shape of the femur than the rest. All the 50 procedures were examined clinically and radiologically. Mean age of the patients was 48 (rang from 35 to 61, SD 7) years at time of the surgery. Mean follow-up time was 54 (range from 45 to 61, SD 5) months. Thirty male and 14 female patients were operated on; one female and five male patients had bilateral surgery in two stages. Patients' distribution according to diagnosis was: primary osteoarthritis (OA) in 22, avascular femoral head necrosis in 18, OA with mild dysplasia in 6, post-traumatic OA in 3 and OA secondary to Perthes disease in 1. All procedures were performed by the same surgeon, in the routinely used supine position, from anterolateral approach, with minimally invasive technique. Any intra- or postoperative complications were recorded.

The Proxima™ stem is made of forged titanium alloy, with a Duofix™ HA (porous coating and hydroxyapatite) surface coating. Nine sizes of standard as well as high-offset stems for each side are available. Cementless Duraloc™ porous coated cups (Depuy) with 10° lipped polyethylene liners and 28 mm metal heads were used in all cases.

The indication was hip osteoarthritis or avascular necrosis in young and active patients who were not appropriate candidates for a resurfacing procedure. The following elements were considered contraindications to implantation of a Proixima stem: stem size 1 or 2 for patients with body weight over 100 kg, severe hip dysplasia, previous hip osteotomy or other acquired femoral distortion, cortical index less than 3, severe osteoporosis.

The clinical status of the patients was documented with the Harris Hip Score (HHS) [Harris, 1969]. Low molecular weight heparin was administered for 42 days postoperatively for thromboembolism prophylaxis. Partial weight bearing using crutches was recommended for four weeks post operatively, thereafter full weight bearing with canes was allowed for two additional weeks.

Pre- and post-operative radiographs were taken with identical settings for each patient. Implant migration was assessed according to Martell et al [Martell et al., 1993]. Implant stability was evaluated according to Engh et al [Engh et al., 1987], based on the radiological features of the bone-implant interface. Criteria for radiological loosening of the implant were defined as a radiolucent zone greater than 3 mm, or a horizontal and/or vertical migration greater than 2 mm with an adjacent radiolucent zone [Kim et al., 2003]. Stem alignment was rated as normal if its deviation from the axis of the femoral shaft was 5° or less. A deviation of 6 to 10° was rated as "varus" or "valgus"; a deviation exceeding 10° was rated as "severe varus" or "severe valgus".

### 3.2. Results

Mean preoperative HHS value was 39 (range: 11 to 71; SD 13). Mean postoperative HHS was 78 at six months (range: 44 to 94; SD 14), 90 at twelve months (range: 52 to 99; SD 13) and 87 at fifty four months (range: 51 to 95; SD 13). We had two complications: an intraoperative fracture was treated by open reduction and fixation with a plate. One patient had dislocation as a result of socket malposition, therefore only the socket's position was adjusted in a revision surgery as the stem had been properly implanted. We did not observe any infection, deep vein thrombosis or pulmonary embolism.

The alignment of the Proxima™ stem on the immediate post-operative radiograph was found to be in severe varus position on two occasions (Fig. 3); nine stems were implanted in varus, and 39 in neutral position. During the follow-up period, no signs of either clinical or radiological loosening were detected.

At the latest follow-up examinations, all respondents stated that they would undergo the operative procedure again. Ninety five percent of the patients were completely satisfied with the outcome of the surgery; the patient who had an intraoperative periprosthetic fracture and the other patient who had a dislocation were satisfied as well.

### 3.3. Discussion

The number of cases and the length of follow-up are not extensive enough to draw a final conclusion in comparison to traditional arthroplasty procedures. However, it is sufficient to conclude that this procedure greatly differs from standard femoral implantation; therefore a number of factors may be usefully discussed.

#### *3.3.1. Head-neck resection*

Attention should be paid to the level of the head-neck resection. A crucial bony surface for fixation of the stem is lost if the cutting plane is more oblique than optimal, i.e. if it is close to the traditional cutting plane. On the medial side the resection should always start at the head-neck junction and run more distally while proceeding laterally, thus creating a wider entrance for the stem (see paragraph 3. below). Ender et al have reported in conclusion of a five-year follow-up of 120 CUT® short-stem implantations, that out of the 11 revision cases, seven femoral necks had ben resected either too diagonally (traditionally) or too widely [Ender et al., 2007].

#### *3.3.2. Positioning*

Inadequate hit force during the "round the corner" broaching can result in a varus position of the stem. As no intramedullary guidance is available for the Proxima™ stem due to its metaphyseal location, a varus position is more likely to occur, especially when a minimally invasive approach is used, as visualization of the femoral axis is difficult. It is imperative to perform intraoperative axis measurements during sequential broaching. Until proper experience is acquired the use of fluoroscopy is advisable. Ghera and Pavan reported a study on

65 Proxima™ stem implantations, in which 44 stems were found to be in neutral position, 15 in varus and 6 in valgus [Ghera & Pavan, 2009]. Gilbert et al found that from 34 Mayo® short stems implanted, 14, 19, and 11 cases were neutrally aligned, in varus and in valgus position, respectively [Gilbert et al., 2009]. In our series 2 of 50 Proxima™ stems at the beginning of the learning curve were found to be in severe varus (Fig. 3), 9 in varus and 39 in a neutral position, which seems to be comparable with the previous reports.

### 3.3.3. *Stem sizing*

The "round the corner" broaching technique was developed to save bone stock in the lateral segment of the metaphysis. However, it can happen that the broach of the planned size would not fit into the resected part of the femoral neck (Fig. 4).

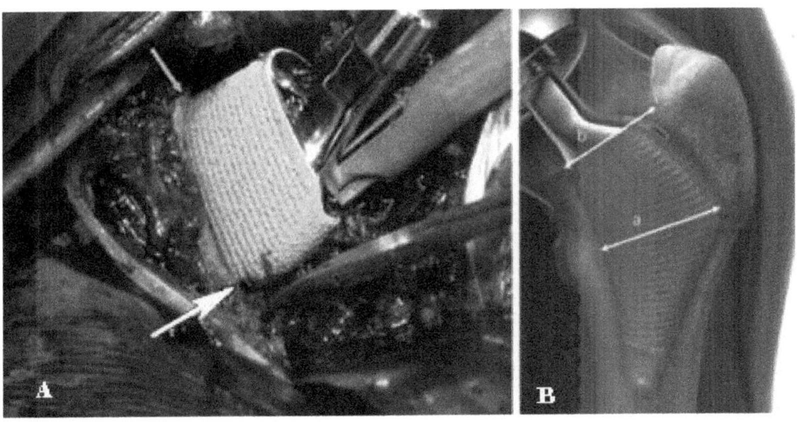


**Figure 4.** Fitting of the Proxima™ stem into the proximal femoral metaphysis. "Round the corner" technique is used to protect the soft tissues and bone stock, and take advantage of the lateral flare. (a) Intraoperative picture; the cortical bone of the neck is in contact all around with the largest diameter of the stem (arrows) (b) the measured width of the stem (a)is wider than the entrance (b).

In this situation, the following solutions are possible depending on the bone stock quality:

**a.** When the cancellous bone is weak, the neck in the lateral aspect of the resection plane should be gently enlarged until the stem of the desired size can be implanted. An undersized stem in a weak cancellous bone tends to tilt into varus, and may sink deeper than expected. The deep position of the stem then needs to be corrected by a longer neck, which raises the biomechanically disadvantageous torque force on the short stem (Fig 3).

**b.** When the cancellous bone is hard, implantation of a Proxima™ stem smaller than the calculated size of the metaphysis is acceptable. Even if the stem does not reach the lateral cortex, the strong and compact cancellous bone can hold the femoral component firmly (Fig. 5).

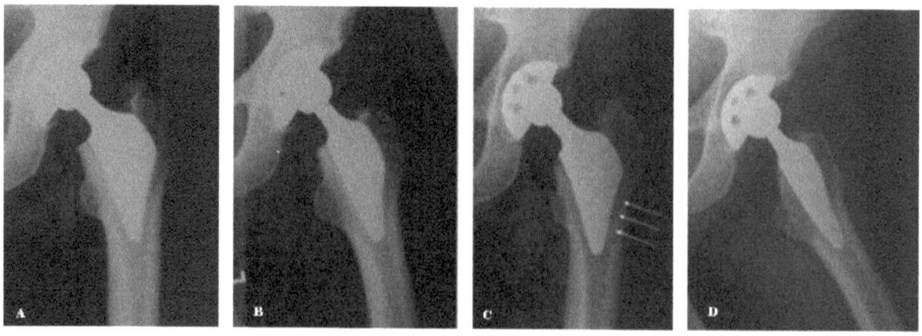


**Figure 5.** AP and lateral radiographs of a Proxima™ stem in a hard cancellous bone (a-b) immediately after operation (c-d) 24 months post op. The stem is fixed by strong and compact cancellous bone, without loosening.

### *3.3.4. Cortical index*

Calculation of the cortical index: Cortical index = (10 × (a-b))/a, where a is the outer diameter of the femur and b is the inner diameter of the medullary cavity 10 cm below the level of the lesser trochanter (Fig. 6).

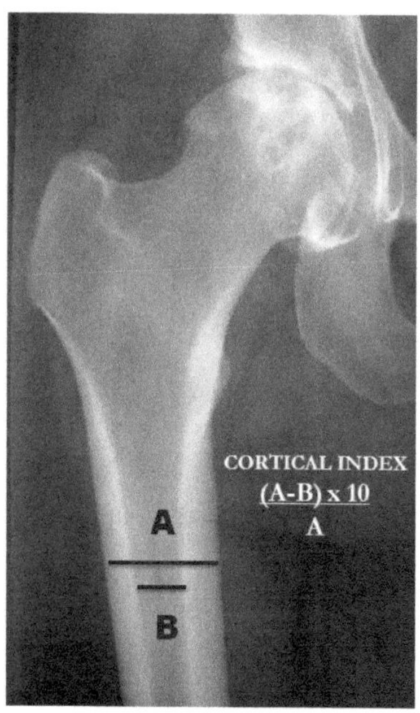


**Figure 6.** Calculation of the cortical index. Cortical index = (10 × (a-b))/a, where a is the outer diameter of the femur and b is the inner diameter of the medullary cavity 10 cm below the level of the lesser trochanter.

Short-stem hip implantation is contraindicated when cortical index scores are less than 3; in this situation a cemented stem is advisable. If the cortical index is between 3 and 4, an oversized Proxima™ stem would be suggested; if the cortical index exceeds 4, a normal sized Proxima™ stem could be used.

Among the 50 Proxima™ stem implantations, the only intraoperative complication was a spiral femoral shaft fracture. The stem sank deeper into the femoral shaft than the identical sized broach, causing an infraction, which resulted in a complete spiral shaft fracture during the repositioning maneuver. The cortical index of the affected hip was 3.75; the mean cortical index of the other cases was 6.07.

## 4. Conclusion

Bone-saving hip arthroplasty using metaphyseal stems is gaining importance because the increasing number of young patients, and hip resurfacing is not always indicated. In the last decade, the practice of hip arthroplasty has changed; younger age-group is more frequently undergo surgery because of the need for a better quality of life. The success of non-cemented total hip arthroplasty relies on osteo-integration of the implants. Prerequisite is primary stability, which can be achieved by the fixation principle of "press-fitting" [Morscher et al., 2002]. Clinical studies investigating the migrational behavior of femoral components have shown that the failure rate of uncemented stems correlates with migration [Krismer et al., 1999]. Sychterz found that in vivo bone loss was most extensive in the proximal-medial region [Sychterz et al., 2002]. Following traditional arthroplasty procedures, bone density measurement has shown a bone loss of 16 to 30% [Kim et al., 2003; Schmidt et al., 2002; Sychterz et al., 2002]. Engh's post mortem investigation has found 7 to 52% bone loss around non-cemented femoral components with osteo-integration [Engh et al., 1992]. DXA measurements by Kishida et al. proved that two years after resurfacing procedures 12% raise in bone density developed in the Gruen 7 zone [Kishida et al., 2004].

The previously mentioned facts, along with the experiences obtained from revision surgeries (technical difficulties caused by bone loss due to loosening) and the high cost of the solutions, have led to a change at the level of primary arthroplasty principles to a more preventive approach. As for the material of the prosthesis components, highly cross-linked polyethylene, metal-on-metal and ceramic sliding surfaces have advanced. According to component design, short-shaft stems came into prominence for those young and active patients for whom resurfacing of the hip is contraindicated (large avascular necrosis of the head, osteoporosis, obese patient etc.) The very proximal location of these stems retains the chance for an implantation of a non-revision stem during revision surgery. Short-stem prosthesis with a close anatomical fit to the proximal cortex aim to maximize primary stability, particularly in rotation. It is also proposed that the shorter shaft leads to more physiological loading of the femur, thereby limiting potential bone resorption due to stress shielding. Further advantages are the reduction of the risk of thigh pain and facilitating minimally invasive surgery, particularly when using an anterior approach [Renkawitz et al., 2008].

At our department both resurfacing and short-shaft stem are available for young and active patients. Short stem is implanted when indication criteria are sufficient. The advantages and disadvantages of short-stem arthroplasty are reported through the author's experiences with the metaphyseal stems [Tóth et al., 2010]. It provides vertical stability by the wedge shape of the stem together with the addition of a lateral flare and preservation of the femoral neck. The preservation of the femoral neck provides greater torsional stability and reduces distal migration of the femoral stem. The absence of any diaphyseal fixation attempts to achieve proximal load transfer so as to reduce stress shielding and thigh pain. It also attempts to preserve the femoral canal and femoral elasticity, and ease revision.

The number of cases and the length of follow-up time in the short stem literature are not extensive enough to draw a final conclusion in comparison to traditional arthroplasty procedures. However, it is sufficient enough to conclude that this procedure differs, therefore a number of factors may make sense to be discussed.

## Author details

Kálmán Tóth and Gellért Sohár

Department of Orthopaedics, University of Szeged, Faculty of Medicine, Szeged, Hungary

## References

[1] Dabirrahmani, D.; Hogg, M., Kohan, L., & Gillies, M. (2010). Primary and long-term stability of a short-stem hip implant. Proceedings of the Institution of Mechanical Engeneers, Part H, Vol.224, No.9, (n.d.), pp. 1109-1119

[2] Ender, S.A; Machner, A., Pap, G., Hubbe, J., Grashoff, H., & Neumann, H.W. (2007). Cementless CUT femoral neck prosthesis: increased rate of aseptic loosening after 5 years. Acta Orthopaedica, Vol.78, (October 2007), pp. 616-621 (doi: 10.1080/17453670710014301)

[3] Engh, C.A.; Bobyn, J.D., & Glassman, A.H. (1987). Porous-coated hip replacement. The factors governing bone ingrowth, stress shielding, and clinical results. The Journal of Bone and Joint Surgery, British Vol.69, (January 1987), pp. 45-55

[4] Engh, C.A.; McGovern, T.F., Bobyn, J.D., & Harris, W.H. (1992). A quantitative evaluation of periprosthetic bone-remodeling after cementless total hip arthroplasty. The Journal of Bone and Joint Surgery, American Vol.74, (August 1992), pp. 1009-1020

[5] Floerkemeier, T.; Tscheuschner, N., Calliess, T., Ezechieli, M., Floerkemeier, S., Budde, S., Windhagen, H., & von Lewinski, G. (2012). Cementless short stem hip arthroplasty METHA® as an encouraging option in adults with osteonecrosis of the

femoral head. Archives of Orthopedic Trauma Surgery, Vol.132, (August 2012), pp. 1125–1131 Epub 2012 May 1

[6] Ghera, S. & Pavan, L. (2009). The DePuy Proxima hip: a short stem for total hip arthroplasty. Early experience and technical considerations. Hip International: The Journal of the Clinical and Experimental Research on Hip Pathology and Therapy, Vol.19, No.3, (July-September 2009), pp. 215-220

[7] Gilbert, R.E.; Salehi-Bird, S., Gallacher, P.D., & Shaylor, P. (2009). The Mayo conservative hip: experience from a district general hospital. Hip International: The Journal of the Clinical and Experimental Research on Hip Pathology and Therapy, Vol.19, No.3, (July-September 2009), pp. 211-214

[8] Gill, I.R.; Gill, K., Jayasekera, N., & Miller, J. (2008). Medium term results of the collum femoris preserving hydroxyapatite coated total hip replacement. Hip International: The Journal of the Clinical and Experimental Research on Hip Pathology and Therapy, Vol.18, No.2, (April-June 2008), pp. 75-80

[9] Goebel, D. & Schulz, W. (2009). The Mayo cementless femoral component in active patients with osteoarthritis. Hip International: The Journal of the Clinical and Experimental Research on Hip Pathology and Therapy, Vol.19, No.3, (July-September 2009), pp. 206-210

[10] Harris, W.H. (1969). Traumatic arthritis of the hip after dislocation and acetabular fractures: treatment by mold arthroplasty. An end-result study using a new method of result evaluation. The Journal of Bone and Joint Surgery, American Vol.51, No.4, (June 1969), pp. 737-755

[11] Hube, R.; Zaage, M., Hein, W., & Reichel, H. (2004). Early functional results with the Mayo-hip, a short stem system with metaphyseal-intertrochanteric fixation. Orthopäde Vol.33, No.11, (November 2004), pp. 1249–1258

[12] Khanuja, H.S.; Vakil, J.J., Goddard, M.S., & Mont, M.A. (2011). Cementless Femoral Fixation in Total Hip Arthroplasty. The Journal of Bone and Joint Surgery, American Vol.93, No.5, (March 2011), pp. 500-509

[13] d'Imporzano, M. & Pierannunzii, L. (2006). Minimally invasive total hip replacement. Journal of Orthopaedic Traumatology, Vol.7, (2006), pp. 42–50

[14] Kim, Y.H.; Oh, S.H., & Kim, J.S. (2003). Primary total hip arthroplasty with a second-generation cementless total hip prosthesis in patients younger than fifty years of age. The Journal of Bone and Joint Surgery, American Vol.85, No.1, (January 2003), pp. 109-114

[15] Kim, Y.H.; Kim, J.S., Park, J.W., & Joo, J.H. (2011). Total hip replacement with a short metaphyseal-fitting anatomical cementless femoral component in patients aged 70 years or older The Journal of Bone and Joint Surgery, British Vol.93, No.5, (May 2011), pp. 587-592

[16] Kim, Y.H. & Oh J.H. (2012). A comparison of a conventional versus a short, anatomical metaphyseal-fitting cementless femoral stem in the treatment of patients with a fracture of the femoral neck The Journal of Bone and Joint Surgery, British Vol.93, No.6, (June 2012), pp. 774–81

[17] Kishida, Y.; Sugano, N., Nishii, T., Miki, H., Yamaguchi, K., & Yoshikawa, H. (2004). Preservation of the bone mineral density of the femur after surface replacement of the hip. The Journal of Bone and Joint Surgery, British Vol.86, No.2, (March 2004), pp. 185-189

[18] Krismer, M.; Biedermann, R., Stöckl, B., Fischer, M., Bauer, R., & Haid, C. (1999). The prediction of failure of the stem in THR by measurement of early migration using EBRA-FCA. Einzel-Bild-Roentgen-Analyse-femoral component analysis. The Journal of Bone and Joint Surgery, British Vol.81, No.2, (March 1999), pp. 273-280

[19] Leali, A.; Fetto, J., Insler, H., & Elfenbein, D. (2002). The effect of a lateral flare feature on implant stability. International Orthopaedics, Vol.26, No.3, (April 2002), pp. 166–169

[20] Mai, K.T.; Verioti, C.A., Casey, K., Slesarenko, Y., Romeo, L., & Colwell C.W. Jr. (2010). Cementless Femoral Fixation in Total Hip Arthroplasty. American Journal of Orthopedics, Vol.39, No.3, (March 2010), pp. 126-130

[21] Martell, J.M.; Pierson, R.H., Jacobs, J.J., Rosenberg, A.G., Maley, M., & Galante J.O. (1993). Primary total hip reconstruction with a titanium fiber-coated prosthesis inserted without cement The Journal of Bone and Joint Surgery, American Vol.75, No. 4, (April 1993), pp. 554-571

[22] McElroy, M.J.; Johnson, A.J., Mont, M.A., & Bonutti P.M. (2011). Short and Standard Stem Prostheses Are Both Viable Options for Minimally Invasive Total Hip Arthroplasty. Bulletin of the NYU Hospital for Joint Diseases, Vol.69(Suppl 1), (n.d.), pp. S68-76

[23] Molli, R.G.; Lombardi, A.V., Jr, Berend, K.R., Adams, J.B., & Sneller, M.A. (2012). A Short Tapered Stem Reduces Intraoperative Complications in Primary Total Hip Arthroplasty. Clinical Orthopedics and Related Research, Vol.470, No.2, (February 2012), pp. 450–461

[24] Morrey, B.F. (1989). Short-stemmed uncemented femoral component for primary hip arthroplasty. Clinical Orthopedics and Related Research, Vol.249, (December 1989), pp. 169-175

[25] Morrey, B.F.; Adams, R.A., & Kessler, M. (2000). A conservative femoral replacement for total hip arthroplasty. A prospective study . The Journal of Bone and Joint Surgery, British Vol.82, No.7, (December 2000), pp. 52-58

[26] Morscher, E.W.; Widmer, K.H., Bereiter, H., Elke, R., & Schenk, R. (2002). Cementless socket fixation based on the "press-fit" concept in total hip joint arthroplasty. Acta

Chirurgiae Orthopeadicae et Traumatologiae Cechoslovaca, Vol.69, No.1, (n.d.), pp. 8-15

[27] Pipino F. (2000). The bone-prosthesis interaction. Journal of Orthopaedics and Traumatology, Vol 1 No. 1, (December 2000), pp. 3–9

[28] Pons, M. (2010). Learning curve and short-term results with a short-stem CFP system. Hip International: The Journal of the Clinical and Experimental Research on Hip Pathology and Therapy, Vol.20, No. 2, Suppl.7, (May 2010), pp. 52-57

[29] Renkawitz, T., Santori, F.S., Grifka, J., Valverde, C., Morlock, M.M., & Learmonth, I.D. (2008). A new short uncemented, proximally fixed anatomic femoral implant with a prominent lateral flare: design rationals and study design of an international clinical trial. BMC Musculoskeletal Disorders, Vol.9, (November 2008), pp. 147-152

[30] Santori, F.S. & Santori, N. (2010). Mid-term results of a custom-made short proximal loading femoral component The Journal of Bone and Joint Surgery, British Vol.92, No.9, (September 2010), pp. 1231-1237

[31] Sariali, E.; Mouttet,A., Mordasini, P., & Catonné Y. (2012). High 10-Year Survival Rate with an Anatomic Cementless Stem (SPS) Clinical Orthopedics and Related Research, Vol.470, No.7, (July 2012), pp. 1941-1949 (Epub 2012 Mar 9.)

[32] Schmidt, R.; Muller, L., Kress, A. Hirschfelder, H., Aplas, A., & Pitto, R.P. (2002). A computed tomography assessment of femoral and acetabular bone changes after total hip arthroplasty. International Orthopedics, Vol.26, No. 5, (n.d.), pp. 299-302 (Epub 2002 Jun 28.)

[33] Steens, W.; Skripitz, R., Schneeberger, A.G., Petzing, I., Simon, U., & Goetze, C. (2010). [Cementless femoral neck prosthesis CUT--clinical and radiological results after 5 years]. Zeitschrift für Orthopädie und Unfallchirurgie, Vol.148, No.4, (August 2010), pp. 413-419 (Epub 2010 Aug 16.)

[34] Sychterz, C.J.; Claus, A.M., & Engh, C.A. (2002). What we have learned about long-term cementless fixation from autopsy retrievals. Clinical Orthopedics and Related Research, Vol.405, (December 2002), pp. 79–91

[35] Synder, M.; Drobniewski, M., Pruszczyński, B. & Sibiński, M.(2009). Initial experience with short Metha stem implantation. Ortopedia Traumatologia Rehabilitacja, Vol.11, No.4, (July-August 2009), pp. 317-323

[36] Tóth, K.; Mécs, L., & Kellermann, P. (2010). Early experience with the Depuy Proxima short stem in total hip arthroplasty. Acta Orthopedica Belgica, Vol.76, No.5, (October 2010), pp. 613-618

[37] Thomas, W.; Lucente, L., Mantegna, N., & Grundei, H. (2004). [ESKA (CUT) endoprosthesis.] (in German) Orthopäde, Vol.33, No.11, (November 2004), pp. 1243-1248

[38] Walker, P.S.; Culligan, S.G., Hua, G., Muirhead Allwood S.K., & Bentley G. (1999). The effect of lateral flare feature on uncemented hip stems. Hip International, Vol.9, (1999), pp. 71-80

[39] Westphal, F.M.; Bishop, N., Puschel, K., & Morlock, M.M. (2006a). Biomechanics of a new short stemmed uncemented hip prosthesis, an in-vitro study in human bone. Hip International: The Journal of the Clinical and Experimental Research on Hip Pathology and Therapy, Vol.16, Suppl.3, (n.d.), pp. 22-30

[40] Westphal, F.M.; Bishop, N., Honl, M., Hille, E., Püschel, K., & Morlock, M.M. (2006b). Migration and cyclic motion of a new short-stemmed hip prosthesis – a biomechanical in vitro study. Clinical Biomechanics (Bristil Avon), Vol.21, No.8, (2006), pp. 834–840 (Epub 2006 Jun 27.)

# Chapter 7

# All Ceramic Tripolar THA to Prevent Dislocations in Risky Patients

Jean-Yves Lazennec, Adrien Brusson and
Marc Antoine Rousseau

Additional information is available at the end of the chapter

## 1. Introduction

Dislocation remains one of the most common complications after total hip arthroplasty (THA), especially for ceramic-on-ceramic prostheses. Suboptimal implant positioning, muscular insufficiency, significant lower limb discrepancies, and neurological problems are standard causes for THA dislocations or subluxations [1-3]. Instability may also be linked to 2 specific mechanisms, lever-out (with impingement) and shear-out (without impingement).

Microseparation and edge loading of the femoral ball head on the insert are relevant issues for hard-on-hard bearing surfaces, either ceramic on ceramic or metal on metal [4-5]. Tripolar polyethylene (PE) THAs have been extensively used for more than 20 years in Europe [2, 6-7], and clinical data demonstrate that they provide significant improvement in hip stability. Significant concerns nonetheless remain about PE wear and osteolysis. Recent developments in ceramic matrix composites and the introduction of Biolox Delta® with improved fracture toughness have further reduced the risk of fracture and also extended the design flexibility of the material. A novel tripolar all-ceramic bearing for hip prostheses (Ceram-Concept, Newark, DE, USA) has been designed and developed to deal with the problems described above. The tripolar delta ceramic (TDC) THA combines the functional advantages of the tripolar PE THA with the tribological advantages of ceramic bearings.

## 2. The concept

The orientation of the cup in terms of anteversion and inclination has significant consequences on the joint's range of motion and resistance to dislocation [8]. The position of the rotation center in the cup-ball head system affects joint stability: it has been shown that an inset of the rotation center of a few millimeters increases the peak resisting moment against dislocation [9][10]. This benefit in terms of stability has a disadvantage, however: it decreases the range of motion of classical ball-insert systems. The TDC joint allows the center of rotation to be located much deeper inside the insert without significant negative impact on the range of motion [10] [11].

The first all-ceramic tripolar joint was a 22/32 combination including a 22-mm head, a 22/32-mm mobile ceramic head secured with a PE ring, and a 32-mm internal diameter ceramic acetabular insert. Another possibility is a 26/36 combination, including a 26-mm head, a 26/36-mm mobile ceramic head (or "intermediate component" or "bipolar head"), and a 36-mm ceramic acetabular insert. All components were manufactured from Biolox Delta ceramic matrix composite, Ceramtec, Germany.

Tripolar hip prostheses have two bearing surfaces: the outer bearing surface, between the acetabular cup and the intermediate component (bipolar head), and the inner bearing surface, between the intermediate component and the femoral head component (Figures 1-2). The outer surface of the intermediate component is a portion of a solid sphere, the center of which is identical to the center of the acetabular insert during joint loading. The center of the inner bearing surface of the intermediate component (bipolar cup) corresponds to the center of the femoral head and is designed to be inset from the center of the outer bearing surface of the intermediate component (i.e., the center of the acetabular component).

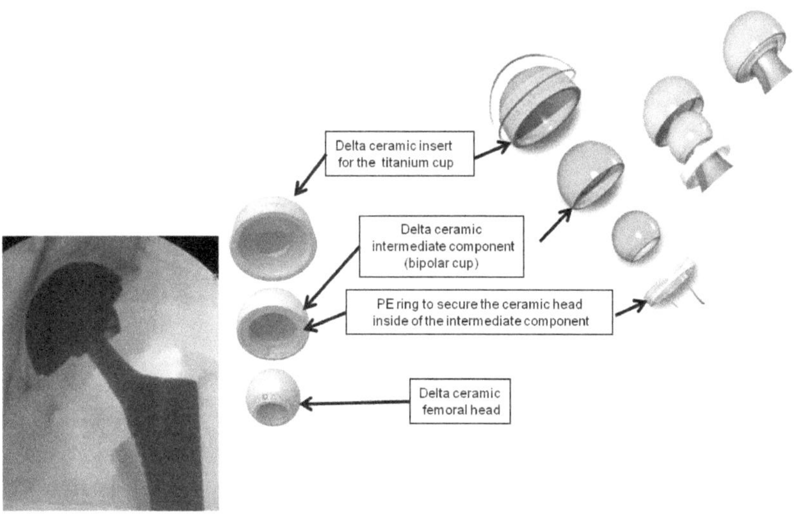


**Figure 1.** Tripolar hip prostheses have two bearing surfaces: the outer bearing surface, between the acetabular cup and the intermediate component (bipolar head), and the inner bearing surface, between the intermediate component and the femoral head component

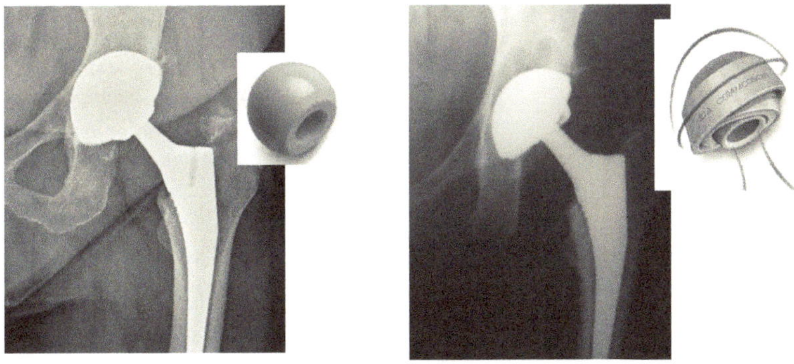

« classical » ceramic on ceramic THA
( 32 mm head diameter )

« tripolar » ceramic on ceramic THA
( « intermediate » cup 32 mm ;
22,2 mm femoral head diameter )

**Figure 2.** Comparison between a conventional ceramic –ceramic prosthesis and a tripolar delta ceramic prosthesis : Implantation procedures for metal-back or acetabular insert placements or for femoral adjustment are the same. The only originality of the tripolar system is the interposition of a "double femoral ball head" or " bipolar head" on the femoral taper.

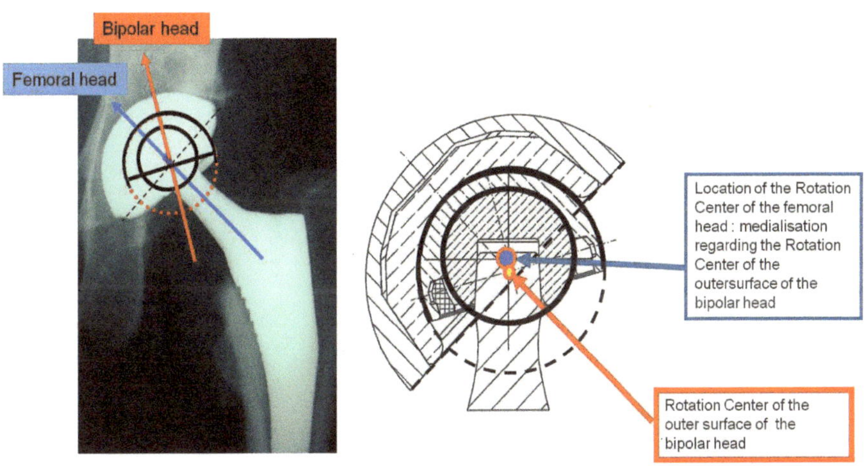


**Figure 3.** The outer surface of the intermediate component (bipolar head) is a portion of a solid sphere, the center of which is identical to the center of the acetabular insert during joint loading. The center of the inner bearing surface of the intermediate component corresponds to the center of the femoral head and is designed to be inset from the center of the outer bearing surface of the intermediate component (i.e., the center of the acetabular component).

This geometric arrangement thus creates a certain amount of eccentricity between the acetabular component and the femoral head component (Figure 3). If the centers of rotation of the femoral head and of the outer surface of the bipolar head are not aligned when TDC joint loading begins, the intermediate component starts to align itself: the bipolar head (i.e., the intermediate component) can, through the two bearing ceramic delta surfaces, act as a self-adjusting cup and deal with the variations of femoral head and acetabular orientation (Figure 4).

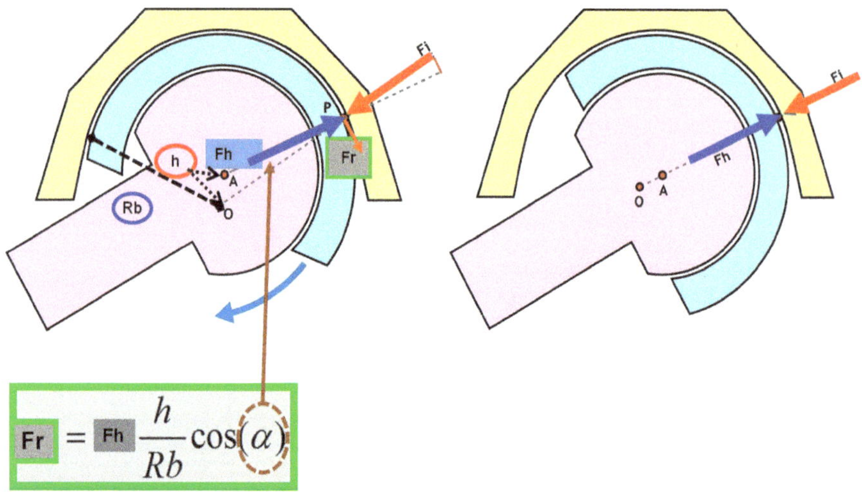


**Figure 4.** Mechanism of adaptation of the bipolar head in the TCD joint : the non alignment of the rotation centers for the femoral head (A) and the bipolar head (O) induces a self adaptation of the bipolar head. Fh is the contact force which acts on the head at point P. This force is applied on the femoral head through the femoral neck. If friction is neglected, it is necessarily aligned with its centre A. Fi is the reaction force of the acetabular insert upon the bipolar head. If friction is neglected, it is necessarily aligned with its centre O.If Fr and Fi are not mutually in equilibrium, they create a resulting force Fr. The resultant force Fr inducing the adjustment of the bipolar head can be calculated ( h is the value of the medialisation of the femoral head center ( O A distance ) ; Rb is the radius of the bipolar head ; alpha is the angle between Fh et Fi ).

## 3. Preclinical studies

### 3.1. Evaluation of the mechanical performance of the femoral head and the bipolar head

The mechanical reliability of this device was evaluated by a qualification program according to the criteria defined by CERAMTEC and the standards for marketing authorization. Standard qualification programs were performed on the 22.2-mm ball head and the standard XLW 32/41-mm cup insert. A new program, based on a ball head qualification program, was set up for the bipolar head (intermediate component). Specifications of the bipolar component (diameter, roundness, clearance, etc.) are identical to those for the 32-mm ceramic ball head (Figure 5).

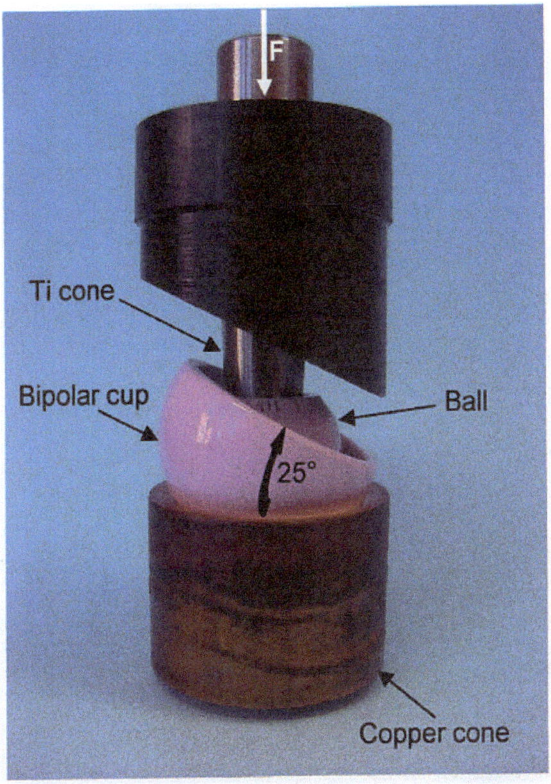


**Figure 5.** Experimental protocol for burst tests on tripolar delta ceramic ( TDC ) implants.

The bipolar component has particularly high resistance to fracture, as shown in Table 1 [9].

| Static Test (kN) | Avarage value | Minimal value |
|---|---|---|
| Avarage value required 46 kN<br>Minimal value required 25 kN | 129 | 58 |
| **Post fatigue Test** | **Average value** | **Minimal value** |
| Avarage value required 46 kN<br>Minimal value required 20 kN | 91 | 82 |

**Table 1.** Evaluation of the intermediate component: static and post-fatigue tests

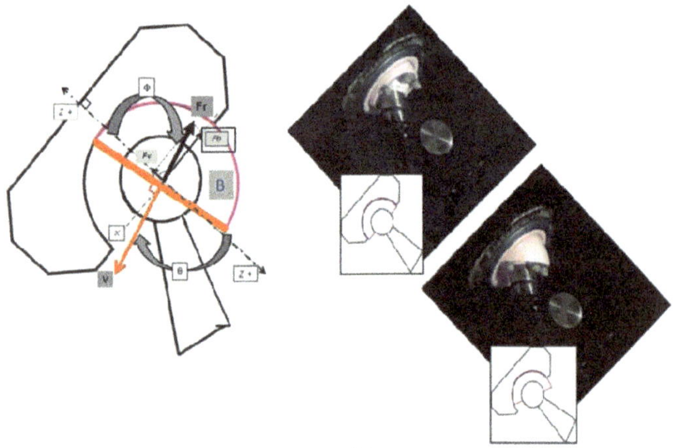


(a)

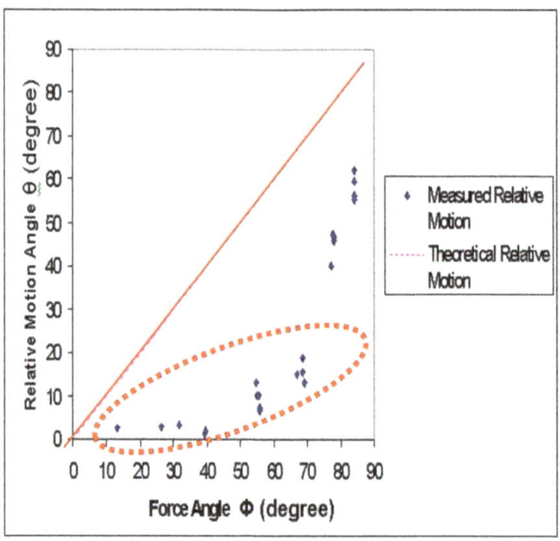


(b)

**Figure 6.** a) *In-vitro* investigation of the relative motion of the intermediate component for shear-out situations. In shear-out situation, dislocation is supposed to occur without impingement between the acetabular cup and the femoral component. When the direction of the total joint contact force (Fr) goes beyond the edge of the acetabular cup, dislocation occurs. The implementation of an experiment with the tripolar system is more complex than with a classical THA. A series of tests was conducted to record the position of the intermediate component with a motion analysis system. The resultant force on the intermediate component is defined as $F_r$. The vertical force applied to the intermediate component is defined as $F_v$; the horizontal force is defined as $F_h$. The center of the inner bearing surface of the intermediate component (i.e., the center of the femoral head component) is designed to be inset from the outer bearing surface of the intermediate component (i.e., the center of the acetabular component), thus creating a certain amount of eccentricity between the acetabular component and the femoral head component. Theoretically, when the loading on the joint arc surface is not in line with the centers of the arc, self-alignment of the intermediate component will be initiated. Shear-out situation was simulated by applying different magnitudes of $F_h$ while keeping $F_v$ at a fixed value. For a given $F_v$, as the magnitude of $F_h$ increased, the direction of the resultant force $F_r$ moved toward the edge of the acetabular cup and eventually beyond the edge chamfer. The angle between the direction of Fr and the negative z-axis is defined as Φ; the angle between the direction of the normal vector (V) of the bipolar component (B) and the positive Z-axis is defined as θ. The angle Φ between the resultant force Fr and the negative z-axis was calculated experimentally from the force data recorded by load cells. Reflective markers were rigidly glued to the rim of the intermediate component representing the plane of the bipolar head whose orientation was to be measured. Positional data of the markers implanted on the bipolar component were recorded by motion analysis cameras. Since $F_h$ and $F_v$ were applied in x-z plane, the motion angle between the normal vector of the measured plane and the positive z-axis (θ) was plotted against the resultant force angle (Φ). (b) The dash line 1 represents the θ vs. Φ curve in an idealized theoretical situation (suction force ignored, frictionless). In the ideal situation the normal vector of the intermediate component at any time should seek alignment with the direction of the joint contact force. Dots represent the measured θ vs. Φ curve. Qualitatively, θ increases with the increase of Φ. The rotation of the intermediate component in x-z plane is correlated with the direction of the resultant contact force. At Φ below 40 ° (when the direction of the load was not much deviated from the aligned center-shaft), there was a "toe" area which meant the intermediate component remained in its original horizontal position and did not react to the change of direction of the resultant force $F_r$.This was due to the effects of surface adhesion and friction : the rotation moment formed by the offset contact forces must first overcome the resistance of suction and friction before it can effectively rotate the intermediate component. As Φ went beyond the toe region, the slope of the experimental curve gradually increased ; the slope of the curve is not exactly superimposable to that of curve 1 because of the suction force and friction.

### 3.2. Biomechanical tests

- Two typical scenarios (lever-out and shear-out) that can lead to dislocations were investigated. The studies provided evidence that the relative motion of the intermediate component is closely related to the eccentricity between this component and the femoral head [11-12].

We compared the adaptation in impingement situations with lever-out loading between a standard ceramic joint (32-mm ball head/ceramic insert) and the TDC, with a 32-mm self-adjusting cup.

- The variable for assessing dislocation stability was torque during subluxation (resisting moment) against levering the head out of the cup [13]. With the standard system (ceramic ball and socket), dislocation appears as soon as there is contact between the femoral neck and the acetabular insert because of the moment applied. This dislocation by impingement is directly related to range of motion.

The mechanism with the TDC system is different, as are the steps involved. First, the ball head alone rotates. In a second stage, contract forces cause rotation of the bipolar head. Finally, the ball head and the bipolar head rotate together [14]. The moment that must be applied to the joint to obtain luxation is higher than for the conventional system: the increase of this peak resisting moment has been measured at 18.71%

Shear-out loading has also been investigated: the direction of the normal vector (V) of the intermediate component (bipolar head) expresses its relative motion. Adaptation was explored by evaluating the orientation of V in various directions and at various magnitudes of the force to the TDC joint. The orientation of the resultant force (Fr) on the bipolar head is expressed by the angle Φ (Figure 6). Until that angle reaches 40°, the intermediate component remains in its original position, not reacting to the change of direction of this Fr force.

At that point, the intermediate piece adapts and the curve expressing the orientation of vector V changes abruptly.

### 3.3. Tribological tests

- Simulator studies were carried out under ISO standard conditions, but also under microseparation conditions that replicated head/cup rim contact at heel strike.
- Microseparation is most appropriate for the evaluation of ceramic bearings, as the experimental conditions are optimal for reproducing clinical wear rates and wear mechanisms, including stripe wear, as found on standard ceramic-on-ceramic retrievals. The aim of the tribological tests was to assess the wear characteristics under standard and swing phase microseparation between 200 and 500 µm for a total of 5 million cycles with the Leeds II Physiological Anatomical hip joint simulator [15].
- Under standard conditions, wear was very low on both the tripolar and the conventional ceramic-on-ceramic bearings. The wear of the tripolar all-ceramic hip was less than 0.01 $mm^3$/million cycles, which is the detection limit for wear measurement, and the conventional ceramic-on-ceramic bearing produced a wear rate of 0.04 $mm^3$/million cycles. The difference between these very low wear rates is not clinically significant.
- Under microseparation conditions, wear performance differed significantly. In a previous study, conventional Biolox Delta components were tested under microseparation conditions in the same simulator with reported wear rates of 0.32 $mm^3$/million cycles during bedding-in (0-1 million cycles) that then fell to a steady state wear rate of 0.12 $mm^3$/million cycles (1-5 million cycles) [8, 12]. Furthermore, stripe wear appeared on the standard Biolox Delta heads and increased the surface roughness Ra from <0.005 µm to between 0.02 µm and 0.13 µm.
- Testing of the TDC joint showed no macroscopic visual evidence of wear. Wear was less than 0.01 $mm^3$/million cycles (i.e., below the detection limit for wear measurement). No stripe wear was observed; the surface roughness of the ball heads and the outer and inner surfaces of the bipolar head were smoother at the end of the test, indicating that they had undergone a polishing effect.
- The design of the TDC joint with its mobile ceramic head prevented edge loading of the head on the edge of the cup, so significantly reduced wear under these severe, but clinically relevant microseparation conditions [15].

Dislocation tests have been performed to evaluate the resistance of the PE ring in securing the ball head inside the intermediate component. Results were similar to those for similar PE rings that have been used for more than 18 years in standard double-mobility hip joints. The average maximum load for clipping the PE ring was 151.1 N before the tests; it rose to 175.5 N after 5 million cycles of microseparation. The increase in clipping resistance is due to the water load of the ring that occurs in the course of 5 million cycles. The wear volume of the PE rings could not be accurately quantified as it was within the systematic error of the soak control ring. The back side of the PE rings showed no damage, with only a light polishing effect observed in places [9].

## 4. Clinical data

Clinical results come from the first 2000 consecutive cases in a multicenter study. No specific learning curve was necessary: the surgeons did not change their implantation procedures for metal-back or acetabular insert placements or for femoral adjustment. The only originality of the system is the interposition of a "double femoral ball head" on the femoral taper. Positioning the femoral head on the taper is simple, as the intermediate cup is easily secured in a second step with the PE ring (Figure 7,8,9) [10].

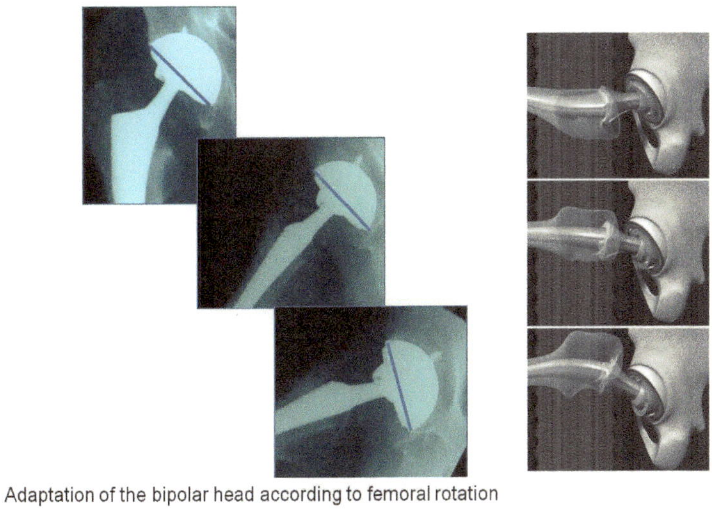


**Figure 7.** Adapted of the bipolar head according to femoral rotation

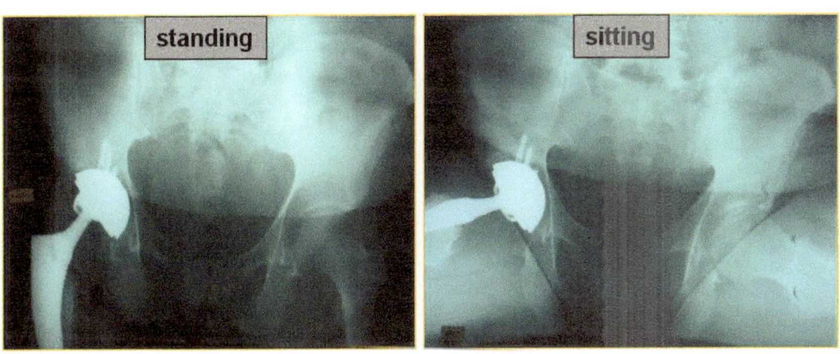


**Figure 8.** Adaptation of the bipolar head according to standing and sitting position

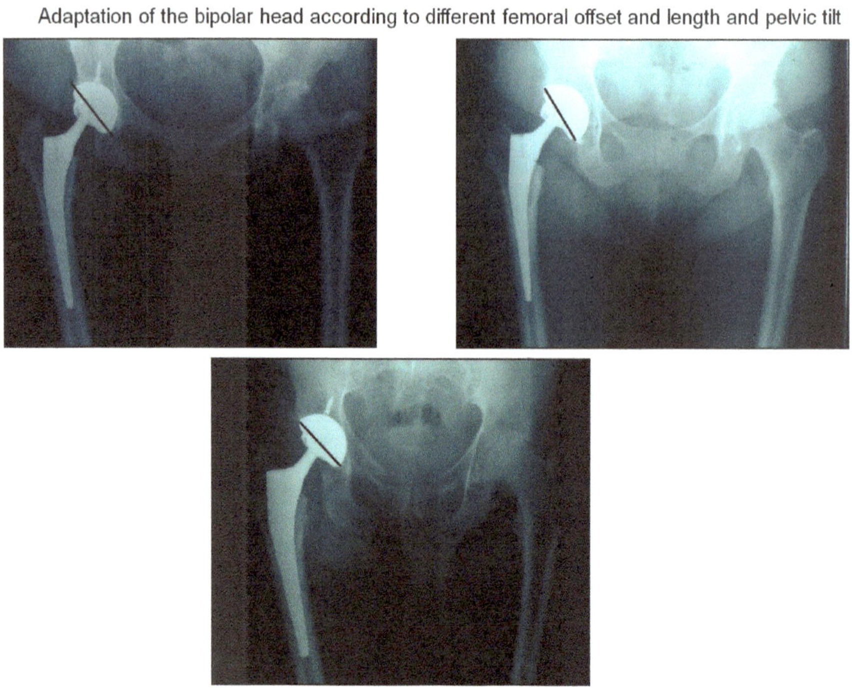


**Figure 9.** Adaptation of the bipolar head according to different femoral offset and length and pelvic tilt

In our experience, indications for this device are risk of instability, stiff coxarthrosis, osteonecrosis, revisions, oblique pelvis or significant rotational problems, neurological disorders, and some patient problems (alcoholism and psychiatric disorders). The Harris hip score indicates that clinical changes are similar to those with standard THA. The dislocation rate was 0.6%, despite a posterior approach in 87% of the cases. The main explanations were inadequate reconstitution of femoral neck length and/or offset. In a few cases (1.2%), patients described some occasional and irreproducible loud noise from the hip area, similar to that described for standard PE double-mobility systems. Experience with the double mobility PE joints has related this noise to sudden relocation of the intermediate component. The phenomenon is completely different from squeaking in terms of sound characteristics and mechanical aspects. A specific radiologic protocol allowed us to use the EOS® low dose imaging system to observe the adaptation of the intermediate component in standing and sitting positions. The mobility of the intermediate component is consistent with earlier studies and with experimental data. In some patients with significant lower-limb anatomic abnormalities, the tripolar system has been a successfully used as a salvage procedure to resolve cases with complex instability (Figure 10).

| | | Bipolar cup | Acetabular cup |
|---|---|---|---|
| standing | Frontal inclination | 18° | 32° |
| | anteversion | - 46° | 45° |
| sitting | Frontal inclination | 41° | 36° |
| | anteversion | 43° | 42° |

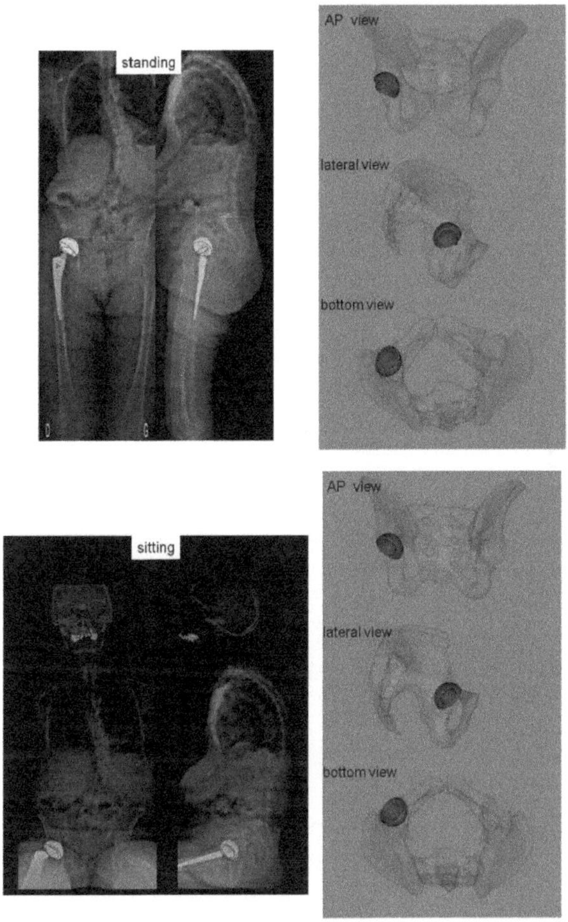


**Figure 10.** EOS imaging in standing and sitting position. In this case, the scoliosis including a significant pelvic rotation induces a specific adaptation of the intermediate component (bipolar head). One can observe the adaptation of the bipolar head with retroversion in standing position to compensate the hyperanteversion of the femoral neck. The orientation of the bipolar head is significantly different from the acetabular cup anteversion. In sitting position, the adjustment is different and the 2 cups anteversions are equivalent.

## 5. Conclusions

The use of the tripolar all-delta-ceramic joint appears to be an interesting alternative for optimizing THA function where, as in some cases, no ideal solution can be found for acetabular implantation. The self-adaptation of the intermediate cup can be demonstrated: the additional outer-bearing surface motion creates a second adjustable acetabulum. Its effectiveness against dislocation and microseparation can be explained and documented experimentally. The tripolar ceramic joint provides significant resistance to wear and stripe wear. Nevertheless, it cannot compensate for suboptimal THA implantation resulting in excessive shear-out laxity due to shortening of the head-neck length or lack of femoral offset [3, 16].

## Author details

Jean-Yves Lazennec[1], Adrien Brusson[2] and Marc Antoine Rousseau[1]

1 Department of orthopedic and trauma surgery, La Pitié-Salpétrière hospital. Paris, France

2 Department of Anatomy, université Pierre et Marie Curie, Paris, France

## References

[1] Jolles, B.M., P. Zangger, and P.F. Leyvraz, Factors predisposing to dislocation after primary total hip arthroplasty: a multivariate analysis. J Arthroplasty, 2002. 17(3): p. 282-8.

[2] Lautridou, C., et al., [Survival of the cementless Bousquet dual mobility cup: Minimum 15-year follow-up of 437 total hip arthroplasties]. Rev Chir Orthop Reparatrice Appar Mot, 2008. 94(8): p. 731-9.

[3] von Knoch, M., et al., Late dislocation after total hip arthroplasty. J Bone Joint Surg Am, 2002. 84-A(11): p. 1949-53.

[4] Ishida, T., et al., Detailed wear mapping of retrieved second-generation metal on metal THR. Annual Meeting of the Orthopaedic Research Society, 2006. Poster No: 1656.

[5] Stewart, T.D., et al., Long-term wear of ceramic matrix composite materials for hip prostheses under severe swing phase microseparation. J Biomed Mater Res B Appl Biomater, 2003. 66(2): p. 567-73.

[6] Grigoris, P., M.J. Grecula, and H.C. Amstutz, Tripolar hip replacement for recurrent prosthetic dislocation. Clin Orthop Relat Res, 1994(304): p. 148-55.

[7] Leclercq, S., S. el Blidi, and J.H. Aubriot, [Bousquet's device in the treatment of recurrent dislocation of a total hip prosthesis. Apropos of 13 cases]. Rev Chir Orthop Reparatrice Appar Mot, 1995. 81(5): p. 389-94.

[8] Lazennec, J.Y., A. Brusson, and M.A. Rousseau, Hip-spine relations and sagittal balance clinical consequences. Eur Spine J, 2011. 20 Suppl 5: p. 686-98.

[9] Lazennec, J.Y., et al., Two ceramic bearing surfaces with a self adjusting cup: a new application of delta ceramics to reduce the risk of dislocation and subluxation bioceramics and alternative bearings. Bioceramics and alternative bearings in joint arthroplasty, 2005. 10th Biolox Symposium

[10] Lazennec, J.Y., et al., All ceramic tripolar Total Hip Arthroplasty: experimental data and clinical results, in Bioceramics and alternative bearings in joint arthroplasty, F. Benazzo, F. Falez, and M. Dietrich, Editors. 2006, Steinkopff. p. 5-9.

[11] Chen Q, et al., Motion of the intermediate component of an eccentric tripolar T.H.P. Annual Meeting of the Orthopaedic Research Society poster 498, 2005. Poster 1181

[12] Krein, S.W. and E.Y. Chao, Biomechanics of bipolar hip endoprostheses. J Orthop Res, 1984. 2(4): p. 356-68.

[13] Bader R, et al., iomechanical study of resistance to dislocation of the ceramic-ceramic delta tripolar joint. Biomaterialen, 2004.

[14] Chen, Q., et al., Technical note: validation of a motion analysis system for measuring the relative motion of the intermediate component of a tripolar total hip arthroplasty prosthesis. Med Eng Phys, 2005. 27(6): p. 505-12.

[15] Jennings, L.M., et al., Wear and friction characteristics of the tripolat all ceramic hip prosthesis. Annual Meeting of the Orthopaedic Research Society poster 498, 2006.

[16] Toni A., S.A., Ceramic on ceramic: long term clinical experience ed. B.i.j. arthroplasty. 2001: Thieme

Chapter 8

# "Neck-Sparing" Total Hip Arthroplasty

Lee E. Rubin, Scott A. Ritterman and
Timothy McTighe

Additional information is available at the end of the chapter

## 1. Introduction

Advanced arthritis of the hip joint can lead to profound changes in quality of life. Debilitating pain, stiffness, and altered gait biomechanics all affect the ability to stay mobile and maintain gainful employment; these concerns are magnified in younger patients with hip disease. While symptomatic hip arthritis typically affects older patients, there is a growing subset of active patients in their 30s, 40s, and 50s who are affected and were previously thought of as, "too young for a hip replacement." Over the last several decades, advances in hip replacement surgery are allowing us to rethink that position.

A total hip replacement is one of the most reliably successful procedures in orthopaedics. Long term data has shown that with a well positioned modern prosthesis we can give our patients reliable pain relief that has a very high chance (>80% in most cases) of lasting over twenty years[ 1, 2]. While this may be very comforting to a 75 year old retired patient with relatively low functional demands, twenty year survival will not suffice for patient in their 30s with advanced arthritis. For this reason in the past, many surgeons were reluctant to perform joint replacement surgeries in young patients for fear of condemning them to multiple revisions over a lifetime of use.

Recent literature on the revision-free survival rates for modern hip implants have shown remarkable success, with 10-year survival rates of 100% for a variety of press-fit, uncemented femoral stem designs at a mean time of 8.2 years from surgery.[ 3] A 2012 award-winning study from the American Association of Hip and Knee Surgeons showed 100% survival for cross-linked polyethylene bearing surfaces at 10 year follow-up[ 4]. Another recent paper, looking at the 10-year analysis of various bearing couples, showed respective survival rates of 98.4%, 95.6%, and 87.9% for metal-on-polyethylene, ceramic-on-ceramic, and metal-on-metal groups.

[ 5] The outstanding results of modern implants and bearing surfaces have given surgeons new confidence when facing the challenging of hip arthroplasty in a young, active patient.

The ideal hip replacement prosthesis for a young patient has several important elements. It would be easily integrated, forming a long lasting bond with the host bone, yet be easily removed if needed. Another aspect of the modern hip prosthesis that has evolved is the actual design of the femoral implant itself. Several implant designs on the market are 'bone sparing,' meaning that less bone is taken off of the head/neck of the femur. Over the past decade, hip resurfacing was a popular procedure in this regard. In a resurfacing procedure, the femoral neck and much of the head are left in place. A metal cap is placed on the end of the femoral head and a metal cup is placed in the acetabulum. Resurfacing procedures have fallen out of favor recently for several reasons, including the difficulty of placing the prosthesis as well as concerns with metal-on-metal articulations.

## 2. Neck sparing arthroplasty

A "neck-sparing" or "bone-sparing" prosthesis is not a new concept but is one that has been gaining in popularity. This prosthesis is similar in design to other modern prosthesis but preserves more native bone in the femoral neck of the patient during femoral preparation. With a similar idea to the resurfacing, the hope is to allow placement of an implant while leaving a viable option for revision at a later date. These prostheses are proximally porous coated; after the femoral bone cut is made, more femoral neck bone is left in situ, and the proximally coated implant loads and helps maintain this "extra" bone over time. Any modern bearing surface can be utilized by the surgeon. This novel design saves a significant portion of native host bone and will lead to theoretically easier revision surgery when the time comes. A small saw can be slipped around the neck of the prosthesis and the "extra" bone is removed, allowing revision to a primary hip implant rather than the traditional, extensive revision implants currently in use today.

The level of the femoral bone resection varies based on the arthroplasty technique. (Figure 1) A native right proximal hip is visible in Figure 1.1. In hip resurfacing (1.2 A) and "mid-head" resurfacing (1.2 B) (available in Europe), most of the femoral bone is retained. With neck sparing arthroplasty (1.2 C) and conventional total hip arthroplasty (1.2 D), progressively more bone is resected during the operation. With hip revision surgery, native bone is often eroded, leading to an even lower bony resection level (1.2 E). "Neck-sparing" implants allow the surgeon to retain the native bone between cut levels C and D (Figure 1.3), with the concept of native neck bone stock preservation for future revision surgery in the young patient.

The idea of neck retention is not a new concept. Freeman, Townley, Whiteside and Pipino have all advocated saving the femoral neck since the 1980s. Freeman is credited with his classic article "Why Resect The Neck?" as the Godfather of neck retention[ 6]. His stem retained the femoral neck but was a conventional length straight stem that engaged both the metaphysis and diaphysis. The original stem was designed for cement fixation, with subsequent modifi-

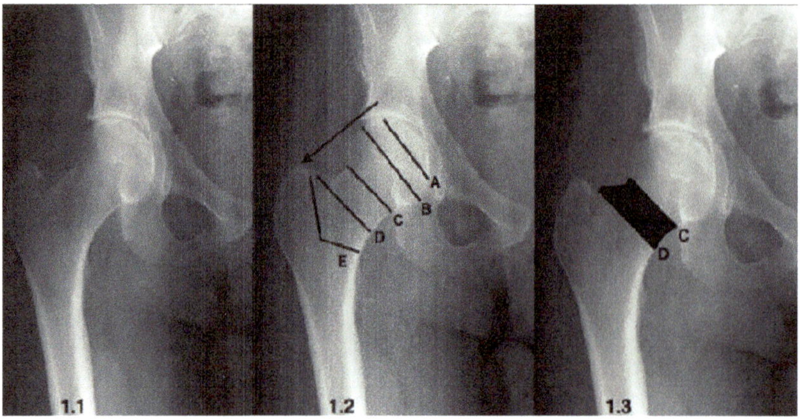


**Figure 1.** 1.1) Native right proximal hip. 1.2) Bone resection levels for hip resurfacing (A), mid-head resurfacing (B), neck-sparing arthroplasty (C), conventional total hip arthroplasty (D), and revision hip arthroplasty (E). 1.3) Illustration of native bone preserved during neck sparing arthroplasty compared to conventional total hip arthroplasty.

cation to introduce a cementless style stem that was of the same stem length and geometric shape with HA coating, as seen in Figure 2.

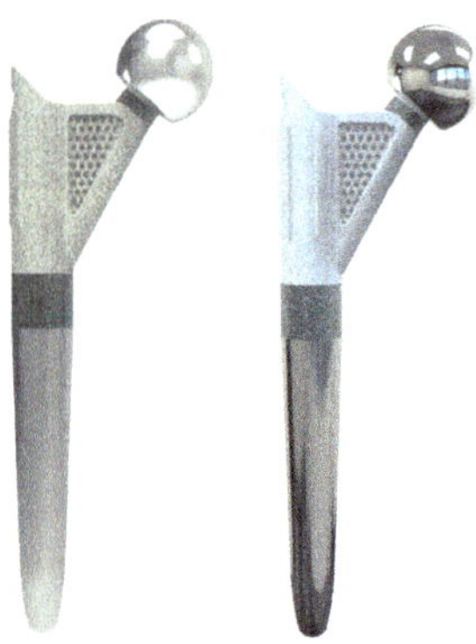

**Figure 2.** Freeman Femoral Stems. Left: Cemented Right: Cementless

Townley and Whiteside also designed conventional length straight stems that retained the femoral neck, but it was Professor Pipino who first advocated the short curved neck sparing stem to be stabilized by fit and fill of the femoral neck as a cementless press fit stem in 1979. He is also credited with term "tissue-sparing," referring to both saving hard and soft tissue as a surgical strategy. His Biodynamic hip prosthesis was implanted from 1983 to 1996 (Figure 3 Left), until it was replaced by the modified CFP hip stem (Figure 3 Right) Pipino reported outstanding results of his stem design, with 97% satisfactory radiographic results and an implant survival rate of almost 100% at 25 years.[ 7]

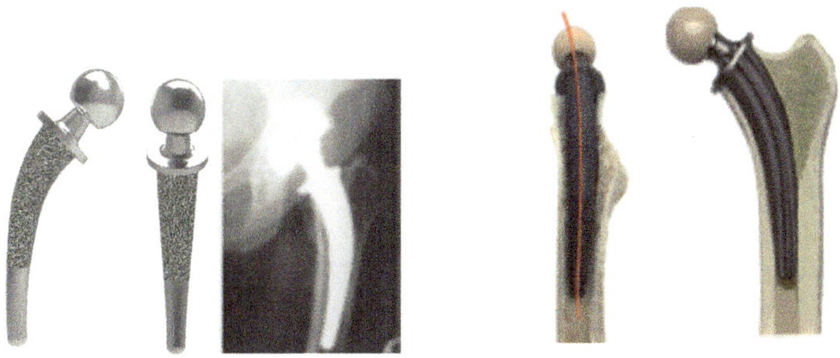

**Figure 3.** Left: Biodynamic c.c. stem by Howmedica, Right: CFP Stem by Link.

The CFP prosthesis stem is made of titanium alloy, a material better suited for cementless fixation than cobalt-chromium alloy. The left and right stem versions with built-in anatomical anteversion were adapted to the normal anatomy of the proximal femur. The left and right stems were available in six stem sizes along with two stem curvatures; the stem featured bilateral longitudinal ribs to increase surface contact and oppose torsional forces.

To promote osseointegration, the CFP stem has a 70 μm microporous surface with the exception of the short distal portion. In addition, the microporous surface is provided with a special 20 μm hydroxyapatite (calcium phosphate) coating which does not seal the surface but keeps the porous structure intact.

## 3. Biomechanics of neck sparing stem designs

The natural trabecular pattern of the bone and the trabecular orientation provide support against the natural functional loading, thus creating the necessary functional stability of the individual bone areas within the proximal femur. (Figure 4) The femoral neck and the adjoining medial aspect of the femur in the calcar region show the strongest bone structure with a high load capacity to support the stem. (Figure 5)

Femoral neck retention reduces both torsional and bending moments (forces) at the stem / bone interface. In accordance with Wolff's Law, the reduction of stresses relative to the natural situation would cause bone to adapt itself by reducing its mass, either by becoming more porous (internal remodeling) or by getting thinner (external remodeling).

In Figure 6, The neck on the left has been resected at the conventional level; in the one on the right the neck has been retained. Because the difference in the height of resection the length of the moment arms, the varus- turning moment increases by a factor of four when the neck is

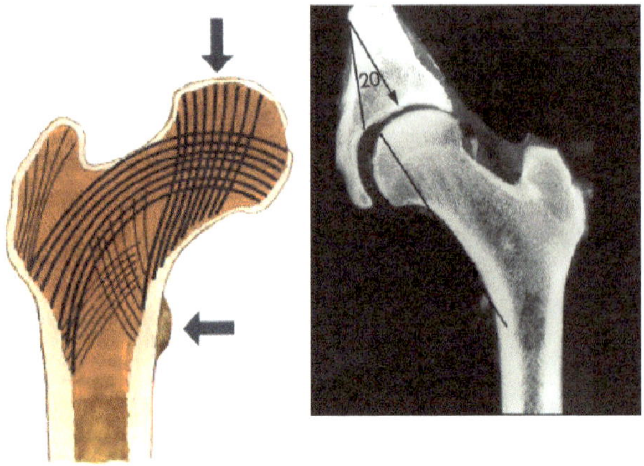


**Figure 4.** Trabecular bone patterns

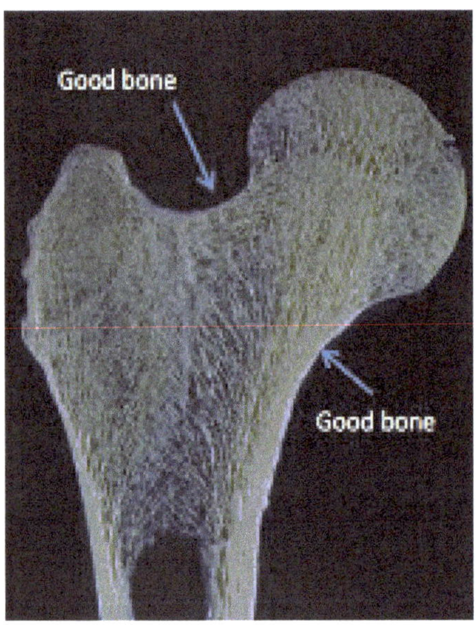


**Figure 5.** Cross section of the proximal femur

resected (Figure 7). At the same time the area of bone available for supporting the vertical component of the resultant of the forces acting on the implant is almost tripled

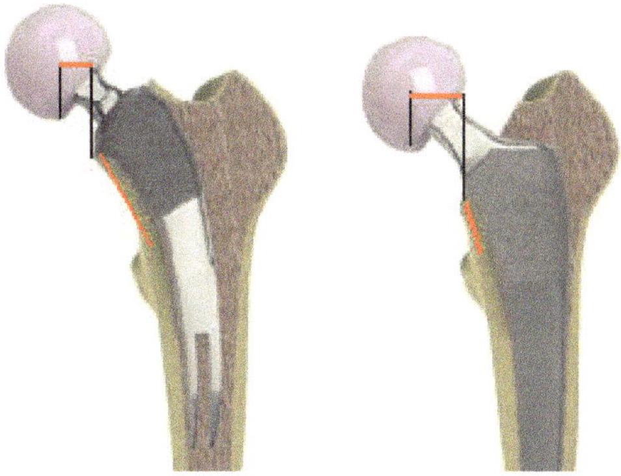

**Figure 6.** Illustrations comparing neck retention to conventional neck resection bending moment.

The anterior-posterior directed component of the resultant force is represented by an arrow. Neck resection generates a significant torsional moment.

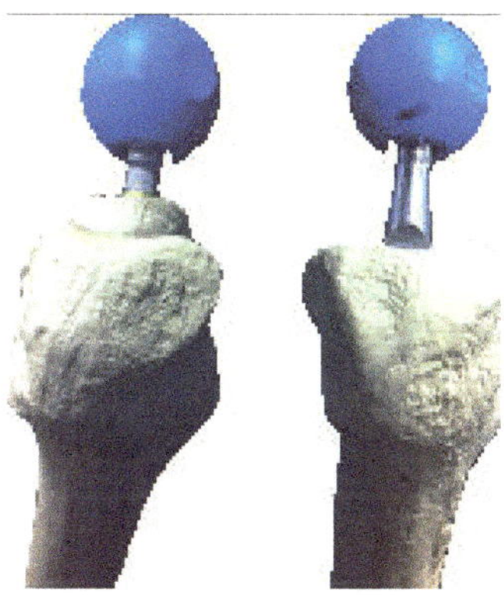

**Figure 7.** Varus /Valgus turning moment in neck retention vs. conventional neck resection

It is important to remember that not all neck-sparing stems are not all short neck stabilized stems. Historically, neck sparing stems were not short curved neck stabilized by design (Figure 8).

To-date, most neck-sparing stems have been somewhat disappointing in their long-term ability to stimulate and maintain the medial calcar. For that reason, a new short stem neck stabilized design approach was undertaken to improve proximal load transfer and to create a bone or tissue sparing stem that would be simple in design, amenable to reproducible technique and provide for fine tuning joint mechanics while stimulating and maintaining ongoing, in-vivo compressive loads to preserve the medial calcar.

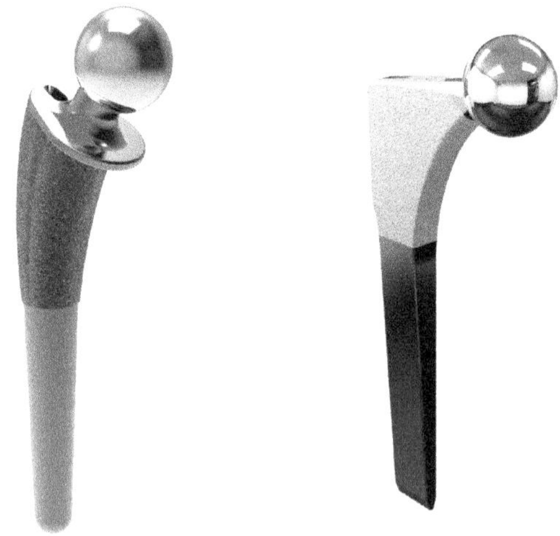

**Figure 8.** Left: Townley Platform Stem. Right: Whiteside Neck Sparing Stem.

## 4. "Short" hip arthoplasty stems

The use of short stems is growing. Initial short and mid-term follow up studies of a number of these stems suggest that stable, durable fixation and excellent clinical outcomes can be achieved. As a result, a very large number of short stem designs are available. Until recently, there was no classification system for uncemented short stem implants that would allow for comparisons of clinical and radiographic results.

A number of advantages have been argued to justify the design and clinical usage of short stems; Elimination of femoral proximal-distal mismatch, tissue preservation (hard & soft), facilitation of less invasive surgical exposures, less invasive surgical violation into the femoral canal, less violation into the trochanteric bed, improved proximal bone remodeling, less intraoperative blood loss, less postoperative rehabilitation, less instrumentation and less inventory cost.

All of these advantages are worthwhile if they can be proven to be significant benefits to the clinical outcome and increased survivorship of the device. The real question is can these shorter length devices obtain strong and long-lasting stability of the implant without diaphyseal anchoring?

The European experience with certain styles of conservative designs are years ahead of the U.S. experience. So it is reasonable to look towards Europe for both trends and early to mid-term clinical results. Some of these devices are not available in the U. S. and some are new to their clinical experience. As a result, the Joint Implant Surgery and Research Foundation

(JISRF) developed a short stem classification system based off stabilization contact for implant stability.[ 8]

JISRF developed this classification system to help identify, differentiate and catalog short stemmed total hip implants by primary stabilization contact points. Not all short stems generate the same radiographic findings and or clinical results. It is also important to appreciate the specific design and appropriate surgical technique for a given design. We believe this classification system helps to clarify some of the design principles and clinical findings. While there will be subcategories within the main categories, (Examples: Neck plugs versus short curved neck stems) but the primary stabilization point determines the same overall category.

## 5. JISRF classification system for short stems: Implant examples

1. Head Stabilized

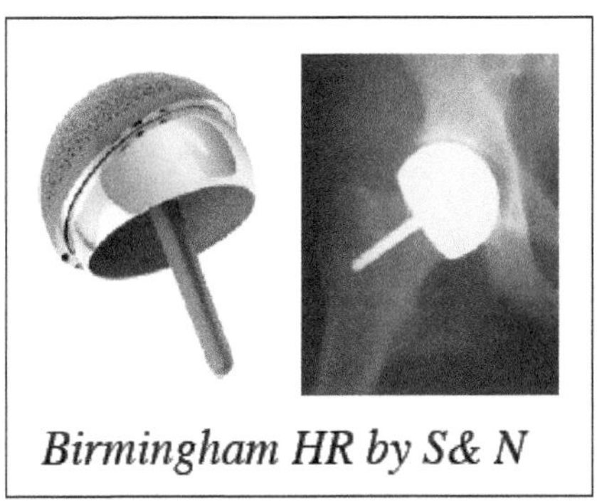


**Figure 9.** Hip Resurfacing Arthroplasty and "Mid-Head" Resurfacing Arthroplasty (Birmingham System, Smith and Nephew)

2. Neck Stabilized, Figure 11:

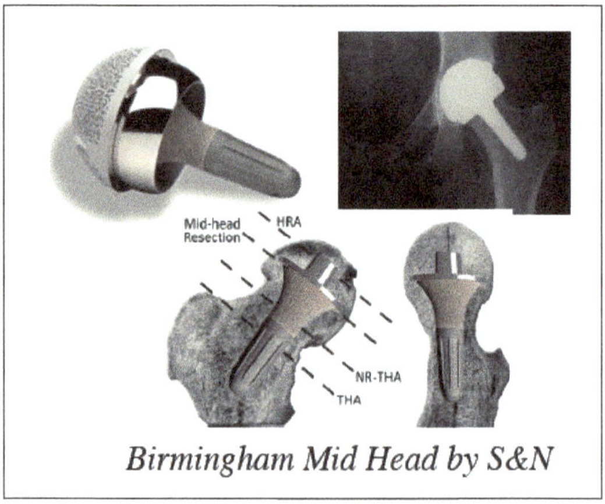


**Figure 10.** Hip Resurfacing Arthroplasty and "Mid-Head" Resurfacing Arthroplasty (Birmingham System, Smith and Nephew)

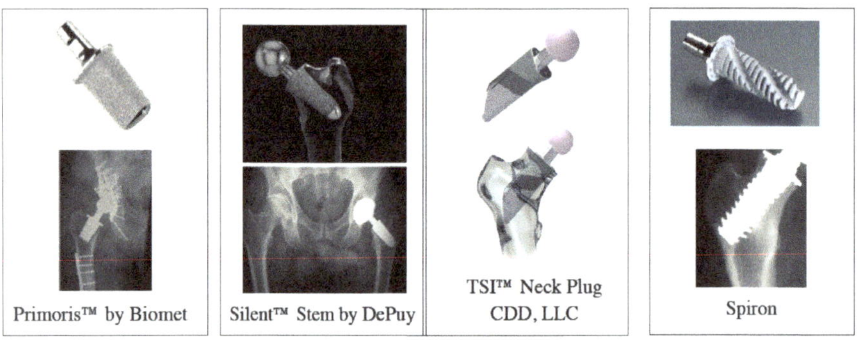


**Figure 11.** Metaphyseal Stabilized

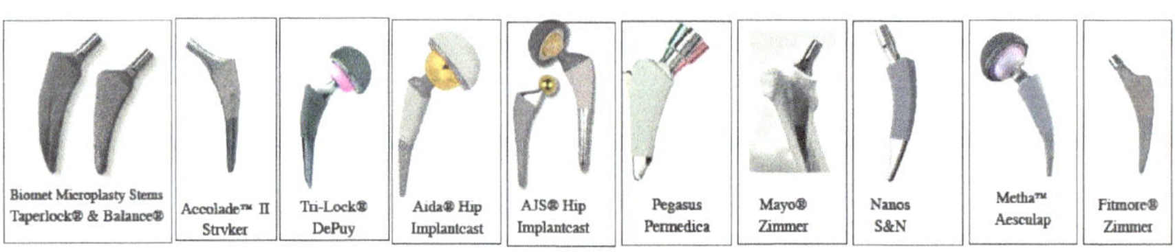


**Figure 12.** Conventional (Metaphyseal/Diaphyseal) Stabilized: Traditional Arthroplasty Stems

## 6. Current design rationale for a modular, short, curved neck stabilized stem

### Stem Design:

The TSI™ Stem is a simple short curved trapezoidal neck sparing design that is tissue conservative (hard & soft) and features a number of unique and novel elements to improve upon short and long-term survivorship. This novel design has been licensed by Concept, Design and Development, LLC., in Chagrin Falls, Ohio to two commercial partners and has been introduced into the Australian market as the MSA™ Stem and the United States as the Apex ARC™ Stem. (Figure 13)

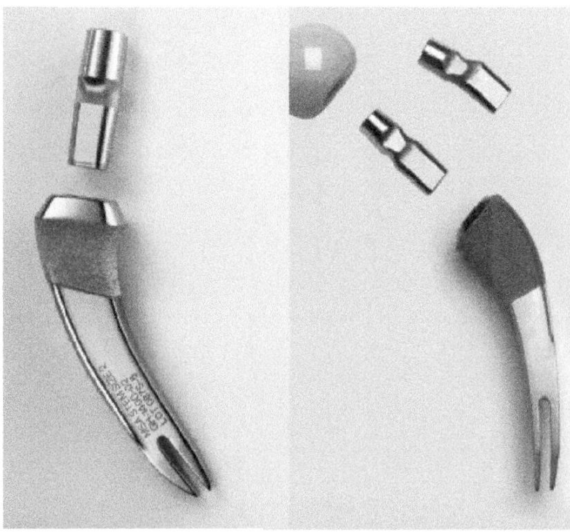

**Figure 13.** Left: The MSA™ Stem; Right: The Apex ARC™ Stem

The basic curvature of the stem comes from the historical work of Thompson and Müeller. A side-by-side comparison of the Mueller rasp and the ARC™ stem are seen in Figure 14. The medial curve and overall stem length are almost identical.

This simple, yet novel, stem design allows for considerable tissue conservation of both hard and soft tissue. Native bone is preserved in Gruen zones 7, 3,4,5 and zone 1, as seen in Figure 15.

The medial curve reduces the need to remove lateral bone, where one can risk damage to the musculature and increased bleeding by removal of cancellous bone in the greater trochanter (Figure 31). The stem shape is based on a curved trapezoidal design that is intrinsically stable within the cylindrical femur. The torsional stability is enhanced by a lateral "T-Flange" feature, however, this has proven to be too aggressive in the small female profile and has been removed on the size 0 stem.

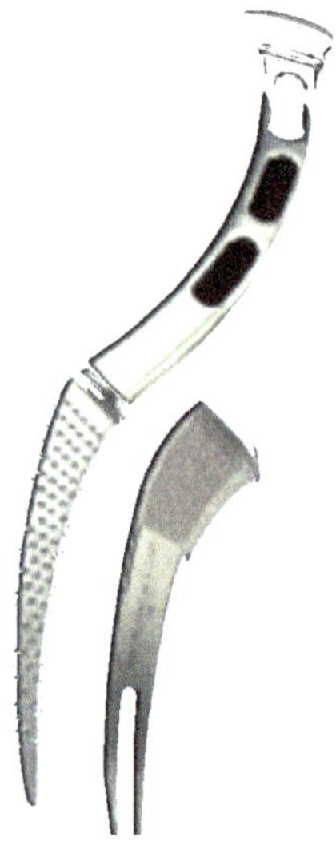

**Figure 14.** Image of historic Mueller proximal femoral rasp (left) placed adjacent to modern TSI neck-sparing arthroplasty implant (right).

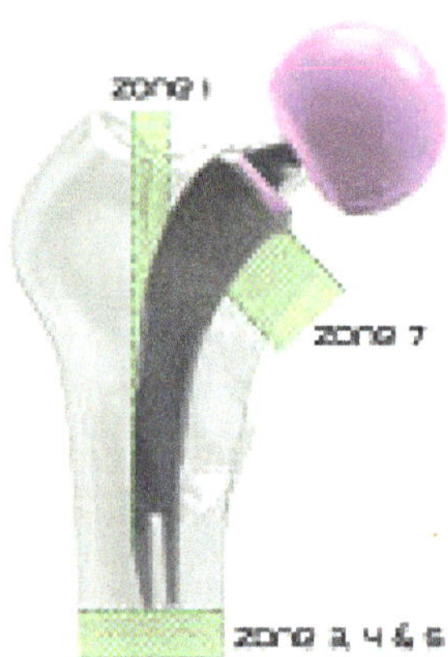


**Figure 15.** Image demonstrating areas of bone preservation maintained with neck-sparing arthroplasty, including Gruen Zones 1, 3, 4, 5, and 7.

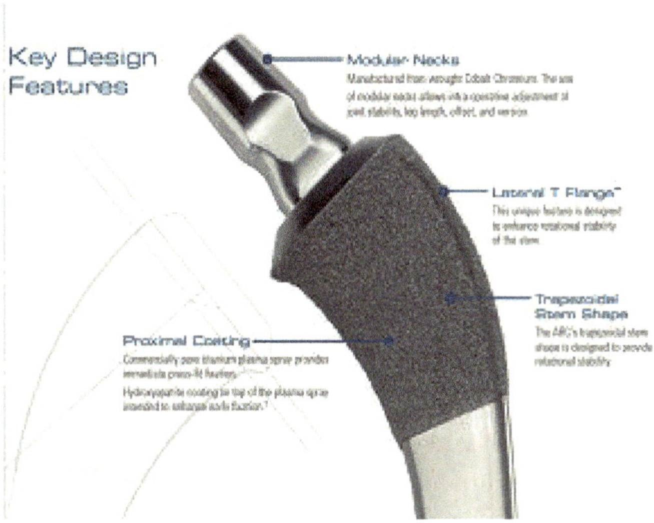


**Figure 16.** Key Design Features of the ARC™ stem.

A porous titanium coating is applied circumferentially to the upper third of the stem and is a combination of commercially pure titanium applied first using a plasma spray process after which a thin layer of hydroxyapatite (HA) is also applied using a plasma spray process. The proximal portion of the stem also has a patent pending novel conical flair element that is design to off load compressive loads to the medial calcar. (Figure 17) This very unique feature has demonstrated positive stress transfer in both FEA modeling and now clinical observations.

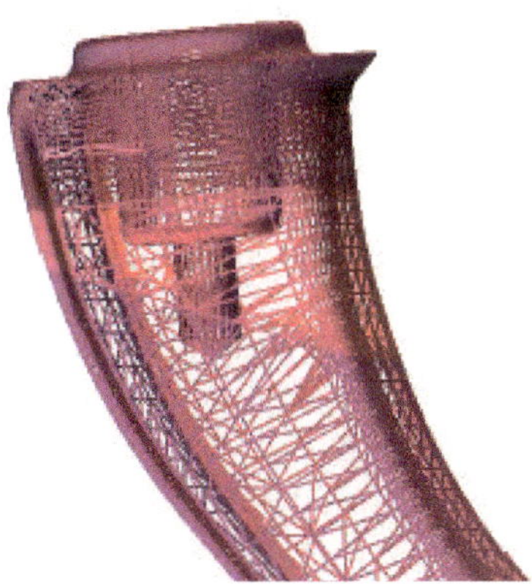

**Figure 17.** Medial Flare seen on the lateral profile in 3-Dimensional stem rendering

A lateral distal relief of 11º reduces any distal tip contact with the lateral cortex if the stem is in a slight varus position. The sagittal slot reduces distal stiffness reducing the potential of distal load transfer and reduces hoop tension in type A bone by allowing stem to pinch in.

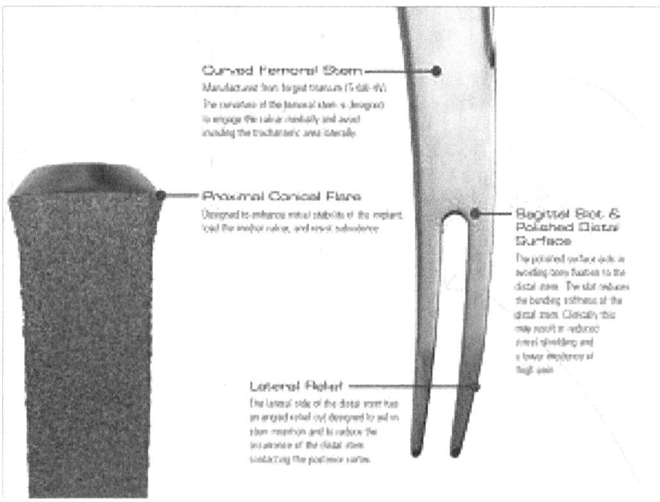


**Figure 18.** Additional Design Features of the ARC™ stem.

The TSI™ neck stabilized stem with a modular cobalt-chrome neck has demonstrated a reduction of maximum principal tensile stress in the neck stabilization stem was 35% less than that of a monoblock taper style design. (Figure 19) With regards to potential failure mode, the neck sparing feature with a short cobalt-chrome modular neck has basically eliminated potential fatigue failure of the neck, as opposed to other recent titanium modular neck designs that have demonstrated catastrophic fatigue fractures.[ 9]

## 7. Stress in the femoral component

The ring of cortical bone saved in the neck sparing stem has significant bio-mechanical advantage. Pipino refers to this as a "tension band." (Figure 20) The principal stress measured in the femoral component was lowest for model with cortical neck ring intact compared to the monoblock conventional cementless stem. (Figure 21)

The stress in the distal femur slightly reduces with the TSI neck sparing stem and reduces even more if the cortical rim remains intact. This data supports the concept that the medial conical flair does offload compression to the proximal femur especially if the cortical ring is intact.

The short TSI™ stem demonstrates better loading patterns as compared to Pipino's first stem (Biodynamic), (Figure 22) which was made of cobalt-chrome material. The x-ray on the right

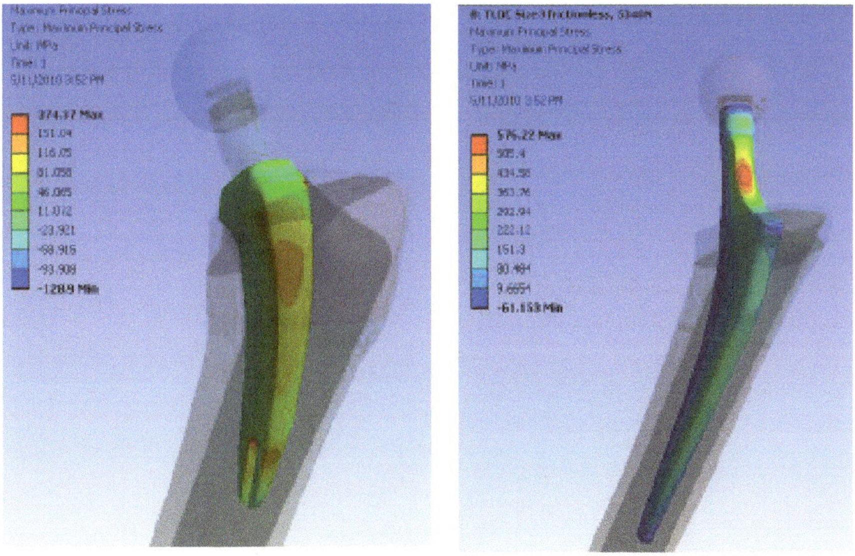

**Figure 19.** Finite Element Analysis of a short neck-sparing arthroplasty stem (left) compared to a monoblock stem (right). Increased areas of stress foci are highlighted in red.

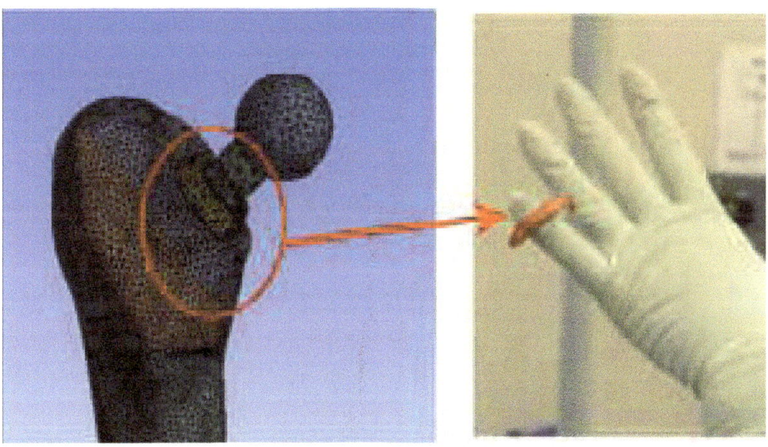

**Figure 20.** Ring of Proximal Femoral Bone

side of Figure 22 is his current stem CFP which still has had some medial calcar bone resporption issues.

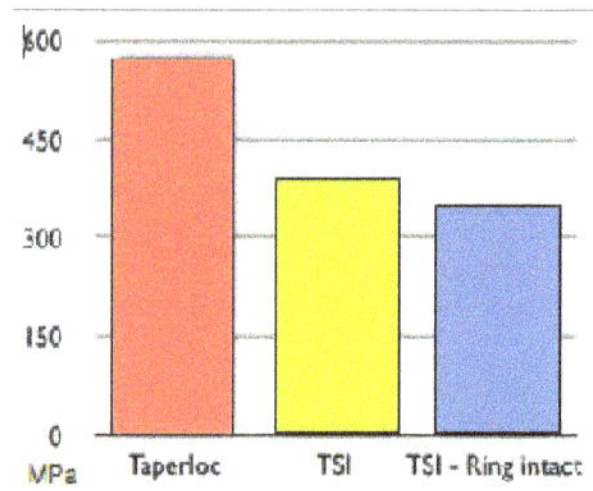


**Figure 21.** Assessment of proximal femoral stress with axial loading

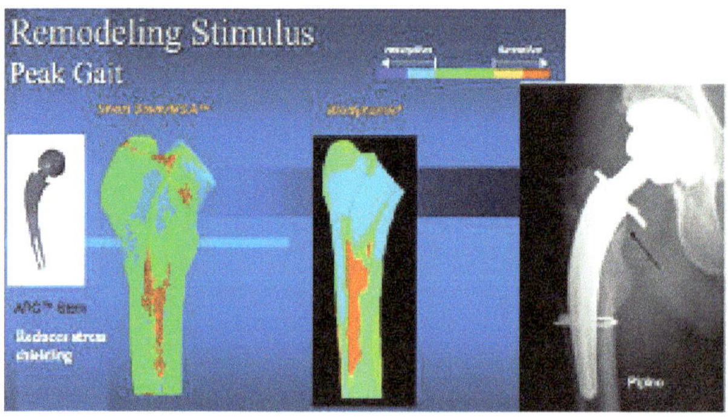


**Figure 22.** FEA Modeling of ARC™ (Left) compared with the Biodynamic stem (Right), showing normalized loading of the medial calcar on the left, and decreased loading on the right.

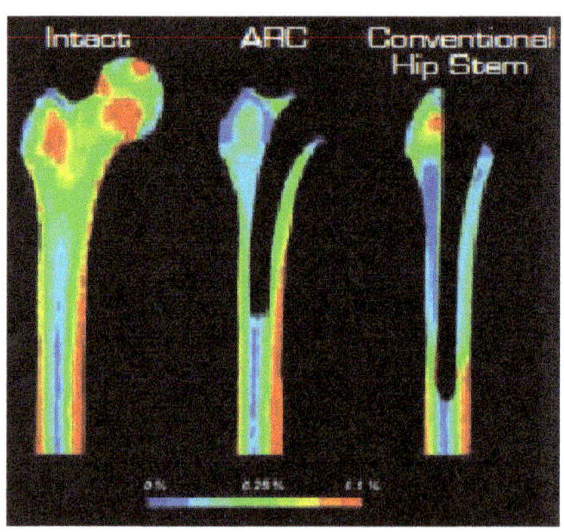


**Figure 23.** FEA Modeling of an intact femur (left), the ARC™ stem (Center) and a long, extensively coated press-fit stem (right), demonstrating improved proximal strain patterns compared to the AML style conventional cementless stem.

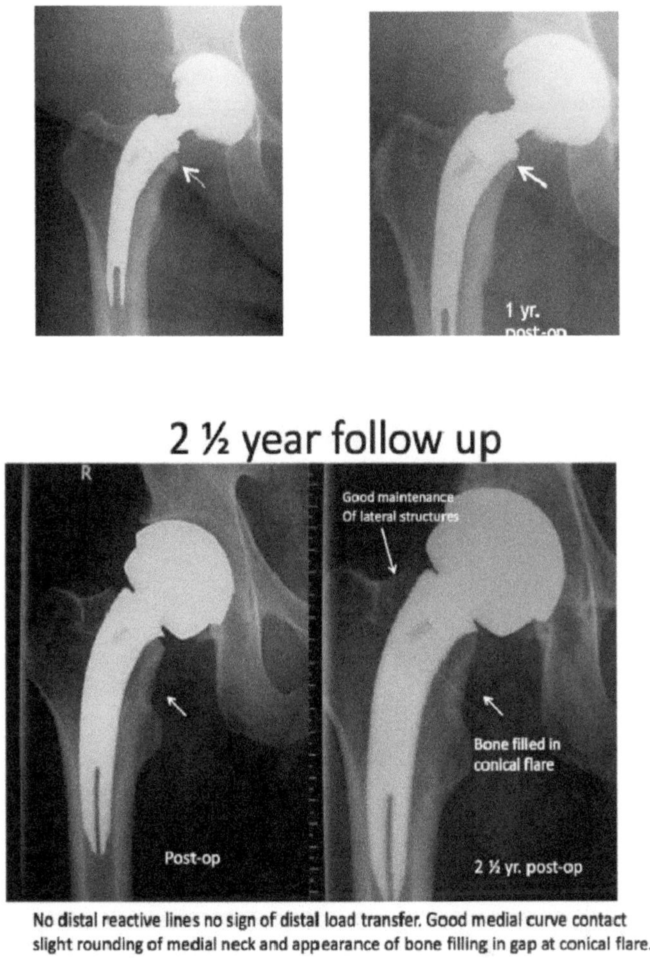


Prof. Ian Woodgate, Sydney, Australia

**Figure 24.** A and B: Clinical case examples of favorable bone remodeling from the ARC™ stem

## 8. Proximal neck modularity

Target Restoration of hip mechanics is aided by proximal neck modularity, especially focued on femoral offset, neck length, and combined version. Using monoblock femoral stem designs, restoration of hip mechanics is difficult to address. Often, accomplishing intra-operative joint stability comes with an increased risk for over-lengthening..

Neck Modularity allows intraoperative fine tuning of joint mechanics, reducing risk of impingement and mitigating risk of accelerated wear and dislocation. This priniciple also aids in access in the event of acetabular revision. Monoblock hip stems are based on proportionality of design. As the stem gets bigger, the neck gets longer. Unfortunately, this scenario is not consistent with the variability seen with proximal femoral geometry, and is illustrated with the radiographs seen in Figure 25.

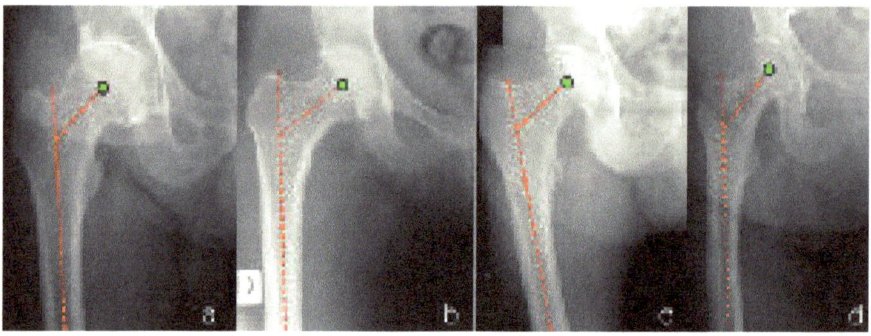


**Figure 25.** Anatomic variations commonly associated with primary osteo-arthritis patients using a monoblock stem: a: large canal, short neck, low offset, b: thin canal, long neck, high offset, c: large canal, short neck, high offset, d: thin canal, long neck, low offset

Femoral head center location data (Figure 26) shows that a wide variety of offsets and lengths are required to properly balance the soft tissues, but there is often little correlation between head center and stem size. A significant number of small stem diameters (10 or 11.5 mm) required large >45 mm femoral offsets.

One only has to review actual usage data on modular necks to validate the need of proximal modularity. A review of ARC™ Modular Neck Experience (Figure 27) on 1,640 stems implanted from April 2010 to August 2012 demonstrated that a significant variety of stems were selected by surgeons while using the device to fine-tune the biomechanics of the hip joint in vivo.

## 9. Clinical utilization and outcomes

**Case One:** A 29 year-old man presented with the acute-onset of debilitating pain in his left hip from osteonecrosis with collapse secondary to chronic steroid use for immunosuppression of severe lupus. (Figure 28). His symptoms developed over 4 weeks and were incapacitating, requiring the use of two crutches and high doses of long-acting narcotic for comfort.

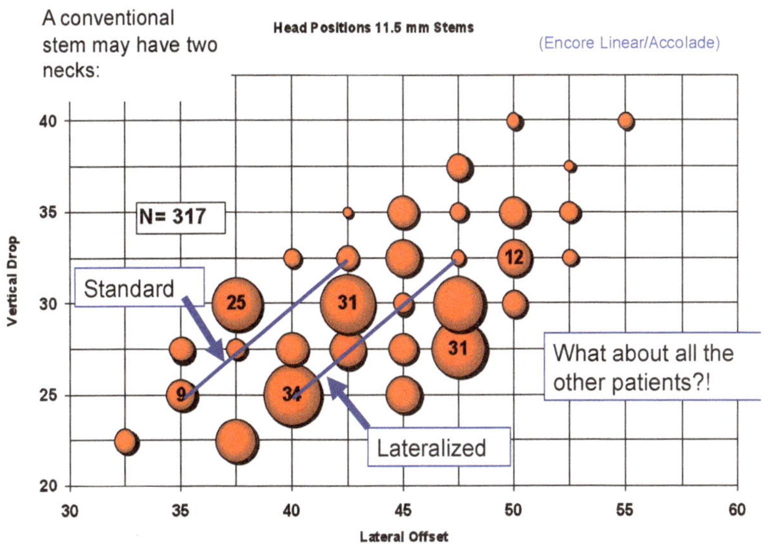


**Figure 26.** Femoral head location data, mapping a relationship of femoral implant sizing related to vertical drop (vertical axis) and lateral offset (horizontal axis). Most conventional femoral stems are available only in "standard" and "lateral" offsets, which do not match the variety of combined values seen in native anatomy.

Neutral Neck Standard = 33%
Neutral Neck Long = 3% new size
**Total Neutral Necks = 36%**

8°Varus/Valgus =19%
8°Varus/Valgus Long = 3%
**Total 8°Varus/Valgus = 22%**

12°Varus Valgus =17%
12°Anteverted/Retroverted = 30% new size
**Angled Necks Total = 47%**

**Figure 27.** ARC™ modular neck utilization data, from April 2010 to August 2012.

He was treated with total hip arthroplasty using a neck sparing implant and a ceramic on cross-linked polyethylene bearing surface couple. The implants were inserted via the direct anterior approach with a "bone-sparing technique" allowing retention of 1.5 cm of his proximal femoral bone, with anatomic restoration of his hip center of rotation (Figures 29 and 30). His postoperative course showed complete resolution of his pain with elimination of narcotic use, dramatic improvement in his hip function, and he was able to begin returning to work as a professional chef after less than 8 weeks of recovery.

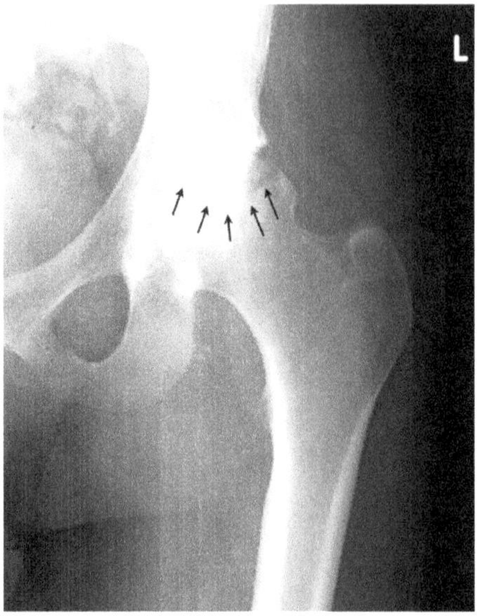


**Figure 28.** Left Hip Joint with AVN and acute collapse of the dome of the femoral head, indicated by arrows.

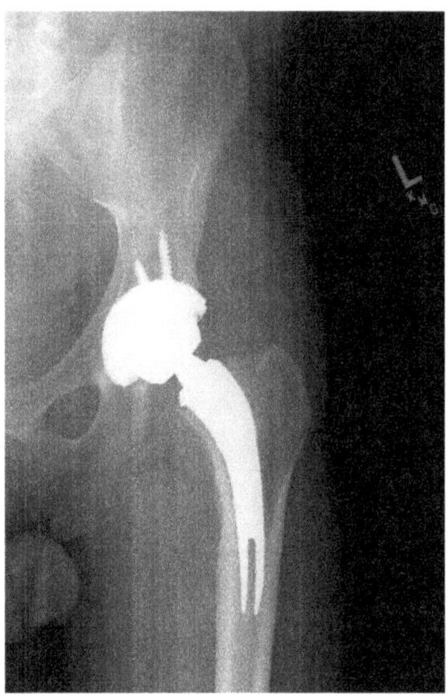


**Figure 29.** Postoperative AP Left Hip, Showing ARC™ "neck-sparing" arthroplasty in an anatomic position with restoration of hip alignment, offset, and position.

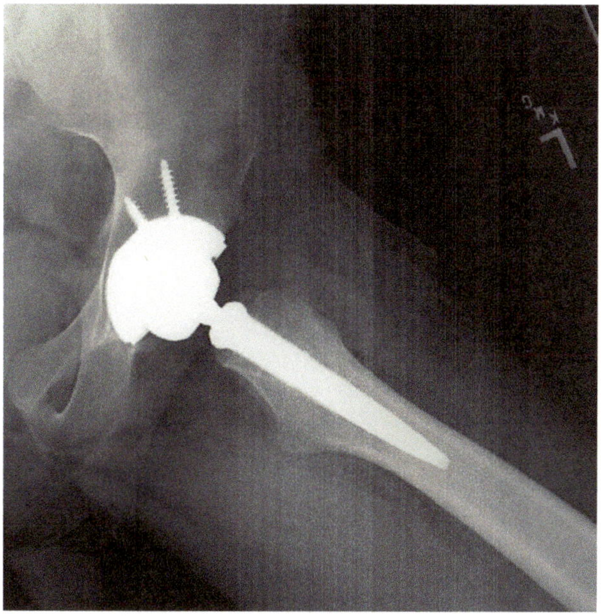

**Figure 30.** Postoperative Lateral Left Hip demonstrating anatomic prosthesis positioning.

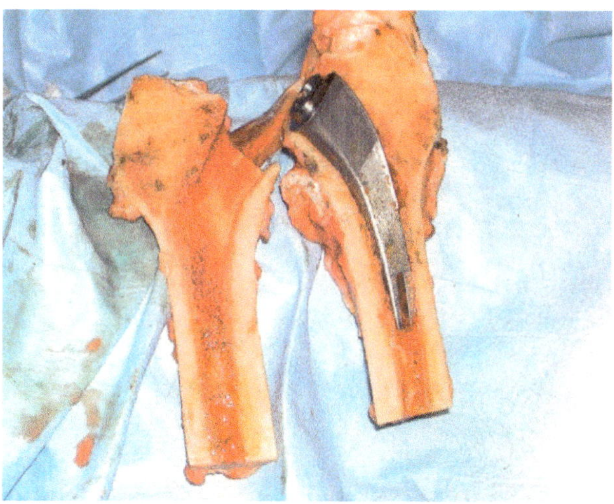

**Figure 31.** Coronal cross-section of cadaveric left proximal femur, demonstrating neck-sparing prosthesis position along medial calcar, with retained femoral neck and conservation of native trochanteric bone visible.

**Case Two:** A 32 year-old man presented for evaluation after having been previously diagnosed with advanced bilateral osteonecrosis of his proximal femoral heads. His management had already included a comprehensive medical and metabolic workup to assess for causes for the avascular necrosis, but none had been elucidated. He denied any known exposure to high dose corticosteroids and had no history of alcohol intake. He had previously undergone core decompression procedures at an outside institution on both the right hip (18 months prior) and the left hip (14 months prior) in the recent past, without any significant improvements in his clinical function or symptoms. He underwent simulateneous, bilateral neck-sparing THA, and is walking normally once again after a brief course of rehabilitation. The specific details of his case were described in detail elsewhere.[ 10]

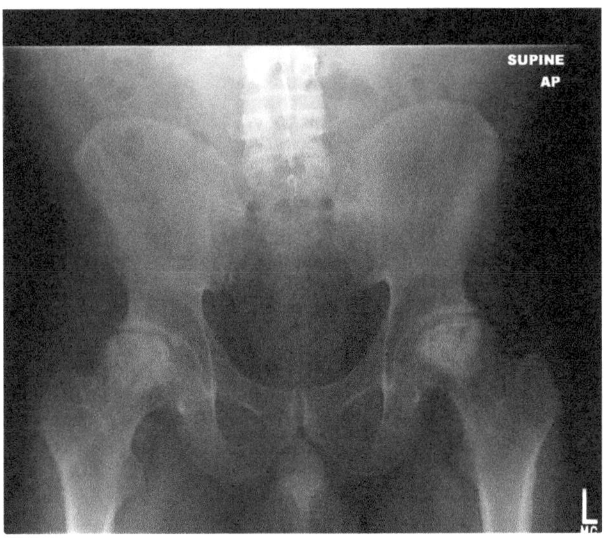


**Figure 32.** Preoperative AP Pelvis of a 32 year-old male with severe, bilateral, osteonecrosis with associated femoral head collapse and secondary arthrosis.

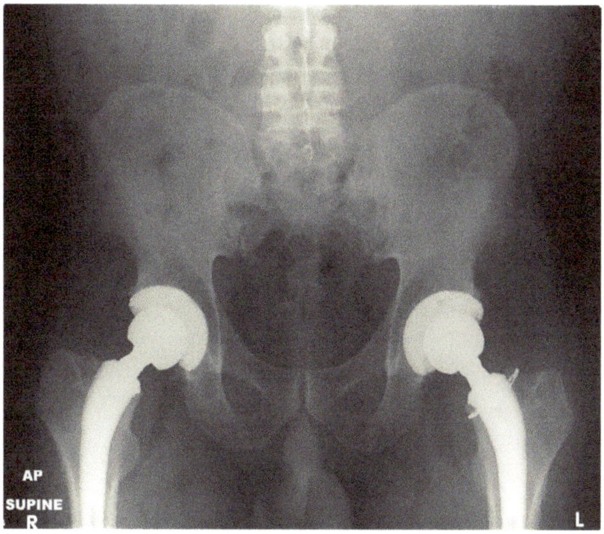


**Figure 33.** Postoperative AP Pelvis

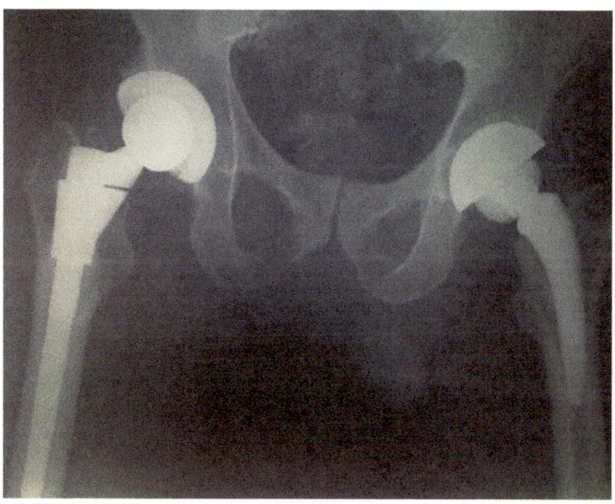

**Figure 34.** Comparison of historic versus modern femoral stem modularity. Right hip: S-ROM Prosthesis, 1984; Left Hip ARC™ Stem, 2012. (Image Courtesy Louis Keppler, MD and JISRF.)

## 10. Short-term results of TSI and ARC™femoral stem

Since the introduction of these modular, short, neck-sparing femoral stem designs, the early results of implant utilization have been tracked by their manufacturers and JISRF.[ 11]

With 1,970 stems implanted worldwide, There have been only 8 stem explants, and an overall femoral stem survival of 99.5% at 29 months. There were 2 traumatic and 1 chronic dislocations, 2 cases of aseptic loosening, 2 infections, and 1 neck/stem disassociation. 10 cases had a leg length discrepancy greater than 7mm. 6 cases had an iatrogenic calcar fracture, and 3 required wiring. 6 patients had subsidence more than 5mm. There were 3 neck exchanges, with 2 performed for cup revisions. There were 3 intra-operative femoral perforations, and 5 cases that of intra-operative calcar fractures resulting in stem bail-out. There have been no known cases of pseudotumors, no elevated peripheral metal ion levels, and no known occurrence of modular neck fracture.

## 11. Conclusion

Over the next several decades we will continue to see improvements in implant fixation, bioengineering of bearing surface designs, and prosthesis design that will allow us to reliably replace hip joints in younger and more active adult patients. The design of the "neck-sparing" products and bearing surfaces mentioned herein have certainly played a large part in achieving this goal, but continued improvements and careful outcomes monitoring will be needed over the next few decades.


## Acknowledgements

Rubin and Ritterman: Unrestricted educational grant from Joint Implant Surgery and Research Foundation. McTighe: Ownership interests, patents, and licensing fees related to Concept, Design, and Development (CDD) and TSI Stem designs.


## Author details


Lee E. Rubin[1], Scott A. Ritterman[2] and Timothy McTighe[3]

*Address all correspondence to: lrubin@universityorthopedics.com

1 Division of Adult Reconstruction, Warren Alpert Medical School of Brown University, University Orthopedics, Inc. Providence, Rhode Island, USA

2 Brown University and Rhode Island Hospital, Providence, Rhode Island, USA

3 Joint Implant Surgery and Research Foundation (JISRF), Chagrin Falls, Ohio, USA 1

## References

[1] Moussa, H, Pierre, B, Jacques, D, et al. Alumina-on-Alumina Total Hip Arthroplasty A Minimum 18.5-Year Follow-up Study." J Bone Joint Surg Am (2002)., 84(1), 69-77.

[2] Neumann, L, Freund, K. G, & Sorenson, K. H. Long-Term Results of Charnley Total Hip Replacement." J Bone Joint Surg Br (1994). B (2): 245-251., 76.

[3] Polkowski et alTotal Hip Arthroplasty in the very Young Patient." Journal of the American Academy of Orthopaedic Surgeons. (2012)., 20, 487-497.

[4] Engh, C. A, & Hopper, R. H. Huynh C et. al. A prospective randomized study of cross-linked and non cross-linked polyethylene for total hip arthroplasty at year follow-up. Journal of Arthroplasty (2012). S): 2-7., 10.

[5] Milosev, I, Kovac, S, & Trebse, R. et. al. Comparison of ten-year survivorship of hip prosthesis with use of conventional polyethylene, metal-on-metal, or ceramic-on-ceramic bearings. J Bone Joint Surg Am (2012)., 94(19), 1756-1763.

[6] Freeman, M. A. Why resect the neck? J Bone Joint Surg Br (1986)., 68(3), 346-9.

[7] Pipino, F, & Keller, A. Tissue-sparing surgery: 25 years' experience with femoral neck preserving hip arthroplasty. Journal of Orthopaedics and Traumatology. (2006)., 7(1), 36-41.

[8] Stulberg, S. D, Keggi, J, & Keppler, L. et. al. A classification system for short stemuncemented total hip arthroplasty. Poster Presentation at the International Society for Technology in Arthroplasty. Sydney, Australia, October (2012)., 4-6.

[9] Mctighe, T, & Brazil, D. Memorandum: Modular Necks. Reconstructive Review (2012)., 2(2), 98-101.

[10] Rubin, L. E, Tuttle, J. R, & Ritteman, S. A. Simultaneous bilateral direct anterior total hip arthroplasty utilizing a modular neck-sparing arthroplasty femoral stem. Reconstructive Review (2012)., 2(2), 68-71.

[11] Mctighe, T, Keggi, J, & Keppler, L. et. al. The First 1,200 (1,790) U.S. Short Curved Neck Stabilized Stems. Poster Presentation at the International Society for Technology in Arthroplasty. Sydney, Australia, October (2012)., 4-6.

Chapter 9

# Optimization of Tuberosity Healing in Prosthetic Reconstruction of Proximal Humerus Fractures

Moby Parsons

Additional information is available at the end of the chapter

## 1. Introduction

Achieving successful clinical outcomes after hemiarthroplasty for 4-part proximal humerus fractures remains a sobering challenge for even the experienced shoulder reconstruction surgeon or traumatologist. Despite what appears to be secure tuberosity fixation at the time of wound closure, serial postoperative radiographs often reveal progressive displacement and/or resorption of the greater tuberosity.[1-3] This results in a situation akin to a posterior-superior rotator cuff tear, where most patients cannot generate sufficient cuff strength to stabilize the humeral head against the superior pull of the deltoid. Secondary mechanical consequences, including shoulder weakness, superior instability and trapezial substitution can compromise outcomes both in terms of shoulder function and pain in such circumstances.[4, 5] Stiffness and cuff dysfunction frequently render the functional results only fair and many patients must accept a limited goals end result.[6-8]

It is well established that restoration of shoulder function after hemiarthroplasty for fracture depends on successful tuberosity healing in combination with proper reconstruction of the head-tuberosity and head-shaft relationships.[1, 7-9] In the native proximal humerus, the edge of the articular cartilage of the superior head is directly adjacent to the cuff insertion and the two are nearly confluent. The dome of the head is about 5-8 mm above the supraspinatus footprint. Restoring this confluence between the cuff insertion and the prosthetic head while maintaining appropriate tuberosity offset relative to the center of rotation is essential for proper cuff mechanics. Restoring proper head height, medial offset, posterior offset and retrotorsion is also critical to achieving soft tissue balance that will provide both strength and stability.

Despite the introduction of fracture-specific prostheses, translating successful anatomical reconstruction into shoulder function is not guaranteed by the theoretical solutions these newer designs propose for complex fracture treatment. Realistically, outcomes after hemiarthroplasty for fracture are a blend of appropriate prosthesis selection and use, optimal management of tuberosity fixation, respect for the biology of fracture healing and application of an appropriate rehabilitation protocol that does not jeopardize these other aims. As follows is a discussion about principles for optimizing tuberosity reduction, fixation and healing using horizontal cable cerclage in combination with a press-fit, porous coated fracture-specific prosthesis. This technique can be applied in the setting of hemiarthroplasty or reverse shoulder arthroplasty for fracture.

## 2. Why does failure of tuberosity healing occur?

As with fractures in other bones, successful union of the tuberosities after humeral hemiarthroplasty requires an optimal biological and mechanical environment for bone healing. Failure occurs for several potential reasons alone or in combination. Firstly, aggressive mobilization techniques during exposure may devascularize and further destabilize the tuberosities by stripping periosteal attachments. These periosteal attachments are critical to the blood supply of the greater tuberosity when the posterior circumflex humeral artery has been severed by the fracture pattern. This is generally the case when fracture severity warrants prosthetic reconstruction. Secondly, violation of the rotator interval capsule during exposure and head retrieval disrupts the remaining bridge of tissue that links the tuberosities. This further destabilizes the tuberosities by dissociating the transverse force couple that counteracts their individual deforming forces.

Thirdly, thermal damage from cement may further damage the endosteal blood supply of the humerus, and cement blocks the marrow cavity and areas where the fracture fragments may interdigitate. Fourthly, conventional suture fixation constructs often fail to achieve sufficiently rigid fixation to permit healing. Poor bone quality and fracture comminution increase the likelihood of suture loosening, which occurs early in the postoperative period. Finally, prosthesis designs that do not provide an adequate template for recreation of the cortical shell of the proximal humerus and those that do not allow direct fixation of the tuberosities to the body of the prosthesis will invite a degree of micromotion that is not compatible with fracture union.

## 3. Features of the EPOCA prosthesis

For fracture hemiarthroplasty, the author prefers the EPOCA Shoulder System (Synthes, Westchester, PA). The EPOCA shoulder prosthesis has several features that make it an ideal choice for use in reconstructing proximal humerus fractures. The design of the humeral prosthesis is based on extensive anatomical studies with the goal of restoring the normal structural relationships between the head, tuberosities and shaft.[10] The rationale behind the design of the EPOCA system is that aspects of the proximal humeral anatomy that are highly variable across the population should be adjustable while those aspects with minimal variation should be standardized. Features with a high variation include head radius, size of the humeral medullary canal, medial offset and tuberosity offset. Features with a low variation include neck-shaft angle and the ratio of head height to radius. To this end, the system offers 5 stem sizes (6 - 14mm in 2 mm increments) and 10 head diameters (40 – 58 mm in 2 mm increments). There are also standard (115 mm) and long (215 mm) stem lengths. Independent adjustment of medial and posterior offset can be achieved by a dual eccentricity (Eccenter) that allows the head to be placed in an infinite number of X-Y positions within a 6 mm orbit relative to the humeral component. This ensures precise reconstruction of the proximal humeral anatomy and center of rotation.

The EPOCA stem comes in both a press fit and cemented option (Figure 1). The former has porous coating on the proximal half, the roughness of which may help promote tuberosity adherence and security. The tapered wedge geometry has a prominent calcar design that helps the stem self-center, self-rotate and self-lock as it is inserted. Thus, even in a fracture situation, a press-fit stem can be used and achieve excellent stem stability without the need for cement fixation.

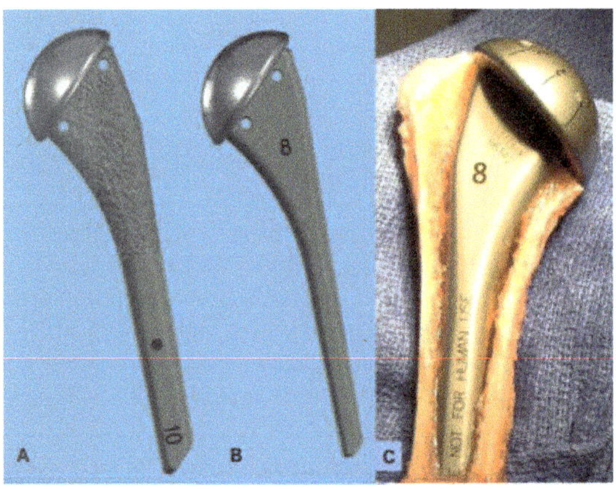


**Figure 1.** The EPOCA stem comes in press-fit, porous coated (A) and smooth, cemented (B) options. Both have a tapered wedge geometry with a prominent calcar design that promotes metaphyseal fill (C). Medial and lateral holes in the proximal stem allow cerclage directly through the prosthesis rather than around its medial calcar portion. These features permit use of the press-fit stem in the setting of fracture due to the rotational stability afforded by the stem geometry.

The proximal body of the stem has both a medial and lateral hole through which cables can be passed for tuberosity cerclage (Figure 1). This construct improves rotational stability of the cerclage fixation compared to cables or sutures passed around the calcar section of the prosthesis. In the latter case, the fixation is not directly linked to the stem so that the tuberosities can still move independently of the prosthesis when the arm is rotated about the axis of the humerus. By passing fixation through the stem of the prosthesis, the tuberosities are compressed directly to the stem so that the construct rotates as a single unit during arm rotation. The improved stability of this fixation obviates the need for multiple other sutures, specifically vertical sutures between the shaft and bone-tendon junction that tend to result in the common mistake of tuberosity over-reduction.

## 4. Preoperative planning

When the decision to operate has been made, the surgeon needs to consider a variety of factors in deciding the best method of treatment for the given fracture pattern. Aspects of the patient's medical and social history are important to consider. The following patients factors may bear on the decision to attempt fixation versus prosthetic replacement: age, hand-dominance, physical demands, expectations, compliance, smoking history, and medical comorbidity.

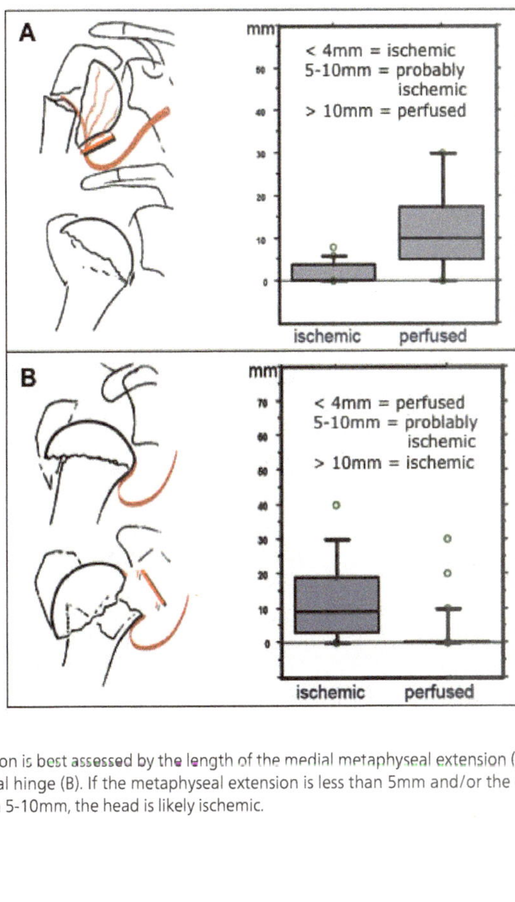


**Figure 2.** Head perfusion is best assessed by the length of the medial metaphyseal extension (A) and the displacement of the medial periosteal hinge (B). If the metaphyseal extension is less than 5mm and/or the displacement of the medial hinge is more than 5-10mm, the head is likely ischemic.

It is essential when assessing these fractures to have a thorough understanding of the fracture "personality" and this usually demands a CT scan with coronal and sagittal reconstructions that allow for 3-D rendering. Such imaging can be invaluable in determining the location and degree of comminution, the integrity of the articular surface, the exact relationship between the head, tuberosity and shaft, as well as prognostic indicators of head vascularity. In the latter case, the length of the medial metaphyseal extension and the displacement of the medial periosteal hinge are most predictive of head perfusion (Figure 2).

This collective information can help the surgeon determine if fixation is both warranted and feasible. Feasibility depends on factors such as bone quality and comminution, fracture complexity, availability of the necessary implants and surgeon skill. If stable, anatomical fixation is not possible, then prosthetic replacement is warranted. While reverse shoulder arthroplasty has become increasingly popular in this setting, there remains a role for hemiarthroplasty in younger and more physically demanding patients. Of note, the technique described herein can be used for secure tuberosity fixation during reverse arthroplasty for fracture where outcome can also be improved by successful tuberosity healing allowing restoration of active external rotation.

## 5. Surgical technique

The patient is positioned as for a shoulder arthroplasty such that the scapula is supported but the arm can be brought over the side of the bed to expose the humeral shaft. The fracture is exposed through a standard delto-pectoral approach taking the cephalic vein laterally with the deltoid. The anterior deltoid is elevated off the coracoacromial (CA) ligament and a sharp angled lever is placed behind the ligament. This helps "roll" the deltoid laterally to expose the proximal humerus.

The clavipectoral fascia is excised en bloc from the CA ligament proximally to the pectoralis major tendon distally and the conjoint tendon medially to the deltoid laterally. Once this layer has been removed, the humeroscapular motion interface is accessible and adhesions in this interval can be freed using blunt dissection. One must avoid overzealous dissection to prevent stripping of any residual periosteal attachment of the tuberosities to the shaft. A curved ring retractor can then be placed beneath the deltoid and a right-angle retractor beneath the conjoint tendon.

The biceps tendon is then identified and followed proximally. It should be sutured to the pectoralis major tendon to preserve native tension and then tenotomized at the superior aspect of the bicipital groove. Because the bicipital groove and a portion of the anterior greater tuberosity usually remain attached to the lesser tuberosity fragment, it is critical to preserve the rotator interval capsule (Figure 3A). Thus, it should not be routinely divided above the transverse humeral ligament as many conventional techniques recommend (Figure 3B). Preservation of the rotator interval will help stabilize the tuberosity repair by leaving a soft tissue bridge between the anterior and posterior fragments. 1
This helps neutralize the individual deforming forces that lead to loosening and failure

of fixation. In a majority of cases there is a longitudinal split in the supraspinatus tendon where the anterior bundle remains attached to the lesser tuberosity fragment. Maintenance of this attachment is critical to maximize the potential for cuff function postoperatively. Exposure of the humeral head and glenoid can be achieved by extending the longitudinal cuff split medially. This can be repaired side-to-side at the conclusion of the case and does not jeopardize the cuff insertion to the bone.

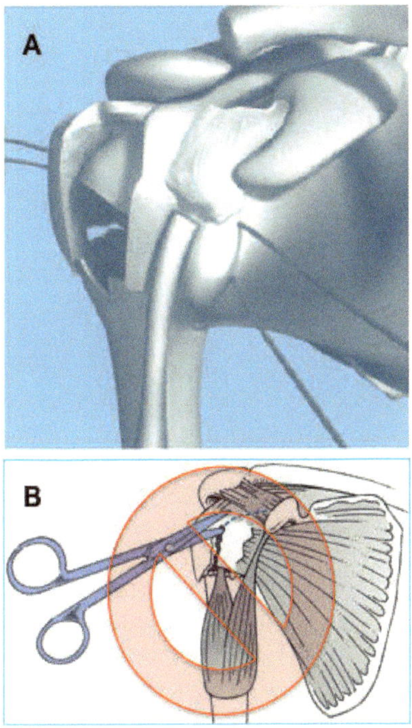


**Figure 3.** In a typical 4-part fracture, the bicipital groove and anterior most portion of the greater tuberosity remains attached to the anterior, lesser tuberosity fragment (A). The anterior bundle of the supraspinatus tendon remains attached to this anterior fragment, separated by a longitudinal split in the tendon at the level of the fracture plane. The rotator interval capsule remains intact and should not be violated as is current convention (B).

Heavy braided suture is placed through the bone tendon interface of each of the subscapularis (SC), supraspinatus (SS) and infraspinatus (IS) tendons. It is essential when placing the posterior sutures that excessive traction is not applied so that soft tissue attachments between the tuberosity and shaft are maintained. Overly aggressive tuberosity mobilization injures the periosteal blood supply and reduces the likelihood of eventual healing. As much as possible, the greater tuberosity should be left in-situ posteriorly.

The humeral head can then be retrieved from the joint through the split in the SS tendon. The head can then be "keyed in" to the shaft to determine the location of the medial metaphyseal extension. The length of this extension is then measured and this length represents the distance above the calcar that the prosthetic head should sit to restore proper head height (Figure 4). This is a simple, reliable and accurate method of determining head height that can be cross-referenced with other accepted methods per the surgeon's discretion. The humeral head is then sized against the prosthetic head trials. One should typically downsize if the native head is in between trial head sizes so as not to overstuff the joint. Cancellousautograft is then harvested from the humeral head for supplemental bone grafting of the tuberosities to aid in restoration of tuberosity offset.

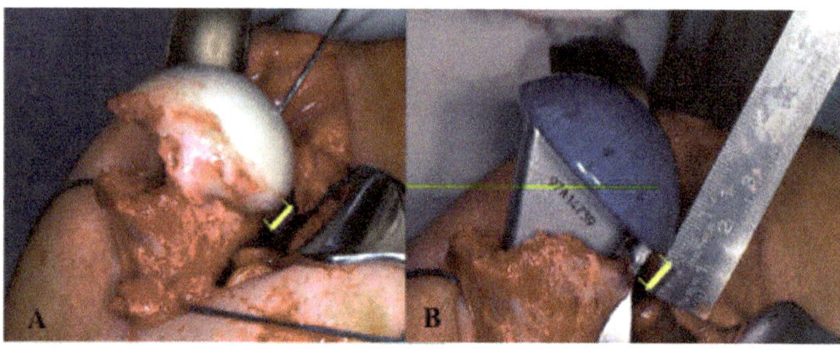


**Figure 4.** The length of the medial metaphyseal extension can be used as an accurate and reproducible method of determining the height at which the prosthesis should be seated to recreate proximal humeral anatomy. The native head can be keyed onto the shaft to determine this height (A). The prosthesis height and medial offset should be set to reproduce the native shoulder anatomy (B).

Prior to stem implantation, it is important to place the cerclage cables through the greater tuberosity in an inside-out fashion (Figure 5) At a level approximately 5 mm below the bone-tendon junction, a 2 mm drill bit is used to make the medial and lateral holes through the tuberosity bone. Again, care should be taken to leave the tuberosity in-situ when these holes are drilled to protect soft-tissue attachments. A Synthes 1 mm needled, beadless cable is then passed through each of the holes. The cable crimp must be taken off before the cable is placed and the crimp saved on the back table so that it is not inadvertently lost. The needle can be bounced off of the curved deltoid retractor and the cable retrieved on the dorsal tuberosity surface. The needle is removed and the cables are then tagged with a hemostat and parked posteriorly for later tuberosity repair.

A distally-angled Fukuda retractor is next placed behind the glenoid to inspect the joint. The root of the biceps should be excised and the glenoid articular surface checked for concomitant fracture. The labrum should be preserved to aid in stability and load distribution. Aggressive capsular releases are not necessary in fracture reconstruction as would be performed during shoulder arthroplasty for degenerative disease, and the temptation to perform a circumferential subscapularis release should be avoided. This will only jeopardize the anterior circumflex humeral artery, which provides vascularity to the anterior tuberosity fragment, and disrupt the important rotator interval "bridge."

The humeral shaft is then exposed by placing the arm in extension, adduction and external rotation. Two blunt Hohman retractors, posteriorly and medially, are used to leaver the shaft anteriorly. If necessary, the medullary canal is opened with the cylindrical starter rasp. Further reaming is not necessary as the EPOCA system uses impaction broaches to prepare the canal. Starting with the smallest broach, proper stem rotation is determined by orienting the laser-etched center line of the broach with a point 8 mm posterior to the deepest point of the bicipital. This point has been shown to correspond to the equatorial plane of the humeral head (Figure 6A & B).[10] The broach is seated to the level that restores the head height according to the pre-determined metaphyseal extension length. Proper retrotorsion of the humeral stem can be confirmed by inserting the 6 mm rod into the broach and measuring roughly 25 degrees relative to the forearm axis with the goniometer.

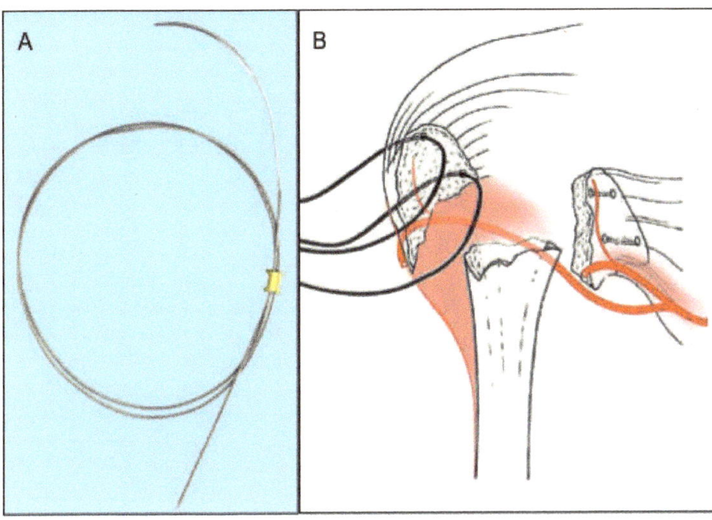


**Figure 5.** The Synthes beadles, needled cable should be used (A); cables should be placed prior to instrumentation of the humeral shaft with care taken not to disrupt periosteal attachments between the tuberosities and the humeral shaft (B).

Progressively larger broaches are introduced until distal (diaphyseal) canal fill is achieved. A curved curette can be used to remove cancellous bone along the medial humeral metaphyseal region to help fully seat the desired broach if necessary. The pronounced calcar design allows the broach to self-center, self-align and self-lock in the proper height and orientation, obviating the need for cumbersome jigs to position the trial stem. Once the stem size has been determined, the trial stem is impacted to the proper height using light progressive taps with the mallet to prevent fracture of the shaft by the wedge-shaped stem.

In a majority of cases, an optimal fit can be achieved allowing the use of a press-fit stem. In the occasional case, one stem size is over-recessed relative to the calcar and the next size too big for the diaphysis. In these cases, the surgeon has two choices. The first is to attempt impaction grafting the smaller stem to the proper height using autograft from the humeral head and the smaller impaction broach. With the diaphyseal portion of the broach inserted only slightly into the canal, small croutons of bone graft can be placed circumferentially around the canal opening and progressively impacted into the metaphysis. This process can be repeated until a snug fit is achieved with the broach. In patients with severely osteoporotic bone, a stable press-fit may not be possible without undue risk of humeral shaft fracture. The second option is to cement the final prosethsis in a conventional manner. In such a case, the final chosen stem will be one size smaller than the broach and trial stem to allow for a circumferential cement mantle.

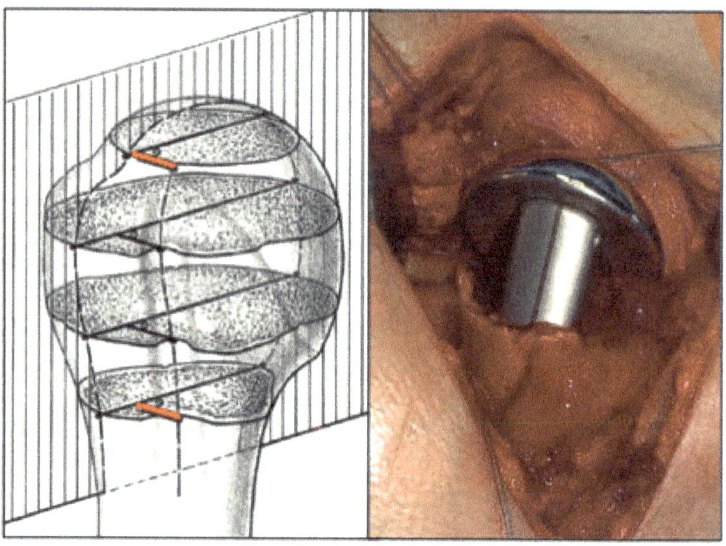

**Figure 6.** The equatorial plane of the humeral head bisects the edge of the articular cartilage adjacent the rotator cuff at a point approximately 8mm posterior to the deepest point of the bicipical groove (A); This is also true in the metaphyseal region and can be used to orient the trial stem into the proper retrotorsion. When the laser etch on the back of the stem is 8mm posterior to the bicipital groove on the proximal aspect of the humeral shaft, the retrotorsion should measure roughly 25-30 degrees relative to the forearm axis (B).

The Eccenter is then placed on the trial stem followed by the trial humeral head. The 2.5 mm hex driver is used to dial the Eccenter with respect to the stem while the head can be manually rotated on the Eccenter. The combined dual eccentricity of this design allows the head to be placed in an infinite number of antero-posterior (AP) and medio-lateral (ML) offset positions within a 6mm orbit (Figure 7A). More importantly it allows independent adjustment of the medial and posterior offset to more accurately restore the patient's native anatomy and center of rotation. Optimal medial offset is achieved by recreating the medial calcar line without step off (Figure 7B). In the AP plane, slight posterior offset is desirable to accommodate the larger greater tuberosity and restore native posterior offset of the humeral head relative to the humeral medullary canal. Once the head position has been chosen, the head and Eccenter can be locked using the 2.0 mm hex driver. The trial prosthesis is then reduced into the joint to confirm a congruent stable fit with the glenoid. After the offset number of the head is recorded, the head is removed and the offset letter of the Eccenter is then recorded so that the construct can be replicated with the final components.

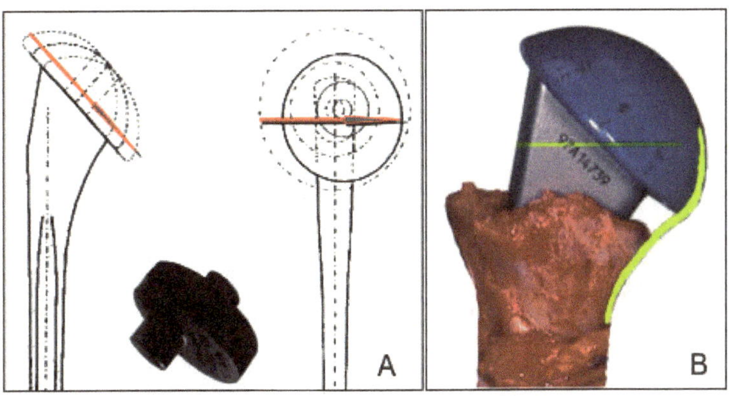


**Figure 7.** The Eccenter in combination with the humeral head provides a dual offset that allows independent adjustment of the medial and posterior offset for optimal head positioning (A); The medial offset should be adjusted to recreate the normal calcar line relative to the humeral shaft (B).

The final component is then assembled using the press and inserted as a monoblock. The diaphyseal portion of the stem is placed into the medullary canal. Prior to fully seating the component, the cables are passed through the medial and lateral holes from posterior to anterior (Figure 8A). The 3 mm retrotorsion bar is then used to cross-check proper rotation and the component is then fully press fit to the pre-determined height.

The prosthesis is then reduced into the glenoid. Two holes are then drilled into the lesser tuberosity fragment using the 2.0 mm drill. These holes should be placed slightly below the bone tendon junction and correspond to positions of the cables exiting the stem. A 14 gauge angiocath can then be inserted from outside to inside through these holes as a transit to shuttle the cables through the bone fragment. Prior to final tuberosity reduction, bone graft from the humeral head is packed around the stem to fill any voids and augment the often fragile cortical sleeve of the tuberosity fragments. A #2 non-absorbable suture is next used to reapproximate the longitudinal SS split. This aids in fine tuning the tuberosity reduction.

Care must be taken not to over-reduce the tuberosities especially distally. Rather than being pulled down and fixed to the humeral shaft with vertical sutures, the tuberosities should be pushed up to restore the native position of the superior rotator cuff insertion relative to the edge of the prosthetic head. Once this position has been optimized, the tuberosities can be securely fixed with horizontal cable cerclage (Figure 8B).

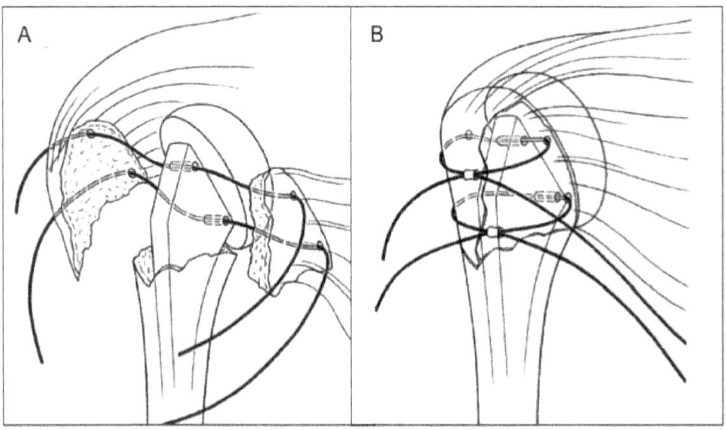


**Figure 8.** The cables should be passed through the prosthesis from back to front before final prosthesis seating. After holes are drilled into the lesser tuberosity fragment, these cables are then passed from inside to outside through the lesser fragment (A). Once the joint is reduced and the tuberosities situated to recreate the proper head-tuberosity relationship, the cables can be tightened and crimped to effect a horizonal cerclage directly to the prosthesis (B).

Both ends of each cable are threaded through their respective crimps, which are positioned over the bicipital groove. The cables are then spaced superiorly and inferiorly on the tuberosities. The superior cable must be placed below the bone tendon junction so that it does not subluxate over the humeral head. To tension the beadless cable, the crimp must be stabilized on one side by either a hemostat or by the accessory locking portion of the Synthes tensioner. The tensioner is then placed on the opposite side and tensioned until a firm embrace is achieved (roughly 20-30 kg). Overtensioning should be avoided so to prevent deforming or crushing the fragile bone and to avoid devascularization. After crimping and cutting the cables to length, the biceps tendon can be used to cover the crimps by a soft tissue tenodesis to the cuff.

Further tuberosity fixation is not necessary and usually only promotes overreduction and 7
devascularization. A single vertical suture, however, can be passed from the shaft around

the superior cable to prevent it from slipping over the head. After copious irrigation, the wound is closed in layers over a drain, followed by a sterile compressive dressing and sling. Postoperative radiographs are obtained in the recovery room to confirm an optimal reconstruction (Figure 9).

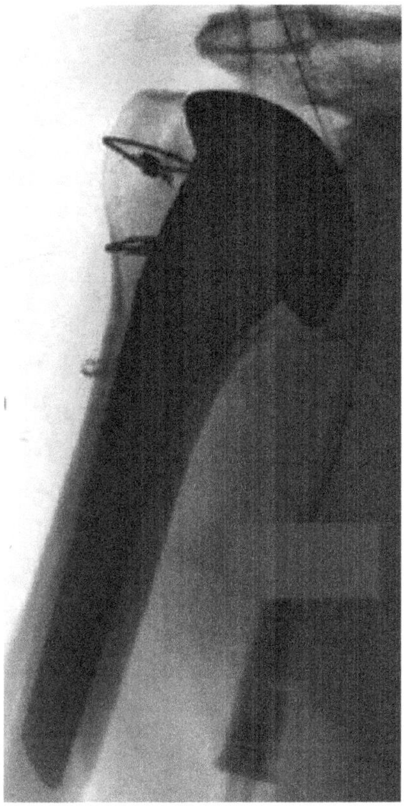

**Figure 9.** Postoperative AP film showing stable tuberosity reduction with anatomical reconstruction of the calcar line, head height and tuberosity height and offset.

## 6. Postoperative protocol

Active use of the arm is avoided for 6 weeks to allow tuberosity healing but passive motion exercises must be started early to maximize postoperative function. Although some advocate no passive motion for several weeks, stiffness remains a significant problem that limits the final outcome of these procedures. Because dense adhesions form in the subacromial space and humeroscapular motion interface, nonoperative and operative treatment of post-surgical adhesive capsulitis in the presence of prosthesis is a substantial challenge that is often marginal in its success. Codman's exercises and positional exercises such as gentle table slides or resting the arm in an abducted position can be started as soon as patients are comfortable. Patients are instructed to steadily increase their passive range on a self-directed basis. Formal physical therapy is often avoided in the early stages to prevent overly aggressive applied stress that might jeopardize tuberosity fixation.

Serial x-rays and clinical status are checked at approximately 2, 4 and 8 weeks postoperatively. Active-assisted range of motion can be added around 6 weeks assuming stable tuberosity fixation. Progressive active range of motion and active use can be started at 8 weeks based on radiographic evidence of tuberosity healing and patient compliance.

## 7. Discussion

Prosthetic replacement for the fractured proximal humerus follows the same biological and mechanical principles that have evolved from experience in fracture fixation in other areas. Surgeons should approach this case with the same tenets and goals as any fracture case and not abandon these principles given the insertion of a prosthesis. Preservation of soft tissue and periosteal attachments is critical to maintaining blood supply to the fracture fragments. Preservation of the endosteal blood supply and avoidance of suture strangulation are also important. Finally, fixation must be sufficiently rigid to reduce micromotion to a level that permits fracture healing. The use of horizontal cable cerclage for tuberosity fixation using the above-described technique in combination with a press-fit, porous humeral stem addresses each of these critical elements to optimize the chance for successful healing in these difficult cases.

Nils et al performed a meta-analysis of fracture hemiarthroplasty outcomes. Although the quality of existing reports was deemed to be insufficient to make formal recommendations about the role of hemiarthroplasty in the fracture setting, the authors did note that "tuberosity healing has influenced functional outcome in all series mentioning this parameter."[7] Boileau et al followed 66 patients after hemiarthroplasty for fracture and found tuberosity malposition and migration in 50% of cases leading to unsatisfactory results including superior migration, stiffness, weakness and pain.[1] Greiner and associated found that tuberosity malposition correlates with the development of fatty infiltration of the cuff muscles and this occurrence was significantly associated with poorer clinical outcomes in patients after hemiarthroplasty for fracture.[11] Huffman and colleagues studied the biomechanics of tuberosity malposition in 4-part fractures and determined that inferior placement (tuberosity overreduction) has a significant negative impact on the mechanical advantage of the deltoid during shoulder abduction.[5]

Taken together, these reports demonstrate that complications related to failure of tuberosity reduction and fixation are frequent, have a negative impact on normal shoulder kinematics, and result in inferior outcomes for pain and function. This fact has remained true despite advances in the development of fracture-specific prostheses, improved suture material and purportedly improved suture constructs. Borowsky and colleagues recently reported on failure modes of suture repair and found that tuberosity migration occurs early and in many cases was over 1 centimeter.[2] Given the frequency of clinical reports of tuberosity migration, it seems clear that currently accepted methods of suture repair fail to achieve a biological and mechanical environment that is suitable for bone healing, particularly in osteoporotic bone. Cable cerclage on the other hand has 4.8 times the circular embracing strength of conventional suture material and does not succumb to creep as suture material is proven to do.[12] Cables also have a prone track record in fracture fixation in long bones, such as periprosthetic fractures, and in fixation of trochanteric osteotomy in revision hip arthroplasty. Thus, their application to tuberosity fixation has a solid mechanical and clinical foundation.[13] Krause et al retrospectively compared cable fixation to nonabsorbable suture fixation and found that consistently better radiographic and functional results were achieved when cables were used with the Epoca stem. [12]

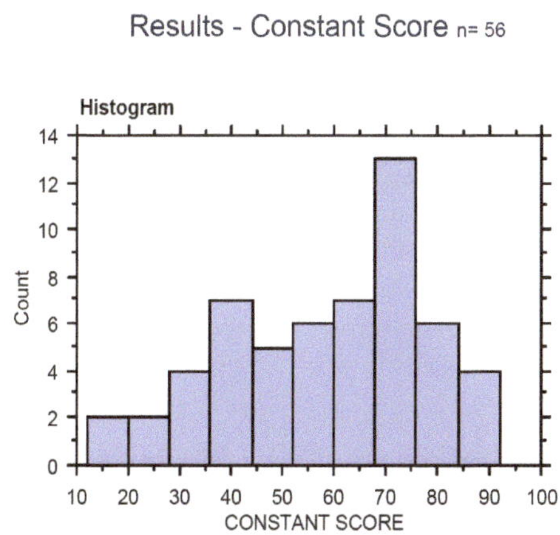


**Figure 10.** Histogram of Constant Scores in a consecutive series of 56 patients s/p fracture hemiarthroplasty with cable cerclage

The technique described above has been refined through Prof. Ralph Hertel's extensive use of this prosthesis in the fracture setting. Between 1997 and 2002, 60 patients were followed prospectively following humeral hemiarthroplasty for fracture.(R Hertel, unpublished data) The mean age was 68 years (range 39 – 88 years) and there were 26 males and 34 females. Four patients were lost to follow-up leaving 56 patients available for review with an average follow-up interval of 40 months (range 12 – 92 months). Successful tuberosity healing was achieved in 49 patients with displacement or resorption in 7 patients. Five patients underwent an additional operation to refix the tuberosities. A total of 31 patients achieved active forward elevation above 120 degrees. The histogram in Figure 10 demonstrates the range of Constant Scores in this series of patients. These results, while not as favorable as those achieved in arthroplasty for degenerative joint disease, do demonstrate that relatively robust shoulder function can be restored by hemiarthroplasty given tuberosity healing and successful patient rehabilitation. Stiffness remains a problem with neither an optimal preventative strategy nor a reliably effective treatment.

## 8. Technique for the reverse prosthesis

There is growing interest in fracture reconstruction using a reverse prosthesis which may afford better active elevation in cases where tuberosity healing is unpredictable and will potentially be unsuccessful. Even in these cases, however, the surgeon should attempt to achieve stable tuberosity fixation to improve the possibility for rotational movement which aids in positioning the hand in space. Specifically, if active external rotation can be achieved through reattachment of the greater tuberosity, patients may achieve greatly improved the functional outcomes with a reverse arthroplasty.

Similar to primary shoulder arthroplasty, fracture specific systems are now available to address this reverse arthroplasty for fracture. As with primary systems, however, their design does not guarantee successful tuberosity fixation and the principles outlined above still apply to reconstruction with a reverse prosthesis. In addition to the importance of sound technique which preserves the optimal biological conditions for fracture healing, tuberosity fixation with horizontal cable cerclage can also be used to achieve a stable reconstruction with a reverse prosthesis. In such cases, the technical steps are essentially identical to those outlined for primary fracture hemiarthroplasty. Figure 11 demonstrates cable cerclage of the tuberosities in a fracture reconstruction using a reverse prosthesis.

As the indication of reverse shoulder arthroplasty for fracture and fracture sequel has gained more traction and as experience with this technique has grown, clinical studies are now available to report on the outcomes of this procedure including comparative studies with conventional hemiarthroplasty. Boyle and colleagues compared 313 fracture hemiarthroplasty patients to 55 fracture reverse patients and found that Oxford Shoulder Scores at 5 years postoperatively were superior in the reverse group.[14] Young et al, however, we unable to realize any gains in range of motion, American Shoulder and Elbow Surgeons Score or Oxford Shoulder Score in patient who underwent a reverse reconstruction compared to those who underwent hemiarthroplasty for fracture cases.[15] Cazeneuve et al reported on 35 patients who underwent reverse reconstruction for fracture or fracture dislocation.[16] Complications including neurological injury, infection, instability and progressive scapular notching led to a complication rate of 24% and stiffness was noted to be a functionally limiting problem. Bufquin et al also reported stiffness with mean active elevation of only 97 degrees and mean active external rotation of only 30 degrees.[17] Tuberosity migration also occurred in 53% of cases. Lenarz and colleagues reported on 30 patients status post reverse arthroplasty for fracture and mean achieved active elevation of 139 degrees and mean active external rotation of 27 degrees with a 10% complications rate.[18]

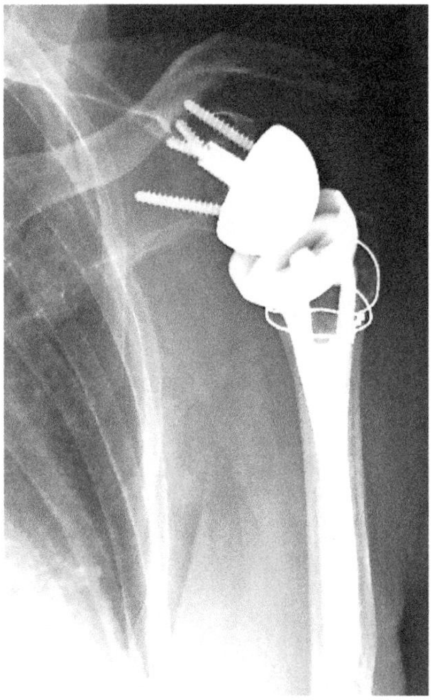

**Figure 11.** AP view showing horizontal cable cerclage tuberosity fixation in reverse arthroplasty for fracture.

Collectively these early outcomes are somewhat sobering relative to the anticipated advantages that reverse shoulder replacement might achieve in fracture cases. They prove the complexity of these cases and the challenges they present to the shoulder reconstruction surgeon. As design modifications continue to improve reverse systems and as experience with reverse arthroplasty in the fracture setting increases, surgeons can hopefully look forward to future advancements in our ability to provide improved function restoration in these difficult cases. Nevertheless, strict adherence to surgical techniques that preserve the biology of fracture healing, that maximize stability of fragment fixation and that permit early rehabilitation to encourage recovery of function are all critical regardless of the theoretical merits of any specific system in terms of biomechanics and design.

## Acknowledgements

The concepts and techniques put forth in this manuscript represent the work of Professor Ralph Hertel, Department of Orthopaedics, Lindenhofspital, Berne Switzerland. He is the principle clinical design surgeon of the EPOCA prosthesis.

## Author details

Moby Parsons

Address all correspondence to: impiv@comcast.net

Seacoast Orthopedics & Sports Medicine, Somersworth, NH, USA

## References

[1] Antuna, S. A., J. W. Sperling, and R. H. Cofield. 2008. Shoulder hemiarthroplasty for acute fractures of the proximal humerus: a minimum five-year follow-up. J Shoulder Elbow Surg 17:202-209.

[2] Berend, K. R., A. V. J. Lombardi, T. H. Mallory, D. J. Chonko, K. L. Dodds, and J. B. Adams. 2004. Cerclage wires or cables for the management of intraoperative fracture associated with a cementless, tapered femoral prosthesis: results at 2 to 16 years. J Arthroplasty 19:17-21.

[3] Boileau, P., S. G. Krishnan, L. Tinsi, G. Walch, J. S. Coste, and D. Mole. 2002. Tuberosity malposition and migration: reasons for poor outcomes after hemiarthroplasty for displaced fractures of the proximal humerus. J Shoulder Elbow Surg 11:401-412.

[4] Borowsky, K., V. Raghuprasad, L. Wear, T. Stevenson, N. Marsden, N. Trent, and A. Bennett. 2010. Failure modes of suture repair of the tuberosities in hemiarthroplasty for four part fracture of the shoulder. 11th International Congress of Shoulder and Elbow Surgery 59.

[5] Boyle, M. J., S. M. Youn, C. M. Frampton, and C. M. Ball. 2012. Functional outcomes of reverse shoulder arthroplasty compared with hemiarthroplasty for acute proximal humeral fractures. J Shoulder Elbow Surg

[6] Bufquin, T., A. Hersan, L. Hubert, and P. Massin. 2007. Reverse shoulder arthroplasty for the treatment of three- and four-part fractures of the proximal humerus in the elderly: a prospective review of 43 cases with a short-term follow-up. J Bone Joint Surg Br 89:516-520.

[7] Cazeneuve, J. F., and D. J. Cristofari. 2010. The reverse shoulder prosthesis in the treatment of fractures of the proximal humerus in the elderly. J Bone Joint Surg Br 92:535-539.

[8] Cazeneuve, J. F., and D. J. Cristofari. 2011. Long term functional outcome following reverse shoulder arthroplasty in the elderly. OrthopTraumatolSurg Res 97:583-589.

[9] Compito, C. A., E. B. Self, and L. U. Bigliani. 1994. Arthroplasty and acute shoulder trauma. Reasons for success and failure. ClinOrthopRelat Res 27-36.

[10] Demirhan, M., O. Kilicoglu, L. Altinel, L. Eralp, and Y. Akalin. 2003. Prognostic factors in prosthetic replacement for acute proximal humerus fractures. J Orthop Trauma 17:181-8; discussion 188-9.

[11] Dimakopoulos, P., N. Potamitis, and E. Lambiris. 1997. Hemiarthroplasty in the treatment of comminuted intraarticular fractures of the proximal humerus. ClinOrthopRelat Res 7-11.

[12] Goldman, R. T., K. J. Koval, F. Cuomo, M. A. Gallagher, and J. D. Zuckerman. 1995. Functional outcome after humeral head replacement for acute three- and four-part proximal humeral fractures. J Shoulder Elbow Surg 4:81-86.

[13] Greiner, S. H., G. Diederichs, I. Kroning, M. Scheibel, and C. Perka. 2009. Tuberosity position correlates with fatty infiltration of the rotator cuff after hemiarthroplasty for proximal humeral fractures. J Shoulder Elbow Surg 18:431-436.

[14] Hawkins, R. J., and P. Switlyk. 1993. Acute prosthetic replacement for severe fractures of the proximal humerus. ClinOrthopRelat Res 156-160.

[15] Hertel, R., U. Knothe, and F. T. Ballmer. 2002. Geometry of the proximal humerus and implications for prosthetic design. J Shoulder Elbow Surg 11:331-338.

[16] Huffman, G. R., J. M. Itamura, M. H. McGarry, L. Duong, J. Gililland, J. E. Tibone, and T. Q. Lee. 2008. Neer Award 2006: Biomechanical assessment of inferior tuberosity placement during hemiarthroplasty for four-part proximal humeral fractures. J Shoulder Elbow Surg 17:189-196.

[17] Krause, F. G., L. Huebschle, and R. Hertel. 2007. Reattachment of the tuberosities with cable wires and bone graft in hemiarthroplasties done for proximal humeral fractures with cable wire and bone graft: 58 patients with a 22-month minimum follow-up. J Orthop Trauma 21:682-686.

[18] Lenarz, C., Y. Shishani, C. McCrum, R. J. Nowinski, T. B. Edwards, and R. Gobezie. 2011. Is reverse shoulder arthroplasty appropriate for the treatment of fractures in the older patient? Early observations. ClinOrthopRelat Res 469:3324-3331.

[19] Lervick, G. N., R. M. Carroll, and W. N. Levine. 2003. Complications after hemiarthroplasty for fractures of the proximal humerus. Instr Course Lect 52:3-12.

[20] Loebenberg, M. I., D. A. Jones, and J. D. Zuckerman. 2005. The effect of greater tuberosity placement on active range of motion after hemiarthroplasty for acute fractures of the proximal humerus. Bull HospJt Dis 62:90-93.

[21] Mighell, M. A., G. P. Kolm, C. A. Collinge, and M. A. Frankle. 2003. Outcomes of hemiarthroplasty for fractures of the proximal humerus. J Shoulder Elbow Surg 12:569-577.

[22] Nijs, S., and P. Broos. 2009. Outcome of shoulder hemiarthroplasty in acute proximal humeral fractures: a frustrating meta-analysis experience. ActaOrthopBelg 75:445-451.

[23] Park, M. S., Y. K. Lee, K. H. Yang, and S. J. Shin. 2003. Management of periprosthetic femoral fractures. J Arthroplasty 18:903-906.

[24] Plausinis, D., Y. W. Kwon, and J. D. Zuckerman. 2005. Complications of humeral head replacement for proximal humeral fractures. Instr Course Lect 54:371-380.

[25] Reuther, F., B. Muhlhausler, D. Wahl, and S. Nijs. 2010. Functional outcome of shoulder hemiarthroplasty for fractures: A multicentre analysis. Injury 41:606-612.

[26] Robinson, C. M., R. S. Page, R. M. Hill, D. L. Sanders, C. M. Court-Brown, and A. E. Wakefield. 2003. Primary hemiarthroplasty for treatment of proximal humeral fractures. J Bone Joint Surg Am 85-A:1215-1223.

[27] Shah, N., H. J. Iqbal, S. Brookes-Fazakerley, and C. Sinopidis. 2010. Shoulder hemiarthroplasty for the treatment of three and four part fractures of the proximal humerus using Comprehensive(R) Fracture stem. IntOrthop

[28] Smith, A. M., R. M. Mardones, J. W. Sperling, and R. H. Cofield. 2007. Early complications of operatively treated proximal humeral fractures. J Shoulder Elbow Surg 16:14-24.

[29] Stiehl, J. B. 2006. Extended osteotomy for periprosthetic femoral fractures in total hip arthroplasty. Am J Orthop (Belle Mead NJ) 35:20-23.

[30] Voos, J. E., J. S. Dines, and D. M. Dines. 2010. Arthroplasty for fractures of the proximal part of the humerus. J Bone Joint Surg Am 92:1560-1567.

[31] Wretenberg, P., and A. Ekelund. 1997. Acute hemiarthroplasty after proximal humerus fracture in old patients. A retrospective evaluation of 18 patients followed for 2-7 years. ActaOrthopScand 68:121-123.

[32] Young, S. W., B. S. Segal, P. C. Turner, and P. C. Poon. 2010. Comparison of functional outcomes of reverse shoulder arthroplasty versus hemiarthroplasty in the primary treatment of acute proximal humerus fracture. ANZ J Surg 80:789-793.

[33] Zyto, K., M. Kronberg, and L. A. Brostrom. 1995. Shoulder function after displaced 5
fractures of the proximal humerus. J Shoulder Elbow Surg 4:331-336.

Chapter 10

# The Evolution of Modern Total Knee Prostheses

Eun-Kyoo Song, Jong-Keun Seon,
Jae-Young Moon and Yim Ji-Hyoun

Additional information is available at the end of the chapter

## 1. Introduction

Many types of prosthesis are used for total knee arthroplasty, and the evolution of knee arthroplasty, which has a history of almost 40 years, involves repetitious cycles of failure and development. During its early stage (1970-1974), instruments of the unicondylar, duocondylar, or hinged types were used, but these were eventually abandoned due to low success rates. A replacement for the total condylar type was successfully developed and became the model for total knee arthroplasty. Recently, unicondylar arthroplasty has produced good results in selected patients, and arthroplasty of the constrained or hinged type have been proven useful for revision surgery or combined surgery, respectively. To solve the problem of the fixed bearing joint, a mobile bearing joint has been developed, and non-cemented fixed knee arthroplasty is receiving renewed attention. Much effort is being expended on the developments of new materials, such as, ceramics and cross-linked polyethylene, on new designs that maximize function and endurance, and on minimally invasive surgery.

## 2. History of the evolution of total knee arthroplasty

### 2.1. Interposition and resurfacing knee arthroplasty

During the late 19th and early 20th century, interposition arthroplasty was attempted using soft tissues. In 1860, Verneuil proposed interposition arthroplasty, involving the insertion of soft tissue to reconstruct the joint surface. Since then, pig bladder, nylon, femoral sheath, anterior bursa of the knee, cellophane, and many other materials have been used, but results have been disappointing. The use of metallic interposition arthroplasty began in the late 1930s. Having obtained successful results for mold arthroplasty in the hip joint, Campbell and Smith-Peterson proposed metal femoral mold arthroplasty[2], and McKeever and MacIntosh proposed hemiarthroplasty of the tibia, but all produced unsatisfactory results in terms of minimizing pain, and high rate of failures of the interposition [3], and thus, these procedures were not widely recognized.

Ferguson [1] attempted resection arthroplasty for ankylosis or severe deformity caused by tuberculosis or infection. This procedure involved resecting cartilage from the knee joint and allowing knee joint movement along the subchondral surface. When too little bone was removed, knees spontaneously fused, and when more bone was removed, knee had good motion but poor stability. Accordingly, these operations were attempted in only the most severe cases because their results were poor.

### 2.2. The hinged prosthesis

In the 1950s, Walldius [4] developed a hinged prosthesis that replaced the joint surfaces of the femur and tibia, as subsequently, modifications of the basic hinged prosthesis design were made by many surgeons. The hinged prosthesis allows the intramedullary stem to align with the artificial knee joint by itself, and is technically easy to perform since all ligaments and soft tissues can be removed due to the mechanical and structural stability of the prosthesis. During the 1950s and 1960s, hinged total knee arthroplasty provided satisfactory results for a longer period of time in more patients than any other knee arthroplasty design used. However, this method could not be widely used since this type of simple hinged prosthesis cannot replace the complex movements of the knee joint and because of a high failure rate due to early loosening caused by overloading the prosthesis and bone contact surface or by infection.

### 2.3. The bicompartmental prosthesis

In 1971, Gunston [5] developed polycentric knee arthroplasty. This was done by adopting the concepts of low friction hip arthroplasty espoused by Charnley. Gunston's knee arthroplasty retained the collateral and cruciate ligaments to help absorb stress, and consisted of relatively flat tibial interposition of high-density polyethylene and a round femoral prosthesis, which replaced the posterior portion of femoral condyles. These components were fixed to bones with bone cement, and replaced the complex movements of 'femoral roll-back'. Polycentric knee arthroplasty was initially successful due to improved mobility and movement range, but the fixation it provided was not sufficient.

Geomedic knee arthroplasty was introduced by Coventry et al. at the Mayo Clinic in 1972[6], and consisted of a polyethylene tibial instrument which was of one structure and was in joint with the femoral condyles. This design was initially devised to sustain the cruciate ligament, but joint mobility was limited because of pathologic posterior cruciate ligament in some cases. The main limitation of this design was rapid and excessive loosening.

Freeman et al.[7] at Imperial College Hospital (London) designed a femoral and tibial prosthesis to work in a 'roller-in-trough' manner by the strength of collateral ligament. The anterior and posterior cruciate ligaments were usually removed, and the tibial prosthesis did not have an intramedullary stem to minimize the risk of infection and to maximize knee joint function for salvage procedures. However, the loosening of the tibial prosthesis became a major drawback.

In the mid 1970s, duocondylar interposition was designed to resemble the anatomic structure of the knee joint [8]. The femoral prosthesis connected with two unicondylar prostheses via an anterior bridge, and formed a joint, which was considerable wider than previous polycentric knee arthroplasties, with two flat tibial instruments. However, the design had the drawbacks of frequent destruction or deformity of the tibial prosthesis.

### 2.4. The tricompartmental prosthesis

In the early 1970s, three types of condylar prostheses were developed, which opened the era of modern knee arthroplasty. First, in 1976, Ranawart et al. [8] at the Hospital for Special Surgery, developed the duocondylar prosthesis; second, Coventry et al.[6] developed the geometric prosthesis; and third, Townley [9] developed the anatomic prosthesis. The condylar prosthesis developed by Ranawart et al. preserved the anterior and posterior cruciate ligaments, provided stability of the knee joint, and used bone cement for fixation to bone. However, the geometric and anatomic types were not produced continuously due to early loosening of fixation. The duocondylar type was further developed to produce the first total condylar prosthesis with a tibial stem by Walker et al. in 1976 [10] at the Hospital for Special Surgery and became the early model for today's posterior cruciate ligament substitution knee arthroplasty. The total condylar prosthesis is a design that removes anterior and posterior cruciate ligaments. The femoral prosthesis, which is made of chrome cobalt, has a symmetric femur with a double curve, which has a flat patellar trochlear groove. The tibial prosthesis is completely made of polyethylene, has good conformity in the flexion and extension states, has anterior and posterior lips in the tibial joint surface, and has eminence in the mid joint surface which provides anteroposterior and mediolateral stability. There is also a stem in the tibial prosthesis, which can endure asymmetric loading. The patellar prosthesis is of the half-ball type and is completely made of polyethylene, with a fixation lug in the middle, which is fixed with bone cement. The features of this early total condylar knee are used in most of today's prostheses. Along with these total condylar prostheses, the duopatellar prosthesis was developed, which preserves the posterior cruciate ligament. This prosthesis is anatomically similar to the normal knee joint with respect to the femoral prosthesis trochlear groove, and forms a joint with a polyethylene patellar prosthesis. The early tibial prosthesis model could be separated into medial and lateral parts, but later a form communicating the bilateral parts was developed. The duopatellar prosthesis was developed into the kinematic condylar prosthesis, which was widely used in the 1980s[11]. Early total condylar prostheses did not allow roll-back in the flexed position and the tibial portion was located posteriorly, which reduced the mobility range when the flexion gap was not balanced. According to early clinical reports, the average mobile angle was 90-100 degrees. To solve this problem, Insall et al. [12] added a cam to the femoral prosthesis and a post to the tibial prosthesis for posterior cruciate ligament substitution knee arthroplasty to accelerate the posterior location of the femoral prosthesis when flexed at about 70 degrees, thus enhancing flexion. These Insall-Burnstein and kinematic interpositions became the foundation of modern knee arthroplasty. Despite the developments of modern joint replacement designs, complications of the femoro-patellar joint were frequent after knee arthroplasty in the 1980s and 1990s, which led to the development of today's knee arthroplasty which increases contact surface in the femoro-patellar joint and prevents lateral displacement of patellar bone.

## 2.5. Unicompartmental knee arthroplasty

Although it has been used since its introduction in 1950s, the results of unicompartmental knee arthroplasty (Figure 1) remain controversial. In the early 1970s, several authors reported unsatisfactory results for unicompartmental knee arthroplasties but over the next decade, better surgical techniques and proper patient selection improved results [13]. Unicompartmental knee arthroplasty can be used in cases with up to moderate arthritis and when diseased is confined to one compartment. Along with Repicci and Eberle's [14] minimally invasive techniques, unicompartmental knee arthroplasty has aroused much interest. As compared with total knee arthroplasty, the unicompartmental knee arthroplasty has the advantage of preserving anterior and posterior cruciate ligaments and of recovering almost the full range of motion of the normal knee joint. It also boasts a small amount of bone loss and theoretically enables easier revision surgery [15]. The recently reported long-term endurance of unicompartmental knee arthroplasty is about 85-95%, which is similar to that of total arthroplasty. Therefore, if patients are properly selected and an adequate technique is used, it may be a good surgical option.

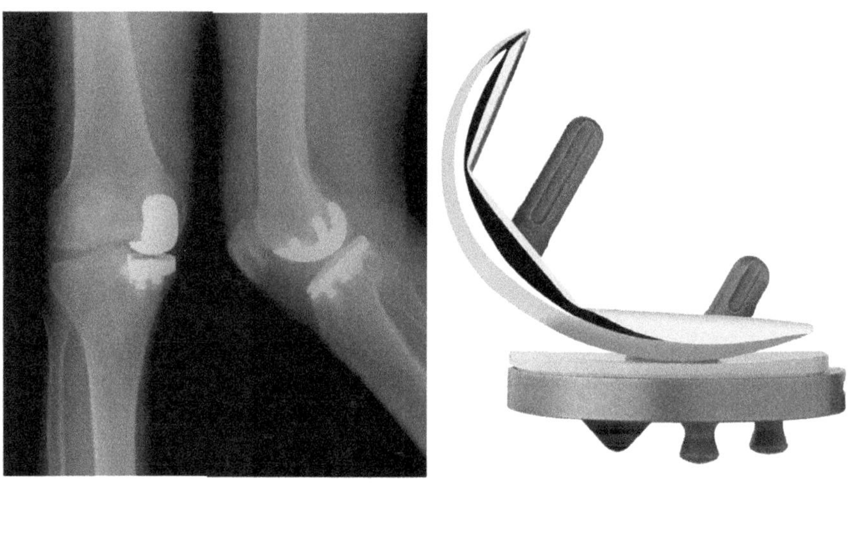

**Figure 1.** Unicompartmental Knee System (Courtesy of Zimmer)

### 2.6. Patellar resurfacing

Patellar resurfacing was described as early as 1955. The first patellar resurfacing materials were metallic components, but this design was limited because of problems concerning metal to cartilage articulation. Subsequently, the polyethylene patellar prosthesis was developed and satisfactory results were obtained. Present day knee arthroplasty became total knee replacement when patellar component was added.

## 3. Spectrum of prosthesis designs

Nowadays, many types of prostheses are used for total knee arthroplasty. However, controversy exists regarding which prostheses are the most appropriate for individual surgeons and specific patients. Therefore, we compare the advantages and disadvantages of each type of interposition knee arthroplasty.

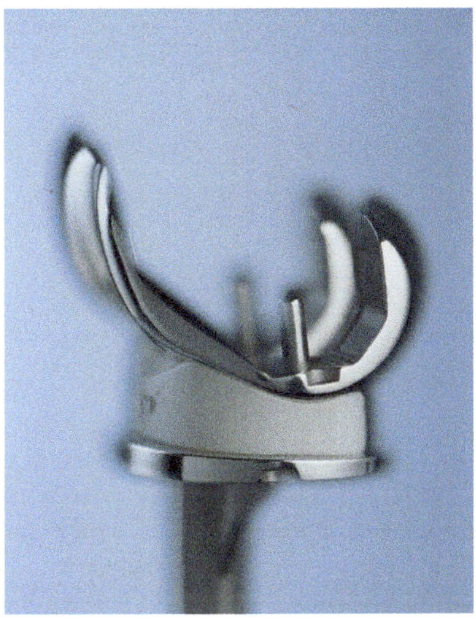

**Figure 2.** Posterior cruciate ligament retention type prosthesis (Courtesy of DePuy)

### 3.1. Posterior cruciate ligament retention versus substitution

All knee arthroplasties require anterior cruciate ligament removal, but retention of the posterior cruciate ligament depends on the type of arthroplasty. The preservation type, in which posterior cruciate ligament is preserved, is considered better than the replacement type for performing functions, such as, climbing stairs, and has the advantage of simplifying revision surgery due to less loss of bone (Figure 2). However, knee joints with degenerative arthritis usually show soft tissue contracture, and when preserving the posterior cruciate ligament, the soft tissue balance is not easy to achieve, which possibly increases the risk of early failure due to polyethylene insert overloading caused by posterior cruciate ligament unbalanced tension [16].

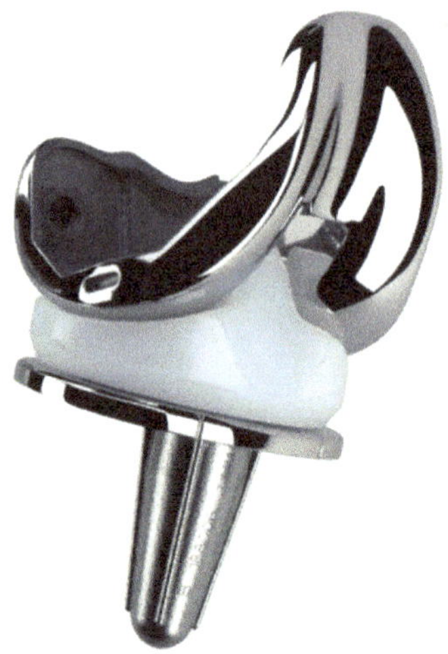

**Figure 3.** Posterior-substitution prosthesis showing that the post-and-cam mechanism offers no restraint to varus or valgus stability (Courtesy of Biomet)

When the posterior cruciate ligament substitution type is used, even degenerative knee joints with relatively severe deformities can achieve ligament balance, and when flexed at 60-70 degrees, the post of the tibial polyethylene contacts the cam of the femoral component and induces posterior placement of femoral bone, which allows relatively satisfactory roll-back and can achieve sufficient knee joint flexion (Figure 3) [17]. However, bone loss at the intercondylar notch makes revision surgery difficult, and fracture may occur intra-operatively or post-operatively in patients with small femurs. From the biomechanical perspective, neither posterior cruciate ligament preservation nor substitution types can totally replace the biomechanics of the normal knee joint. Furthermore, many clinical studies have concluded that there is no significant difference between these two types of prosthesis.

### 3.2. Mobile versus fixed bearing total knee arthroplasty

Traditional fixed bearing knee arthroplasties have produced good clinical results at 10-15 years postoperatively. Unfortunately, problems associated with polyethylene wear can occur in the long-term, especially in young patients. This wear can be reduced by reducing contact stress at the joint surface and by improving the wear characteristics of the material used. Contact stress may be reduced by increasing conformity between the femoral component and the polyethylene insert. The development of mobile-bearing articulating polyethylene surfaces in implants for patients undergoing total knee arthroplasty reflects the efforts made by designers to optimize wear while addressing the complexities of function. However, the trade-off for conformity and free mobile range in fixed bearing knee arthroplasty makes marked improvements in contact stress near impossible. To solve this problem, mobile bearing interposition knee arthroplasty was invented to reduce contact stress but to preserve freedom of movement. In 1986, Goodfellow and O'Connor [18] invented Oxford knee arthroplasty, which is a mobile bearing knee arthroplasty of the bicondylar type (Figure 4), and subsequently, Beuchel and Pappas [19] invented the meniscus sustaining bearing, which boasts low contact stress. However, in the case of the mobile bearing insert, the bearing can be dislocated when flexion extension gaps are inadequate. In Europe, this mobile bearing prosthesis has been used for decades with good clinical results, but recent reports have found no significant differences between this mobile bearing prosthesis and fixed bearing polyethylene.

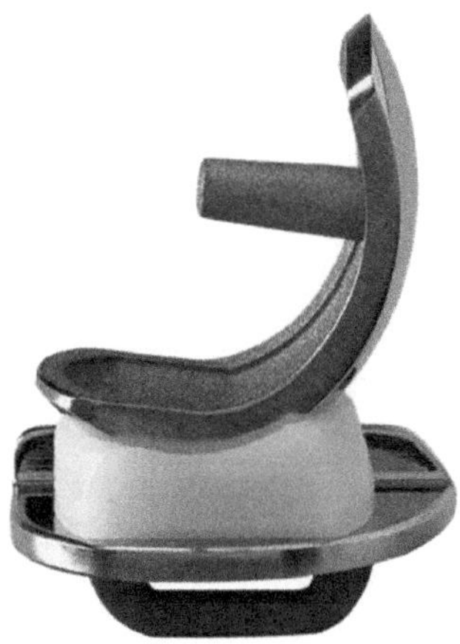

**Figure 4.** Mobile bearing knee prosthesis, which reduces contact stress but preserves freedom of movement (Courtesy of Biomet)

### 3.3. Non-cemented versus cemented knee prostheses

Concern over the long-term tolerance of bone cement fixation led to the development of a non-cemented fixation design in 1980. Hungerford et al. [20] invented the initial porous-coated anatomic design, others include, the Miller-Galante, Miller-GalanteII, Tricon-M, Genesis, and Ortholoc prostheses. These implant designs have a surface topography that is conducive to bone ingrowth. Most are coated or textured so that the new bone actually grows into the surface of the implant. They may also use screws or pegs to stabilize the implant until bone ingrowth occurs. However, because they depend on new bone growth for stability, non-cemented implants require a longer healing time than cemented replacements.

Non-cemented implants, unfortunately, showed higher failure rates than cemented knee arthroplasties due to aseptic loosening and bone loss. In all knee replacement implants, metal rubs against the polyethylene insert, and although the metal is polished and the polyethylene is treated to resist wear, the loads and stresses of daily movements generate microscopic particle debris, which in turn, can trigger inflammatory responses that result in osteolysis or loosening.

Because non-cemented implants have not been used as long as cemented implants, comparisons after long-term use are not possible. However, some studies have shown that non-cemented fixation has success rates comparable to those of cemented fixation [21]. Nevertheless, non-cemented knee arthroplasty has not widely adopted, but recent material developments have resulted in materials that enhance bone ingrowth which has led to the use of non-cemented knee arthroplasty in young patients.

### 3.4. Constrained condylar knee prostheses

Revision total knee arthroplasty is often associated with poorer outcomes due to bone loss and ligament damage, which can result in ligamentous laxity and imbalance. A constrained condylar knee design was developed to resist coronal moments in the plane caused by soft-tissue deficiency. Constrained condylar knee designs have the advantage of allowing changes in the center of rotation during flexion, and thereby, theoretically impart less tangential anterior-posterior stress across the prosthetic interface [22]. An early model of constrained condylar knee design was proposed by Insall et al, although similar to posterior cruciate ligament substitution knee arthroplasty, the polyethylene post is thicker and longer, which provides stability for valgus and varus movements as well as not posterior movements [23]. These early models were developed into Legacy Constrained Condylar Knee (Figure 5)[24]. Excessive constraint is a problem when the LCCK is used and this causes failure by loosening the prosthesis. Thus, in difficult knee arthroplasty cases, usage may be determined during surgery by taking into consideration the need for constraint. For example, in severe valgus knee joints, the LCCK polyethylene insert may be a good candidate, but posterior cruciate substitution tibial bearing is recommended over the constrained type.

### 3.5. Cross-linked polyethylene bearing

The development of arthroplasty design and materials has led to long-term endurance, but the not infrequent need for revision due to polyethylene wear has been a cause of patient dissatisfaction. To reduce polyethylene wear, a cross-linked polyethylene bearing was developed and used in hip replacements in 1990s, and thus, its effectiveness has been proven. Its resistance to wear provides a promising solution for arthroplasty patients, especially today's more active, physically demanding patients. However, in knee arthroplasty, it has neither been widely used nor widely studied. Recently improved resistance in posterior cruciate substitution knees have been reported to lead to cam and post delamination, pitting, cracking or fractures [25].

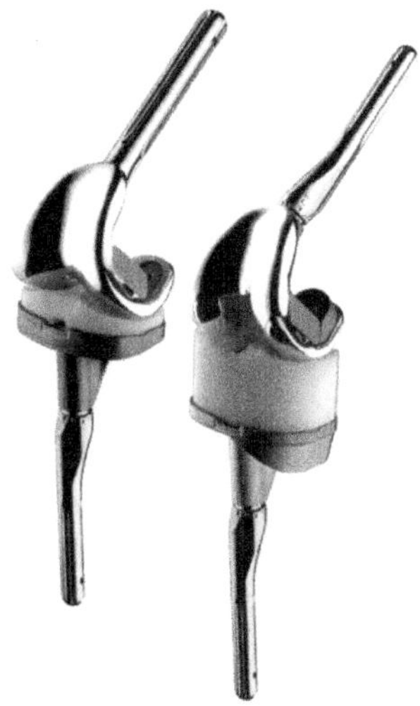

**Figure 5.** The Legacy Constrained Condylar Knee Prosthesis (Courtesy of Zimmer)

### 3.6. High flexion type knee prostheses

Generally, postoperative knee motion range for total knee arthroplasty is less than 120 degrees. Recently, to obtain motion ranges similar to those of the normal knee joint, high flexion femoral prostheses with a thickened posterior portion of femoral prostheis and a wider contact surface with the bearing are being used to reduce contact pressure and wear (Figure 6). To prevent collision between the patellar ligament and bearing at high degrees of flexion, a high flexion bearing with an oblique cutting of the anterior bearing has been developed. Furthermore, many authors have reported that high flexion knee arthroplasty can result in smaller contact loadings and wider ranges of motion than previous knee arthroplasties. For example, Huang et al. [26] found that mean flexion in patients with a high-flexion prosthesis was approximately 10° greater than in patients with a standard posterior stabilized implant. Laskin [27] has also published similar findings. In addition to pain reduction and restoration of function, survivorship is also a decisive contributor to the success of TKA. Thanks to its extended posterior condyle radius, which has been broadened all round, the NexGen CR-Flex system offer a larger contact surface during deep bending, and therefore, spreads contact stress over a large area. However, some authors [28, 29] have reported no increase of flexion when using high-flexion prostheses.

In particular, in a clinical study that used both knee implants, high flexion knee arthroplasty did not show a significant increase in knee joint flexion range. This issue needs to be proven by long-term follow up over 10 to 15 years [30].

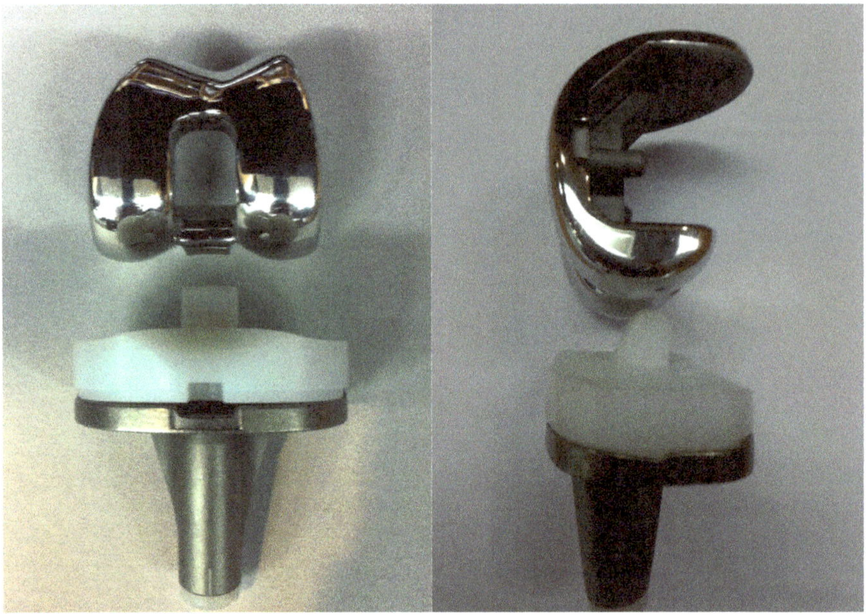

**Figure 6.** High flexion type prosthesis (Courtesy of Zimmer)

### 3.7. Ultracongruent polyethylene bearings

The most important thing to remember when performing posterior cruciate ligament preserving knee arthroplasty is to balance the posterior cruciate ligament and prevent instability by ligament disruption when flexed. For these reasons, deep-dished polyethylene insert (also called ultracongruent insert) was developed. This bearing insert has moderate conformity in coronal and sagittal planes, which can prevent edge loading caused from paradoxical anterior translation due to elevation of the anterior lip of the prosthesis, prevent elevation in flexion, and prevent posterior subluxation (Figure 7). Ultracongruent bearings can reduce cam-and-post wear or fracture that may occur after posterior cruciate ligament substitution knee arthroplasties, and can prevent bone loss at the intercondylar cutting site. This bearing represents a new concept in that it can also maintain the posterior cruciate ligament and provide moderate conformity in total knee arthroplasty. Further long-term clinical follow-up is required along with comparative clinical trials of posterior cruciate ligament preservation, substitution, and sacrificing techniques.

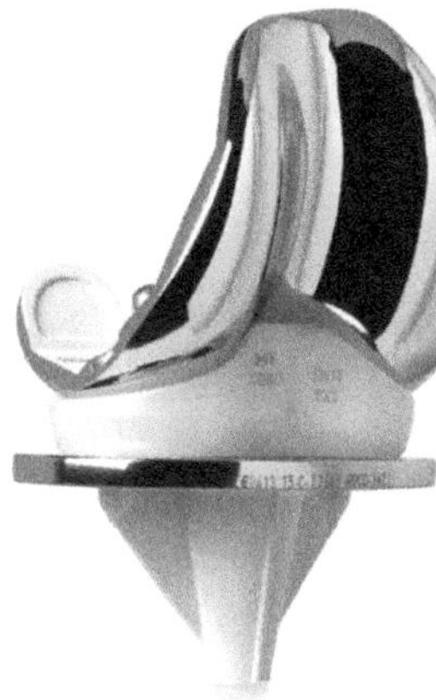

**Figure 7.** Ultracongruent polyethylene bearing (Courtesy of Biomet)

## 4. Conclusion

The history of prostheses evolution follows a repetitive course of development and failure. The continuous and rapid developments of biomechanics and of materials in the 20th century hugely expanded the information available. Furthermore, spectrums of designs are currently being used for total knee arthroplasty.

Most knee replacements are now being performed with PCL-retaining or PCL-substituting prosthesis that have their merits and limitations, as discussed above. New mobile-bearing devices, which address the issue of functional complexity, have been developed and have the potential to prolong implant durability. Nonetheless, prosthesis materials and the historical and current results of different types of prosthesis remain topics of discussion with respect to their indications and contraindications. In the future, the new implant will be developed by applying the pros and removing the cons based on the implant history.

## Author details

Eun-Kyoo Song, Jong-Keun Seon, Jae-Young Moon and Yim Ji-Hyoun

Department of Orthopedic Surgery, Chonnam National University Hwasun Hospital, Hwasun, Korea

## References


[1] Ferguson, W. Excision of the knee joint: recovery with a false joint and a useful limb. Med Times Gaz (1861).

[2] Campbell, W. C. Interposition of vitallium plates in arthroplasties of the knee. Preliminary report. By Willis C. Campbell, (1940). Clin Orthop Relat Res 1988;, 226, 3-5.

[3] MacIntosh DLHemiarthroplasty of the knee using a space occupying prosthesis for painful varus and valgus deformities. J Bone Joint Surg Am (1958).

[4] Walldius, B. Arthroplasty of the knee joint using an endoprosthesis. Acta Orthop Scand (1957). Suppl:19.

[5] Gunston, F. H. Polycentric knee arthroplasty: prosthetic simulation of normal knee movement. J Bone Joint Surg Br (1971). , 53, 272-277.

[6] Coventry, M. B, Finerman, G. A, Riley, L. H, Turner, R. H, & Upshaw, J. E. A new geometric knee for total knee arthroplasty. Clin Orthop Relat Res (1972). , 83, 157-162.

[7] Freeman, M. A, Swanson, S. A, & Todd, R. C. Total replacement of the knee using the Freeman-Swanson knee prosthesis. Clin Orthop Relat Res (1973). , 94, 153-170.

[8] Ranawat, C. S, Insall, J, & Shine, J. Duo-condylar knee arthroplasty: hospital for special surgery design. Clin Orthop Relat Res (1976). , 120, 76-82.

[9] Townley, C. O. The anatomic total knee resurfacing arthroplasty. Clin Orthop Relat Res (1985).

[10] [10] Walker, P. S, Ranawat, C, & Insall, J. Fixation of the tibial components of condylar replacement knee prostheses. J Biomech (1976). , 9, 269-275.

[11] Rand, J. A, Chao, E. Y, & Stauffer, R. N. Kinematic rotating-hinge total knee arthroplasty. J Bone Joint Surg Am (1987). , 69, 489-497.

[12] Insall, J. N, Lachiewicz, P. F, & Burstein, A. H. The posterior stabilized condylar prosthesis: a modification of the total condylar design. Two to four-year clinical experience. J Bone Joint Surg Am (1982). , 64, 1317-1323.

[13] Laskin, R. S. Unicompartmental tibiofemoral resurfacing arthroplasty. J Bone Joint Surg Am (1978). , 60, 182-185.

[14] Repicci, J. A, & Eberle, R. W. Minimally invasive surgical technique for unicondylar knee arthroplasty. J South Orthop Assoc (1999). , 8, 20-27.

[15] Jung, Y. B, & Lee, Y. S. Principles of unicompartmental knee arthroplasty. J Korean Orthop Assoc (2004). , 39, 108-114.

[16] Martin, S. D, Mcmanus, J. L, Scott, R. D, & Thornhill, T. S. Press-fit condylar total knee arthroplasty: 5- to 9-year follow-up evaluation. J Arthroplasty (1997). , 12, 603-614.

[17] Freeman, M. A, & Railton, G. T. Should the posterior cruciate ligament be retained or resected in condylar nonmeniscal knee arthro-plasty? The case for resection. J Arthroplasty (1988). Suppl: SS12., 3.

[18] Goodfellow, J. W, & Connor, O. J. Clinical results of the Oxford knee: surface arthroplasty of the tibiofemoral joint with a meniscal bearing prosthesis. Clin Orthop Relat Res (1986)., 205, 21-42.

[19] Buechel, F. F, & Pappas, M. J. Long-term survivorship analysis of cruciate-sparing versus cruciate-sacrificing knee prostheses using meniscal bearings. Clin Orthop Relat Res (1990)., 260, 162-169.

[20] Hungerford, D. S, Kenna, R. V, & Krackow, K. A. The porous-coated anatomic total knee. Orthop Clin North Am (1982)., 13, 103-122.

[21] Baker, P. N, Khaw, F. M, Kirk, L. M, Esler, C. N, & Gregg, P. J. A randomised controlled trial of cemented versus cementless press-fit condylar total knee replacement: 15-year survival analysis. J Bone Joint Surg Br (2007)., 89, 1608-14.

[22] Kim, Y. H, & Kim, J. S. Revision total knee arthroplasty with use of a constrained condylar knee prosthesis. J Bone Joint Surg Am. (2009)., 91, 1440-7.

[23] Ranawat, C. S, & Sculco, J. P. History of the development of total knee prosthesis at the hospital for special surgery. In: Ranawat CS, editor. Total condylar knee arthroplasty: technique, results, and complications. Berlin: Springer Verlag; (1985)., 3-6.

[24] Easley, M. E, Insall, J. N, Scuderi, G. R, & Bullek, D. D. Primary constrained condylar knee arthroplasty for the arthritic valgus knee. Clin Orthop Relat Res (2000). , 380, 58-64.

[25] Oral, E, Malhi, A. S, Wannomae, K. K, & Muratoglu, O. K. Highly cross-linked ultra-high molecular weight polyethylene with improved fatigue resistance for total joint arthroplasty: recipient of the 2006 Hap Paul Award. J Arthroplasty (2008). , 23, 1037-44.

[26] Huang, H. T, Su, J. Y, & Wang, G. J. The early results of high-flex total knee arthroplasty: a minimum of 2 years of follow-up. J Arthroplasty (2005)., 20, 674-9.

[27] Endres, S, & Wilke, A. Early experience with the NexGen® CR-Flex Mobile knee arthroplasty system: results of year follow-up. Orth Rev (2010)., 2.

[28] Laskin, R. S. The effect of a high-flex implant on postoperative flexion after primary total knee arthroplasty. Orthopedics (2007). Suppl):, 86-8.

[29] Kim, Y. H, Sohn, K. S, & Kim, J. S. Range of motion of standard and highflexion posterior stabilized total knee prostheses: a prospective, randomized study. J Bone Joint Surg Am (2005). A:1470-5., 87.

[30] Endres, S, & Wilke, A. High flexion total knee arthroplasty- mid-term follow up of 5 years. Open Orthop J. (2011)., 14, 138-42.

Chapter 11

# The LP-ESP Lumbar Disc Prosthesis: Concept, Development and Clinical Experience

Jean-Yves Lazennec, Alain Aaron, Adrien Brusson,
Jean Patrick Rakover and Marc Antoine Rousseau

Additional information is available at the end of the chapter

## 1. Introduction

Because of its impairment of patients' personal, social, and professional lives, degenerative disk disease has become an important public health problem with multiple dimensions. The current therapeutic strategy remains controversial and is also a medical and surgical challenge. Conservative treatment, based mostly based on physical therapy, constitutes the first-line approach, but persistent symptomatic disease may be treated surgically in selected patients [1-4]. Lack of pain relief, stiffening of the lumbar spine, non-union, sagittal balance misalignment, bone graft donor site morbidity, and, last but not least, adjacent segment disease are the pitfalls of intervertebral fusion that led to the idea of total disk replacement (TDR) [5-12]. Since 1966 and Fernström's first TDR implantation [13], many designs and concepts have been proposed [14-23]. The devices are usually articulated implants, and their mobility depends on the designs of the bearing surfaces. Ball-and-socket two-piece prostheses have 3 degrees of freedom in every rotation around a single fixed center of rotation. Three-piece devices allow additional translation components, providing 5 degrees of freedom. Articulated TDRs have demonstrated their clinical utility in several patient series. Specifically, the non-inferiority of TDR versus fusion is now generally accepted [18-20, 24]. However, in vitro testing of the two types of implants reveals that both designs have biomechanical advantages and limitations.

Because the healthy human intervertebral disk has a deformable elastic structure with 6 degrees of freedom, elastomeric one-piece intervertebral prostheses might be the most physiological implant for mimicking physiologic levels of shock absorption and flexural stiffness. Designing such a device is challenging, especially when we remember the Acroflex® prostheses: the elastic rubber failed so rapidly in vivo that only 28 were implanted in all [25-26].

The LP-ESP® (lumbar disk prosthesis-elastic spine pad) was developed over a 20-year period. Improvements in technology have made it possible to solve the problem of the bond between the elastic component and the titanium endplates. After successful in vitro and in vivo evaluation, the LP-ESP has been authorized for clinical use in Europe since 2005. The goal of this paper is to present its innovative concept and the clinical results and radiological outcomes over its 7 years of use. In addition to measuring range of motion, we were specifically interested in the quality of the kinematics and thus investigated the mean center of rotation at both the instrumented and adjacent levels. Changes in spinal posture were also a major point of the study.

## 2. Implant design

The design of the LP ESP® prosthesis is based on the principle of the silent block bush (Figure 1). The LP-ESP ® is a one-piece deformable implant including a central core made of silicone gel with microvoids and surrounded by polycarbonate urethane (PCU) securely fixed to titanium endplates. The endplates have five anchoring pegs to provide primary fixation and are covered by a textured T 40 titanium layer (60 μm thick) and hydroxyapatite to improve bone ingrowth (Figure 2).

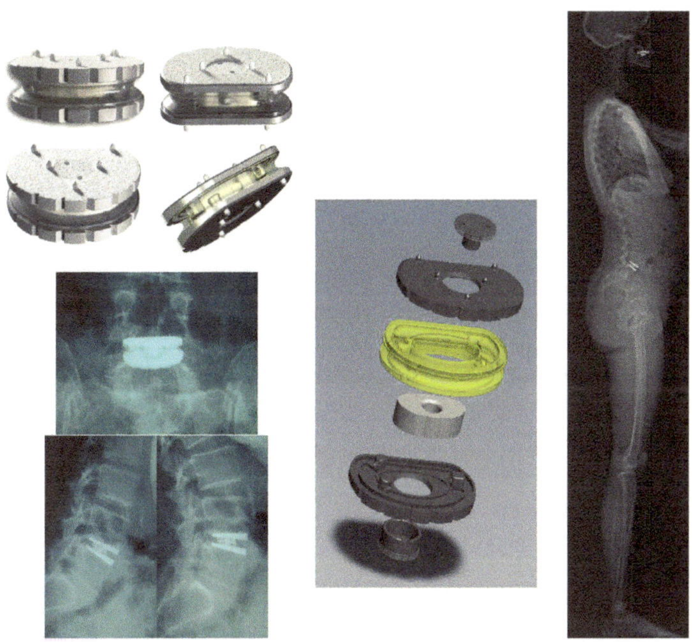

**Figure 1.** The design of the LP ESP® prosthesis is based on the principle of the silent block bush

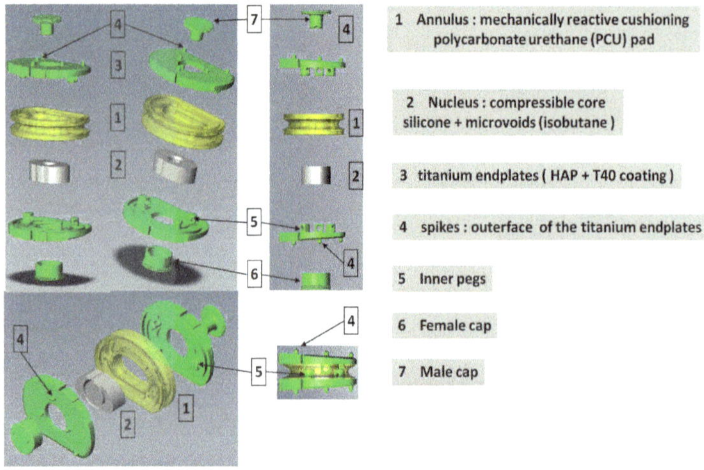


**Figure 2.** The LP-ESP ® is a one-piece deformable implant including a central core made of silicone gel with microvoids and surrounded by polycarbonate urethane (PCU) securely fixed to titanium endplates.

Depending on the size, the titanium endplates differ in thickness and angulation. The prostheses are available in two thicknesses (10 and 12 mm), each with 3 angles of lordosis (7°, 9°, and 11°). Regardless of the model, however, the mechanically active cushion and the mechanical properties of the prosthesis are the same: The differences in thickness of the lordotic angle do not affect the prosthesis's mobility or its cushioning, even shock-absorbing, effect.

Accordingly, the peripheral cushion (that is, the annulus) is securely fixed to the titanium alloy endplates by adhesion-molding technology. This attachment is reinforced by a peripheral groove without the addition of glue. This process of fixation avoids fluid infiltration and the risk of fatigue fractures of the interface, despite the very different mechanical properties of the polymer and the metal endplates. The PCU annulus is stabilized by supplementary pegs located on the internal surface of both metal endplates. The geometry and position of the pegs, between the peripheral groove and the central area of the endplates, were planned to control rotational mobility (Figures 3 and 4 ). The polymer molding was designed to prevent all direct contact between the upper and lower pegs.

The core or nucleus is composed of a compressible silicone structure containing isobutane microbubbles. This core is injected after the annulus surrounding it has been molded. Two titanium caps allow the core to be contained at the moment of the injection. These two pieces are firmly secured to the titanium plates: they also play a mechanical role by their contactless fit, because they contribute to limiting shearing during antero-posterior and medio-lateral translation. The cushioning and compressing effects are obtained on the one hand by the contactless interlocking of the male and female caps and, on the other hand, by crushing the annulus between the two metal plates. The same components limit the shearing effect when the endplates are inclined to the horizontal (Figure 5).

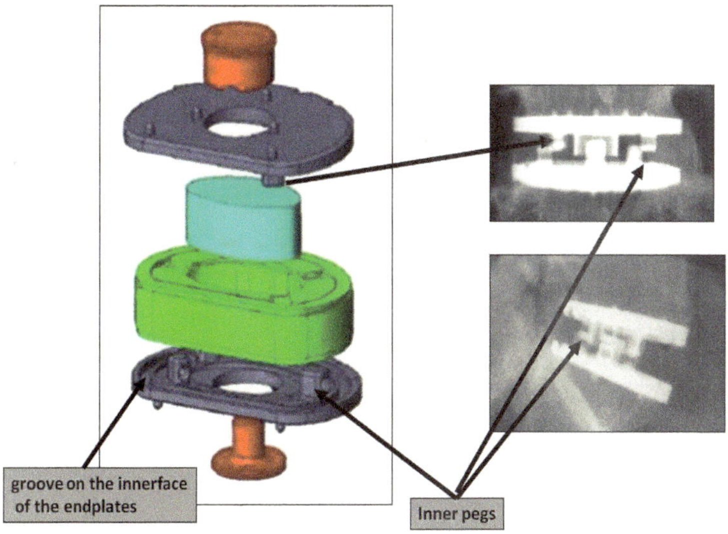


**Figure 3.** The LP-ESP ® is a one-piece deformable implant including a central core made of silicone gel with microvoids and surrounded by polycarbonate urethane (PCU) securely fixed to titanium endplates.

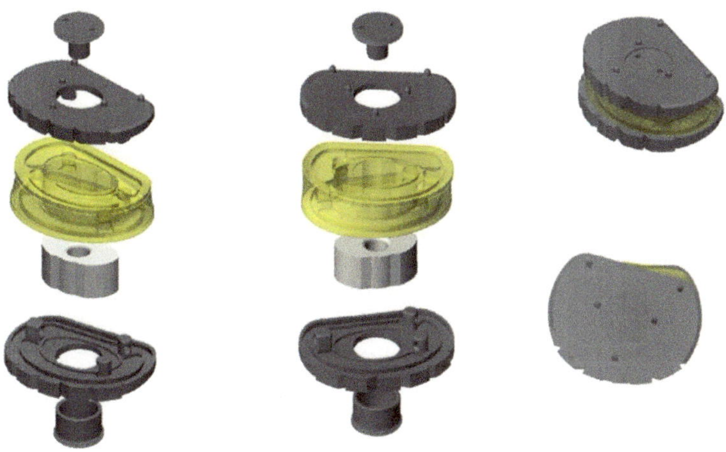

**Figure 4.** The geometry and position of the pegs, between the peripheral groove and the central area of the end-plates, are planned to control rotational mobility

This design and the adhesion-molding technology differentiate the LP ESP prosthesis from other monoelastomeric prostheses, for which the constraints of shearing during rotations or movement are absorbed at the plastic/titanium interface because of the molding technology

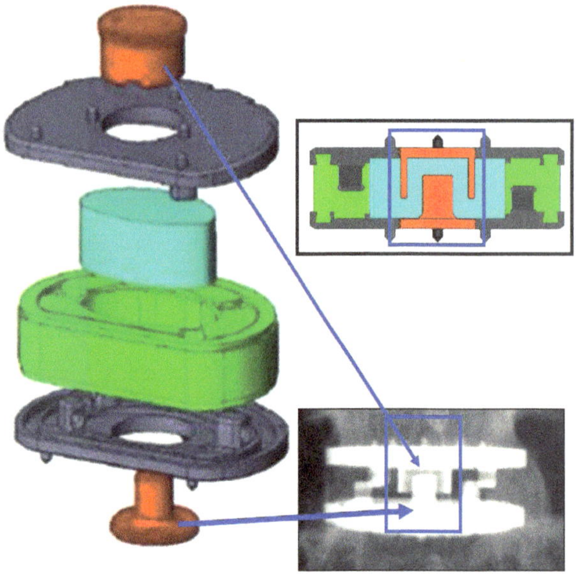

**Figure 5.** The cushioning and compressing effects are obtained on the one hand by the contactless interlocking of the male and female caps and, on the other hand, by crushing the annulus between the two metal plates.

used in their design. The attachment is obtained by the penetration of the polymer through small holes in the endplates. This process creates multiple interfaces and potential fatigue lesions of the anchoring mechanism due to inhomogeneous loading during flexion-extension, lateral inclination, and rotation. Thus, in these designs, the plastic monobloc cushion secured to the titanium plates flows into the space between them during compression, creating an area of friction and wear.

**On the whole, in the LP ESP**, the constraints of the interface between the PCU cushion and its titanium seating are reduced. These are principally constraints of compression:

- between the exterior of the male cap and the interior of the female cap for translations;
- between the pegs for the rotation ;
- between the titanium endplates for flexion.

The principle of the LP ESP® makes it possible to reproduce the anisotropy of the healthy disk, and the design allows modification of the return torque (without modifying the other parameters of the prosthesis. For example:

- bringing the pegs closer together increases stiffness in rotation without modifying either translation or compression;

- diminishing the clearance between the male and female caps increases the stiffness of translation without modifying either rotation or compression;
- modifying the ratio between the small and large diameters of the elliptic form of the cushion changes the ratios of the return torques between flexion/extension and lateral flexion without modifying stiffness in compression or rotation.

## 3. Manufacturing process

The manufacture of this complex implant includes 6 stages, each with its own quality control for each piece:

- Stage 1: Machining titanium (TA6V) plates and male and female caps and 3-dimensional check of each unit.
- Stage 2: Preparation of the annulus made of PCU.
  - Electrochemical treatment of the interior surfaces of the TA6V plates
  - Preparation and quality control of materials including drying PCU granules at 85°C for 4 h to reduce their humidity to less than 0.1%
  - Molding the PCU annulus between the two titanium endplates with a 22-ton vertical injection press (the endplates are pre-positioned in a mold that makes it possible to define the external geometry and to preserve the ovoid-shaped housing of the core).
  - Visual check of each unit, followed by testing compression of the implant without its core.
- Stage 3: Preparation of the core.
  - Placement of the female cap by screwing it in
  - Injection of a silicone-based component through the opening of the male cap
  - Screwing in the male cap as the injection starts
  - Cold polymerization
- Stage 4: Implant checks.
  - dimensional check of each unit,
  - testing rigidity while compressed by an axial load)
  - destructive testing of the first and last pieces of each lot by axial traction of the 2 metal endplates and then visual examination of the polymer parts (annulus and core).
- Stage 5:Two-stage spraying for final preparation of the anchoring endplates:
  - the T40 coating by plasma in a vacuum
  - and the layer of hydroxyapatite by plasma in a controlled atmosphere (inert gas)

Testing is performed as required by the standards:

ASTM F 1185-03 (2009) Standard Specification for Hydroxylapatite Composition for Surgical Implants

ISO 5832-2:1999 Surgical implants-- Metal-based products -- Part 2: Non-alloy titanium

ASTM F 1044: Standard test method for Shear Testing of Calcium Phosphate Coatings and Metallic Coatings

ASTM F 1147: Standard test method for Tension Testing of Calcium Phosphate and Metallic Coatings

ASTM F 1609: Standard Specification for Calcium Phosphate Coating for Implantable Materials.

ISO 13779-1: Hydroxyapatite - Part 1: Hydroxyapatite-based ceramic.

ISO 13779-2: Hydroxyapatite - Part 2: Hydroxyapatite-based coatings.

ISO/CD 13779: Hydroxyapatite - Chemical analysis and characterization of crystallinity and phase purity

- Stage 6: processing in a class 100 clean room workstation
- Stage 7: sterilization by gamma radiation (min: 25 kgray; max: 40 kgray) according to a special validated process

## 4. Design stages

After an initial patent application in 1994 by R. ROY CAMILLE, different avenues of research were explored, with the scientific expertise of the CEA (Commissariat à l'Energie Atomique, Fontenay aux Roses,France) and the industrial expertise of FH Industry for further R & D ( Heimsbrunn, France ).

The preliminary stages involved optimizing the choice of PCU, the development of the attachment of the annulus to the metal endplates without chemical adhesives, the definition of the pegs and caps, and the implementation of reliable techniques for polymer molding and injection.

Biocompatibility tests were performed by BIOMATECH, a subsidiary of NAMSA (Northwood, Ohio, USA).

Human implantation began in 2004 with the first generation of LP ESP® implants, which used endplates without lordosis (40 implantations, all complying with the Huriet Act, which defines French ethical requirements) (Figure 6).

A second generation of implants with lordotic endplates (7°, 9°, and 11°) was introduced in 2005 — LP ESP 1 (Figure 7).

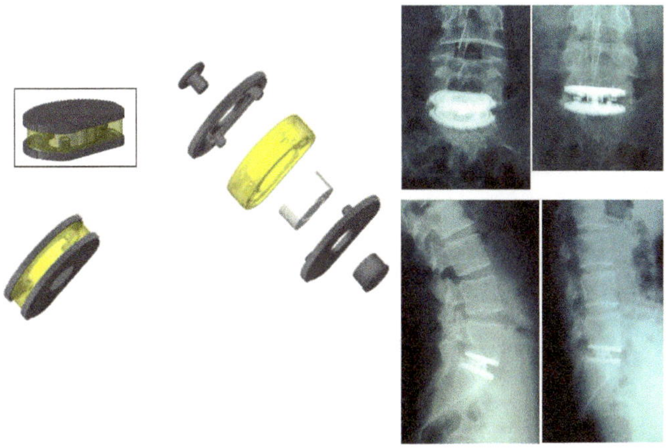

**Figure 6.** First generation of lumbar ESP® ( 2004) : endplates without lordosis

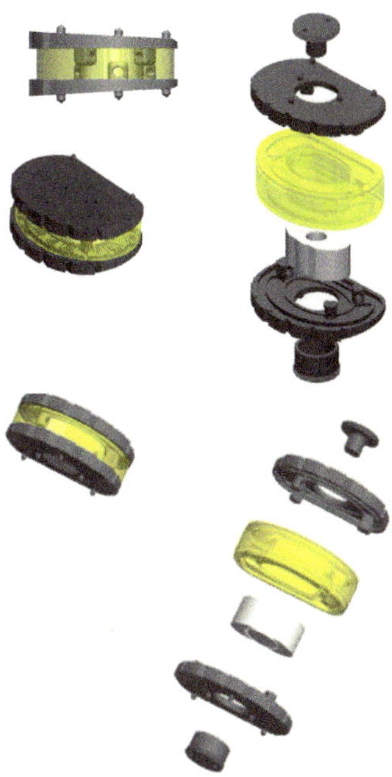

**Figure 7.** Second generation of lumbar ESP® ( 2005) : the shape of the endplates provides lordosis

A final change was made to the PCU annulus in 2006: its periphery is no longer rectilinear but was recessed somewhat during the molding process. This change did not modify the attachment of the cushion of the LP ESP 2® prosthesis but made it possible to reduce its stiffness during compression by 30% without changing its characteristics for flexion/extension, lateral incline, or rotation (Figure 8).

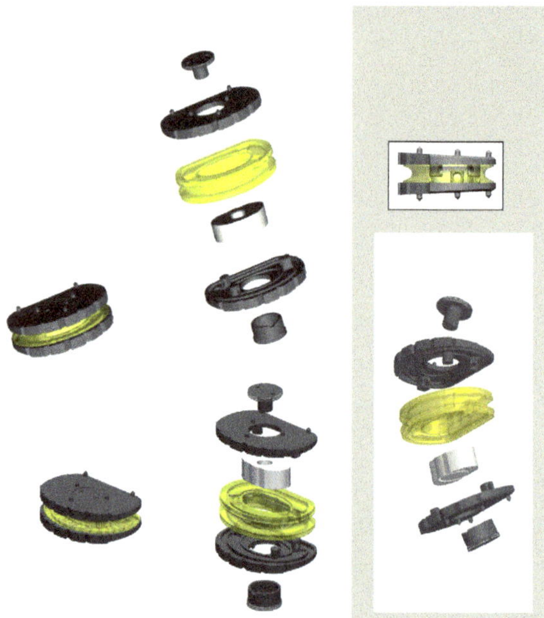

**Figure 8.** Last generation of lumbar ESP® ( 2006) : anterior recess in the PCU annulus to reduce stiffness during compression

This ESP prosthesis received CE marking in 2005, making it the first elastomeric lumbar prosthesis to be validated and authorized for marketing.

## 5. Mechanical properties

The "silent block bush" design of the LP ESP® prosthesis avoids the disadvantage of centers of rotation that are fixed or controlled by the implant design, as observed in disk prostheses based on an articulated design. In addition, in each direction solicited, the prosthesis offers resistance that increases with the amplitude of the movement. In this sense, the LP ESP® cannot be compared to first-generation implants. It meets the mechanical criterion of 6 degrees of freedom and provides a cushioning effect while restoring elastic recovery properties. Its mechanical properties are close to those reported in the literature for the normal disk (see Table 1).

| Pure moments applied in increments up to a maximum value of 10 N-m | References | Level | Natural disk |
|---|---|---|---|
| flexion extension | Panjabi [27] | L4/L5 | 6° |
| | | L5/S1 | 4° |
| | Campana | L1/L2 | 4° |
| | | L4/L5 | 7° |
| | Yamamoto [28] | L1/L2 | 5° |
| | | L4/L5 | 7.5° |
| lateral flexion | Panjabi | L4/L5 | 4° |
| | | L5/S1 | 2° |
| | Campana [29] | L1/L2 | 4.1° |
| | | L4/L5 | 6.1° |
| | Yamamoto | L1/L2 | 5° |
| | | L4/L5 | 5.7° |
| Torsion | Panjabi | L4/L5 | 2° |
| | | L5/S1 | 1° |
| | Campana | L1/L2 | 2.4° |
| | | L4/L5 | 3.4° |
| | Yamamoto | L1/L2 | 2.3° |
| | | L4/L5 | 2.2° |
| axial compression | Gardner- Morse [30] | | 2420 N/mm |
| Variable according to the loading speed, values retained for 0.1 m/s | Virgin [31] | | 3000 N/mm |
| | Kemper [32] | | 1835 N/mm |
| | Bouzakis [33] | | 1700 N/mm |
| Elastic recovery» | | | yes |

**Table 1.** Comparison of the mechanical properties of the LP ESP 2° prosthesis with those of the natural disk

# 6. Biomechanical assessment

The originality of the concept of the ESP® prosthesis led to innovative and intense testing of various sorts.

## 6.1. Structural tests

**a.** Creep tests

After continuous compression to 1250 kN for 2928 hours (122 days), the height loss was 0.2 mm. In the 8 hours following load removal, the residual height loss was 0.1 mm.

**b.** Influence of the pegs included in the PCU annulus to control rotations

Tests were performed for combined compression and rotation: the pegs included in the PCU annulus absorb approximately 50% of the torque.

c. Assessment of the cohesion of the prosthetic cushion and the metal endplates:

The tests were performed for mediolateral and anteroposterior exertion applied to one of the metal endplates, with the other plate attached to the test machine (figure 9). For implants 12- and 10-mm thick, respectively, a force of 450 and 800 N was required to obtain a gap of 1 mm between the 2 endplates in the anteroposterior direction and 550 and 600 N in the mediolateral direction.

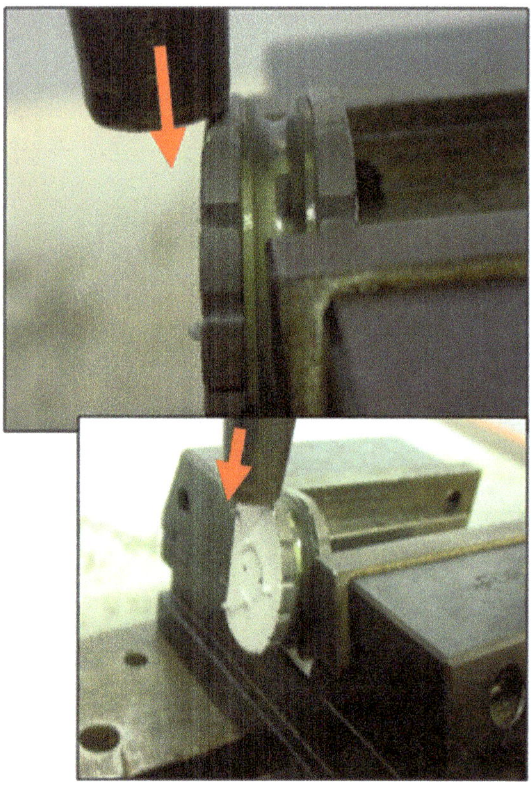

**Figure 9.** Assessment of the cohesion of the prosthetic cushion and the metal endplates: the tests were performed for mediolateral and anteroposterior exertion applied to one of the metal endplates, with the other plate attached to the test machine

**d.** Maximum compression tests

These tests were inspired by the experimental protocol of Virgin [31], who stated that a natural healthy disk is irreversibly injured by a load of 3 to 11 kN. After application of a force of 4,800 N (100 h) and then 9,200 N (64 h), we did not observe irreversible destruction of the implants. Compression tests and then compression-shearing at an angle of 45° were performed on the same samples to obtain successive compressions of 2 mm, 3 mm, and 6 mm. These tests show the implant's excellent tolerance of these compression–shearing mechanisms.

**e.** Tests to validate the final stage of coating on the exterior side of the metal plates

Adding a further final coating of porous titanium and spraying hydroxyapatite on the implant in its permanent form causes its temperature to rise. During the coating process, the disc is cooled by compressed air so that the ambient temperature remains stable at 21°C. Tests were performed to verify the absence of any effect from this rise on the mechanically active cushion in view of the known risk of PCU deterioration at 120°C. These tests demonstrated that the temperature did not reach a level of risk to the PCU.

### 6.2. Fatigue and wear tests

Wear tests were conducted in a 3-axis motion simulator according to the following protocol:

- 10 million cycles of flexion, extension, and lateral tilting
- Frequency = 4 Hz
- Loads of 135 to 1350 N
- Inclination of the prosthesis at 45° to reproduce the sagittal orientation of the disk in functional situations (Figure 10)
- In a demineralized water bath at 37° C

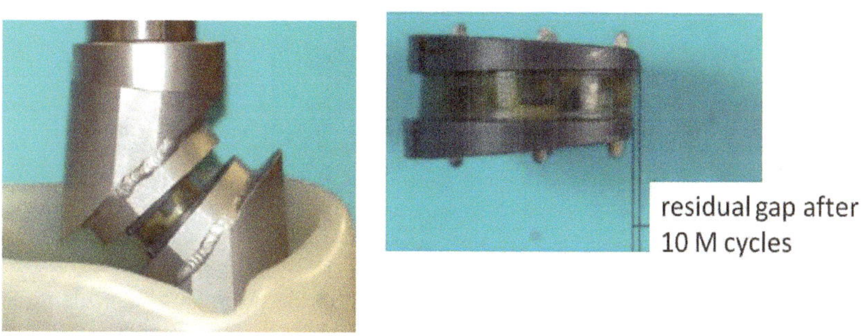


**Figure 10.** Wear tests were conducted in a 3-axis motion simulator (frequency = 4 Hz, loads of 135 to 1350 N), The inclination of the prosthesis was 45° to reproduce the sagittal orientation of the disk in functional situations. The gap between the metal plates was measured after each series of 10 million cycles.

Tests have even been extended to 40 million cycles without any observation of signs of mechanical failure. No loss of cohesion was seen. The residual gap between the metal endplates was 0.55 mm after 20 million cycles and 0.78 mm after 40 million cycles. Loss of mass after 20 million cycles was less than 0.5 % (very low absorption of saline solution and slight degradation of the endplates coating).

### 6.3. Biostability tests

This test was conducted according to the requirements of IS0 standard 10993-13/ biological evaluation of medical devices, Part 13: Identification and quantification of the decay products of polymer-based medical devices.

The biostability of the implant was assessed by analysis of the particles collected during the filtration of the demineralized water bath, after a wear test of 10 million cycles under a load of 1350 N. This study used a scanning electron microscope (SEM LEO1455VP), equipped with an energy-selective spectrometer (EDS OXFORD). No particles from the component materials of the prosthesis were found.

The tests looking for salted out or released matter showed the emission of <1 mg/kg methylene diphenyl 4-4 diisocyanate and of 64.9 mg/kg of 4-4 methylene diamine. These results are consistent with the data in the literature [34].

### 6.4. PCU aging test

The specific PCU used for the LP ESP prosthesis is not oxidized during storage (bionate 80A (DSNM Biomedical,The Netherlands ) according to master file MAF844). Kurz demonstrated that five years of shelf aging has little effect on the mechanical properties of the PCU and concludes that the bionate 80A material has greater oxidative stability than ultra-high molecular weight polyethylene following gamma irradiation in air and exposure to a severe oxidative challenge [35]. Tests were performed after artificial aging in water at 80°C followed by 10 million compression cycles at loads ranging from 150 to 1250 N. In the absence of published standards in the literature, the temperature was determined in comparison with that recommended for aging plastics, including UHMWPE (ASTM standard F 2003: Accelerated aging of ultra-high molecular weight polyethylene after gamma irradiation in air) and the axial load is that recommended by ISO standard 18192 (Intervertebral spinal disk prostheses — Part 1: Loading and displacement parameters for wear testing and corresponding environmental conditions for test) for wear tests. It was not observed significant changes in the stiffness of the implants tested.

No modification of the Fournier transform infrared spectrum or any modification of the mean molecular weight (ASTM standard D 5296) was observed. The chemical composition and organization of the atomic bonds therefore remained identical because oxidation or natural cross-linkage would have modified the atomic organization and thus the spectrum. These results are consistent with the literature [34].

## 7. Biocompatibility tests

They were performed by Biomatech (*Chasse-sur-Rhône, France* ).

All the materials were studied separately and in their final assembly, meeting the specifications for biocompatibility tests described in ISO standard 10993 (Biological Evaluation of Medical Devices).

Cytotoxicity test according to ISO standard 10993-5

Sensitization test according to ISO standard 10993-10

Test of irritation or intradermal reaction according to ISO standard 10993-10; acute systemic toxicity according to ISO standard 10993-11 Chromosomal genotoxicity (Hearts test, and chromosomal anomalies according to ISO standard 10993-3)

The implants also meet the criteria of the FDA's subacute sensitization test (following FDA - Guidelines for Toxicity Tests Chapter IV).

## 8. Clinical results

### 8.1. Evaluation process:

As of today, more than 2000 LP ESP II prostheses have been implanted. No complication related to the materials has been reported. Our clinical experience is based on prospective studies of clinical and radiologic assessment. The time points were 3, 6, 12, and 36 months. The intensity of back pain was evaluated with a Visual Analog Scale (VAS). Disability was assessed with the Oswestry Disability Index (ODI) [36-37, 39]. FDA criteria consider an improvement in the ODI at 2 years equal to or greater than 15% as success. The SF 36 was used to assess global health status [40]; the quality of life dimension of this test (SF-36) is composed of two subscores, the physical component summary (PCS) and the mental component summary (MCS), expressed as percentages [40-44]. The results of this score were compared to data known for a normal population [45]. In addition, the GHQ28 was used to investigate psychological distress [46].

Radiographs of the lumbar spine were prospectively collected for the studies. The time points for the radiological evaluation were 3, 6, and 12 months. The X-ray films were digitalized with the VXR12® scanner (Vidar System Corporation) and analyzed with Spineview® software (Surgiview Corporation, Paris, France), the precision and reliability of which has previously been reported [47]. The analysis was performed by a single observer who was not involved in patient selection, surgical procedures, or follow-up examinations. Kinematics parameters were studied at the level of implantation and the adjacent upper level on the flexion/extension X-rays. Range of motion (ROM) was measured to describe angular mobility quantitatively. As Champain et al. [47] has reported 2° accuracy for the measurement of ROM with Spineview®, we considered that the prosthesis had no motion if the measured range of motion was less than 3°. For mobile levels, the mean center of rotation (MCR) was recorded to assess motion qualitatively, as previously described. An orthogonal coordinate system centered at the posterior superior corner of the lower vertebra, with the X axis along the posterior wall and the Y axis along the endplate, was used to describe the location of the MCR. The percentage of MCRs in a correct or normal location was determined according to the method of Tournier et al [48].

Lateral views in standing position (lumbar spine including femoral heads) were used to assess the sagittal balance indicators, as defined by Duval and Beaupere [49].

- Sacral slope (SS): angle between the endplate of S1 and the horizontal line,
- Pelvic tilt (PT): the angle between the vertical line and the line connecting the center of the S1 endplate to the center of the femoral head. The middle of the line connecting the two femoral heads was used when those were not exactly superimposed;
- Segmental lordosis (SL): the angle between the upper endplate of the superior vertebra and the lower endplate of the inferior vertebra (for L5S1, the upper L5 endplate and the upper S1 endplate).

### 8.2. Clinical results

Clinical outcomes can be assessed from one of our prospective series of 120 patients. The mean operative time was 92 min (standard deviation, SD: 49 min). The mean blood loss was 73 cc (SD: 162 cc).

Analysis of the VAS showed a preoperative baseline of 6.6, a strong decrease to 3.7 points at 3 months, and a stable score of 3.6 through 36 months. The VAS thus decreased by 45%.

The baseline preoperative ODI score was 47.3%; it decreased regularly to 19.5% at 36 months, that is, a reduction of 40%. Overall, 77% of the patients had an ODI score at 36 months that improved by more than 15 points compared with the preoperative score. At 36 months after surgery, 90% of the patients showed an improvement of more than 15% compared with the preoperative value and 83% more than 25% (Tables 2 and 3).

The baseline preoperative GHQ28 score was 64.2; it began to fall at 3 months and remained at 52.2 at 36 months. This indicates an improvement of this psychological score of 18.7%.

The preoperative baseline SF 36 PCS score was 32.3%; it increased to 48.8% at 3 months and reached 56.8% at 36 months, for an increase of 24,5%.

The preoperative baseline SF 36 MCS score was 42.9%; it increased regularly and reached 57.9% at 36 months, for an increase of 15%.

| Mean±SD | PRE OP | 3 MO | 6 M | 12 M | 24 M |
|---|---|---|---|---|---|
| VAS | 6.6±1.7 | 3.7±1.9 | 3.4±2.1 | 3.5±2.3 | 3.4±2.4 |
| ODI (%) | 47.6±14.6 | 30.3±17.6 | 24.5±17.6 | 21.8±16.3 | 20.6±17.3 |
| GHQ 28 | 64.2±15.6 | 52.5±14.7 | 52.7±15.8 | 52.2±15.4 | 50.6±15.4 |
| SF 36 PCS (%) | 32.4±34.8 | 48.4±39 | 51.9±39.3 | 55.6±39.8 | 59±39.2 |
| SF 36 MCS (%) | 42.3±34.0 | 50.8±34.6 | 52.8±35.6 | 53±36.3 | 58.7±34.6 |

**Table 2.** Description of the different evaluations performed

| improvement/preoperative status | 3 M | 6 M | 12 M | 24 M |
|---|---|---|---|---|
| ODI improvement of 15 points | 53 | 69 | 72 | 76 |
| ODI improvement of 15% | 72 | 82 | 85 | 85 |
| ODI improvement of 25% | 59 | 75 | 82 | 83 |

**Table 3.** Improvement in ODI score compared with preoperative score (in % of the population)

## 8.3. Radiological outcome

The radiological results can be analyzed from another prospective series of 41 patients (20 L5S1 and 21 L4L5 implantations) for whom postural and kinematic indicators can be evaluated.

Table 4 summarizes the changes in the radiological indicators of sagittal balance over time. Patients did not have major balance disorders before or after implantation. SS, PT, SL, and DH all changed significantly between the preoperative period and all other time points.

| | Pre-op | 3 months | 6 months |
|---|---|---|---|
| Pelvic incidence (PI) | 54.1° ± 14.6 | | |
| Sacral slope (SS) | 36.5° ± 10.6 | 39.2° ± 5.7 | 40.8° ± 8.5 |
| Pelvic tilt (PT) | 16.7° ± 7.8 | 15.1° ± 6.7 | 13.2° ± 8.2 |
| Segmental lordosis (SL) | 19.4° ± 6.7 | 26.6° ± 5.3 | 27.9° ± 6.9 |
| Discal height (DH) | 28.5% ±10.3 | 50.7% ± 7.4 | 50.3% ± 5.0 |

**Table 4.** Radiological parameters in standing position over time (mean + SD). Changes in SS, PT, SL, and DH were significant between the preoperative measurements and all other time points.

The average range of motion in flexion-extension at the one-year follow-up was 5.0° (SD: 4.8°) (Table 5). The ROM increased significantly from 3 to 12 months, from 3.4 ° to 5.0°. With the 3° cut-off point, 66% of patients demonstrated mobility at one-year. The average ROM for the mobile prostheses was 6.9° (SD: 4.5). The average ROM of the prosthesis was 6.4° (SD: 4.9) at L5S1 and 7.9° (SD: 3.3) at L4L5.

| | 3 months | 6 months |
|---|---|---|
| ROM at the prosthetic level | 3.4° (2.5) | 3.1° (2.8) |
| % of mobile prostheses | 66% | 60% |
| ROM of the mobile prostheses | 4.4° (2.1) | 4.6° (2.8) |
| ROM at the adjacent upper level | 7.5° (5.1) | 7.5° (4.2) |

**Table 5.** Range of motion of the prosthesis and the upper adjacent disk over time. Mean (SD). The instrumented level reached a physiological range of motion similar to the adjacent level above it at between 6 and 12 months.

The MCR was in a normal location for 43% at 3 months, 42% at 6 months, and 87.5% at 12 months. Another prospective series of 74 implants seen at least 2 years after surgery allows analysis of the prostheses with more than 5° of mobility in flexion-extension: the mean mobility at L4L5 was 8.2° and at L5S1, 7.6°, for a global mean mobility of 7.9°. Table 6 compares these values with data from the literature for the same criterion of minimum mobility at 5°.

| Author | Year | Follow-up | Type of Prothesis | L3-L4 ROM | L4-L5 ROM | L5-S1 ROM | Global ROM |
|---|---|---|---|---|---|---|---|
| Gioia [50] | 2007 | 2 | Charité III | 8 | 10.3 | 8 | 8.7 |
| Bertagonil [51] | 2005 | 2 | Prodisc | - | - | - | 6.5 |
| Guyer [52] | 2009 | 2 | Charité | - | 6.5 | 6 | 6.3 |
| | | 5 | | - | 6 | 6.3 | 6.2 |
| David [53] | 1993 | 1 | Charité | 2 | 9.4 | 6.4 | 5.9 |
| Siepe [54] | 2007 | 1 | Charité III | - | 7.2 | 5.9 | 6.5 |
| Zigler [55] | 2012 | 5 | Prodisc | - | - | - | 7.7 |
| Delamarter [56] | 2011 | 2 | Prodisc L | 7.8 | 6.2 | | 7.0 |
| the series | 2012 | 2 | LP ESP | - | 8.2* | 7.6* | 7.9* |

**Table 6.** Mobility described in the literature of implants restoring more than 5° of segmental mobility

## 9. Discussion

The geometry of the LP ESP ® prosthesis allows limited rotation and translation with resistance to motion aimed at avoiding overload of the posterior facet joints. The center of rotation can vary freely during motion. This viscoelastic prosthesis achieves 6 degrees of freedom including vertical translation; it provides a cushion and may allow shock absorption. It thus differs substantially from other current prostheses, which are 2- or 3-piece devices involving 1 or 2 bearing surfaces and providing 3 or 5 degrees of freedom, with no or very little resistance, and no elastic return. A 20-year research program has demonstrated that this concept provides mechanical properties very close to those of a natural disk.

In addition, the biostability of the implant was demonstrated: no particles from the component materials of the prosthesis were found after a wear test of 10 million cycles under a load of 1350 N.

These experimental data should be considered in relation to previously reported results from Nechtow et al. [57] of wear rates of 16.59 ± 0.96 mg/million cycles for ProDisc_ L and 19.35 ± 1.16 mg/million cycles for Charite, and from Grupp et al. [58] of wear rates ranging from 0.14 ± 0.06 mg/million cycles to 2.7 ± 0.3 mg/million cycles for Active L.

Moreover, the size and morphology of the UHMWPE particulates observed in these studies are similar to those described in total hip and knee replacements [59], the osteolytic potential of which is well known.

Seven years after the first implantation, we can document in a solid and detailed fashion the course of clinical outcomes and the radiological postural and kinematical behavior of this prosthesis. The clinical data show early and stable improvement of clinical status, while the radiological data show immediate improvement of local lordosis and discal height at the instrumented level and associated adaptation of the sacral slope. At 3 and 12 months, 66% of cases had physiological mobility at the instrumented level, with secondary self-adjustment of the center of rotation in flexion/extension.

We acknowledge that more studies with more patients and more follow-up would be useful in the future to assess long term reliability. Nonetheless, the series reported here describe the outcomes that might be expected by surgeons and patients over the first 7 years. These encouraging results are basically similar to the clinical results reported by Tropiano [60] et al. with the Prodisc II® and the clinical data of the SB Charite®, as reported by McAffee et al [61]. Although the preoperative radiological parameters showed no major imbalance in spinal posture compared to the global population, SS, PT, and SL improved significantly immediately after implantation. These results are consistent with those reported in literature with articulated prostheses [48, 62, 63].

We note that publications do not appear to report significant sagittal misalignments after prosthetic implantation, whereas lumbar fusion may deleteriously alter the sagittal balance of the spine, including a decrease in the SS and lumbar lordosis [6,7]. The increased segmental lordosis might be related to the lordotic shape of the prosthesis but also probably to the fact that arthroplasty, in contrast to fusion, allows the lumbar spine to find a new balance spontaneously. It has not yet been demonstrated, however, that this self-adaptation of the sagittal balance protects against adjacent level degeneration. Unlike arthrodesis, the preservation or restoration of some mobility with a total disk replacement aims at limiting overload of the adjacent levels.

The optimal ROM after TDR for limiting adjacent segmental disease has not yet been established. Huang et al [64] reported a series of 42 Prodisc I® implantations with 8.7 years of follow-up, and 24% of the junctional levels showed radiological signs of degeneration. In their study, the mean ROM of the disk prostheses adjacent to junctional disease was significantly lower than the mean ROM of the prostheses adjacent to a radiologically normal disk, i.e., 1.6° versus 4.7°. Prevalence of junctional degeneration was 0% among patients with ROM of 5° or more and 35% among those with less than 5°. The authors did not conclude that 5° was the trigger value for avoiding adjacent degeneration, as 65% of patients with less than 5° did not develop adjacent segmental degeneration. In our series, the LP-ESP® device provides mobility levels similar to those with articulated prostheses such as Prodisc, which vary according to the series from 3.8° to 13.2° [62, 64].

We recognize that assessing spinal kinematics with static X-rays in flexion and extension is subject to bias, given the same-day variations due to inconsistent effort during flexion/extension [65]. Nonetheless, flexion/extension X-rays are easily available and cause less irradiation than continuous motion analysis with in vivo fluoroscopy. Quality of movement is also an issue. The LP-ESP is a novel one-piece deformable but cohesive interbody spacer that provides 6 full degrees of freedom about the 3 axes. This allows instantaneous axis rotation change freely, as in the normal disk, while preventing facet overloading.

MCR, initially defined by Pearcy [66], is a pivot point about which a vertebra appears to move and is thought to reflect the quality of movement of a segment. As disk arthroplasty develops, this indicator appears to be an informative parameter for studying the quality of spinal movement imposed by the prosthesis. The coordinates of the MCR for LP-ESP® prosthesis appears similar to those of the natural disk described in literature. After one year of follow-up, we found the MCR in a physiological area in 87.5% of the patients. With the same methods, Tournier et al. [48] reported a normal MCR for 51% of patients receiving the Maverick®, 66% of those with the Prodisc® (both of which have 3 degrees of freedom), and 80% with the SB Charite® (5 degrees of freedom). These results suggest that less constrained prostheses, i.e., those with more than 3 degrees of freedom, are associated with more normal MCR locations. In addition, we observed that the MCR location tends to improve during the first year. However, this must be interpreted while bearing in mind the uncertainty of the MCR measurement reported by Tournier et al., specifically at the L5-S1 level.

## 10. Conclusion

The concept of the LP-ESP® prosthesis is different from that of the articulated devices currently used in the lumbar spine; it allows 6 degree of freedom with elastic return and is intended to respect the spontaneous instantaneous axis of rotation and to reduce facet forces. Our series provide encouraging clinical results about pain, function, kinematic behavior and radiological sagittal balance after implantation of the LP-ESP ®.

## Author details

Jean-Yves Lazennec[1,2,4], Alain Aaron[3], Adrien Brusson[4], Jean Patrick Rakover[5] and Marc Antoine Rousseau[1,2]

1 Department of Orthopedic and Trauma Surgery, La Pitié-Salpétrière Hospital, Paris, France

2 Biomechanics Lab, Arts et Métiers Paritech, Paris, France

3 FH Orthopedics, Heimsbrunn, France

4 Department of Anatomy, Universite´ Pierre et Marie Curie, Paris, France

5 Clinique du Pré, Le Mans, France

## References

[1] Fritzell, P, et al. (2001). Volvo Award Winner in Clinical Studies: Lumbar fusion versus nonsurgical treatment for chronic low back pain: a multicenter randomized controlled trial from the Swedish Lumbar Spine Study Group. Spine (Phila Pa 1976), 2001. 26(23): discussion 2532-4., 2521-2532.

[2] Resnick, D. K, Malone, D. G, & Ryken, T. C. Guidelines for the use of discography for the diagnosis of painful degenerative lumbar disc disease. Neurosurg Focus, (2002)., E12.

[3] Wetzel, F. T, et al. The treatment of lumbar spinal pain syndromes diagnosed by discography. Lumbar arthrodesis. Spine (Phila Pa 1976), (1994)., 792-800.

[4] Thalgott, J. S, et al. Anterior lumbar interbody fusion with titanium mesh cages, coralline hydroxyapatite, and demineralized bone matrix as part of a circumferential fusion. Spine J, (2002)., 63-69.

[5] Moore, K. R, Pinto, M. R, & Butler, L. M. Degenerative disc disease treated with combined anterior and posterior arthrodesis and posterior instrumentation. Spine (Phila Pa 1976), (2002)., 1680-1686.

[6] Kumar, M. N, Baklanov, A, & Chopin, D. Correlation between sagittal plane changes and adjacent segment degeneration following lumbar spine fusion. Eur Spine J, (2001)., 314-319.

[7] Rao, R. D, David, K. S, & Wang, M. Biomechanical changes at adjacent segments following anterior lumbar interbody fusion using tapered cages. Spine (Phila Pa 1976), (2005)., 2772-2776.

[8] Kim, Y. E, et al. Effect of disc degeneration at one level on the adjacent level in axial mode. Spine (Phila Pa 1976), (1991)., 331-335.

[9] Weinhoffer, S. L, et al. Intradiscal pressure measurements above an instrumented fusion. A cadaveric study. Spine (Phila Pa 1976), (1995)., 526-531.

[10] Dekutoski, M. B, et al. Comparison of in vivo and in vitro adjacent segment motion after lumbar fusion. Spine (Phila Pa 1976), (1994)., 1745-1751.

[11] Eck, J. C, Humphreys, S. C, & Hodges, S. D. Adjacent-segment degeneration after lumbar fusion: a review of clinical, biomechanical, and radiologic studies. Am J Orthop (Belle Mead NJ), (1999)., 336-340.

[12] Rahm, M. D, & Hall, B. B. Adjacent-segment degeneration after lumbar fusion with instrumentation: a retrospective study. Journal of Spinal Disorders, (1996)., 392-400.

[13] Fernstrom, U. Arthroplasty with intercorporal endoprothesis in herniated disc and in painful disc. Acta Chir Scand Suppl, (1966)., 154-159.

[14] Cunningham, B. W, et al. General principles of total disc replacement arthroplasty: seventeen cases in a nonhuman primate model. Spine (Phila Pa 1976), (2003)., S118-S124.

[15] Cunningham, B. W, et al. Total disc replacement arthroplasty using the AcroFlex lumbar disc: a non-human primate model. Eur Spine J, (2002). Suppl 2:, S115-S123.

[16] Frelinghuysen, P, et al. Lumbar total disc replacement part I: rationale, biomechanics, and implant types. Orthop Clin North Am, (2005)., 293-299.

[17] Auerbach, J. D, et al. Evaluation of spinal kinematics following lumbar total disc replacement and circumferential fusion using in vivo fluoroscopy. Spine (Phila Pa 1976), (2007)., 527-536.

[18] Awe, O. O, et al. Impact of total disc arthroplasty on the surgical management of lumbar degenerative disc disease: Analysis of the Nationwide Inpatient Sample from 2000 to 2008. Surg Neurol Int, (2011)., 139.

[19] Blumenthal, S, et al. A prospective, randomized, multicenter Food and Drug Administration investigational device exemptions study of lumbar total disc replacement with the CHARITE artificial disc versus lumbar fusion: part I: evaluation of clinical outcomes. Spine (Phila Pa 1976), (2005). discussion E387-91., 1565-1575.

[20] Szpalski, M, Gunzburg, R, & Mayer, M. Spine arthroplasty: a historical review. Eur Spine J, (2002). Suppl 2:, S65-S84.

[21] Goel, V. K, et al. Effects of charite artificial disc on the implanted and adjacent spinal segments mechanics using a hybrid testing protocol. Spine (Phila Pa 1976), (2005)., 2755-2764.

[22] Hochschuler, S. H, et al. Artificial disc: preliminary results of a prospective study in the United States. Eur Spine J, (2002). Suppl 2: , S106-S110.

[23] Galbusera, F, et al. Design concepts in lumbar total disc arthroplasty. Eur Spine J, (2008). , 1635-1650.

[24] Errico, T, Sasso, R, & Mize, e. a. G, Total disc replacement for treating lumbar discogenic back pain: A prospective randomized multicenter study of FlexiCore vs. 360 spinal fusion. Spine J 2008;. (2008). Suppl 1)): , 15S-16S.

[25] Fraser, R. D, et al. AcroFlex design and results. Spine J, (2004). Suppl): , 245S-251S.

[26] Enker, P, et al. Artificial disc replacement. Preliminary report with a 3-year minimum follow-up. Spine (Phila Pa 1976), (1993). , 1061-1070.

[27] Panjabi, M. M, et al. Mechanical behavior of the human lumbar and lumbosacral spine as shown by three-dimensional load-displacement curves. J Bone Joint Surg Am, (1994). , 413-424.

[28] Yamamoto, I, et al. Three-dimensional movements of the whole lumbar spine and lumbosacral joint. Spine (Phila Pa 1976), (1989). , 1256-1260.

[29] Campana, S, et al. Relationships between viscoelastic properties of lumbar intervertebral disc and degeneration grade assessed by MRI. J Mech Behav Biomed Mater, (2011). , 593-599.

[30] Gardner-morse, M. G, & Stokes, I. A. Structural behavior of human lumbar spinal motion segments. J Biomech, (2004). , 205-212.

[31] Virgin, W. J. Experimental investigations into the physical properties of the intervertebral disc. J Bone Joint Surg Br, (1951). B(4): , 607-611.

[32] Kemper, A. R, Mcnally, C, & Duma, S. M. The influence of strain rate on the compressive stiffness properties of human lumbar intervertebral discs. Biomed Sci Instrum, (2007). , 176-181.

[33] Bouzakis, K. D, et al. Loading simulation of lumbar spine vertebrae during a compression test using the finite elements method and trabecular bone strength properties, determined by means of nanoindentations. J Musculoskelet Neuronal Interact, (2004). , 152-158.

[34] Christenson, E. M, et al. Poly(carbonate urethane) and poly(ether urethane) biodegradation: in vivo studies. J Biomed Mater Res A, (2004). , 407-416.

[35] Kurtz, S. M, Siskey, R, & Reitman, M. Accelerated aging, natural aging, and small punch testing of gamma-air sterilized polycarbonate urethane acetabular components. J Biomed Mater Res B Appl Biomater, (2010). , 442-447.

[36] Page, S. J, et al. Scaling of the revised Oswestry low back pain questionnaire. Arch Phys Med Rehabil, (2002). , 1579-1584.

[37] Fairbank, J. C, et al. The Oswestry low back pain disability questionnaire. Physiotherapy, (1980)., 271-273.

[38] Niskanen, R. O. The Oswestry Low Back Pain Disability Questionnaire. a two-year follow-up of spine surgery patients. Scand J Surg, (2002)., 208-211.

[39] Sanjaroensuttikul, N. The Oswestry low back pain disability questionnaire (version 1.0) Thai version. J Med Assoc Thai, (2007)., 1417-1422.

[40] Ware, J. E, & Jr, C. D. Sherbourne, The MOS 36-item short-form health survey (SF-36). I. Conceptual framework and item selection. Med Care, (1992)., 473-483.

[41] Brazier, J. E, et al. Validating the SF-36 health survey questionnaire: new outcome measure for primary care. BMJ, (1992)., 160-164.

[42] Leplege, A, et al. The French SF-36 Health Survey: translation, cultural adaptation and preliminary psychometric evaluation. J Clin Epidemiol, (1998)., 1013-1023.

[43] Mchorney, C. A, Haley, S. M, & Ware, J. E. Jr., Evaluation of the MOS SF-36 Physical Functioning Scale (PF-10): II. Comparison of relative precision using Likert and Rasch scoring methods. J Clin Epidemiol, (1997)., 451-461.

[44] Veresciagina, K, Ambrozaitis, K. V, & Spakauskas, B. Health-related quality-of-life assessment in patients with low back pain using SF-36 questionnaire. Medicina (Kaunas), (2007)., 607-613.

[45] Leplege, A, et al. Manuel de l'utilisateur et guide d'interprétation des scores de la SF-36, ed. P. ESTEM. (2001).

[46] De Mont-marin, F, et al. Validation of a French version of the General Health Questionnaire (GHQ-28) in a diabetic population]. Encephale, (1993)., 293-301.

[47] Champain, S, et al. Validation of new clinical quantitative analysis software applicable in spine orthopaedic studies. Eur Spine J, (2006)., 982-991.

[48] Tournier, C, et al. Total disc arthroplasty: consequences for sagittal balance and lumbar spine movement. Eur Spine J, (2007)., 411-421.

[49] Duval-beaupere, G, Schmidt, C, & Cosson, P. A Barycentremetric study of the sagittal shape of spine and pelvis: the conditions required for an economic standing position. Ann Biomed Eng, (1992)., 451-462.

[50] Gioia, G, Mandelli, D, & Randelli, F. The Charité III Artificial Disc lumbar disc prosthesis: assessment of medium-term results. Journal of Orthopaedics and Traumatology, (2007)., 134-139.

[51] Bertagnoli, R, et al. The treatment of disabling single-level lumbar discogenic low back pain with total disc arthroplasty utilizing the Prodisc prosthesis: a prospective study with 2-year minimum follow-up. Spine (Phila Pa 1976), (2005)., 2230-2236.

[52] Guyer, R. D, et al. Prospective, randomized, multicenter Food and Drug Administration investigational device exemption study of lumbar total disc replacement with

the CHARITE artificial disc versus lumbar fusion: five-year follow-up. Spine J, (2009)., 374-386.

[53] David, T. Lumbar disc prosthesis. Surgical technique, indications and clinical results in 22 patients with a minimum of 12 months follow-up. Eur Spine J, (1993)., 254-259.

[54] Siepe, C. J, et al. Total lumbar disc replacement in athletes: clinical results, return to sport and athletic performance. Eur Spine J, (2007)., 1001-1013.

[55] Zigler, J. E. Five-Year Results of the ProDisc-L Multicenter, Prospective, Randomized, Controlled Trial Comparing ProDisc-L With Circumferential Spinal Fusion for Single-Level Disabling Degenerative Disk Disease. Seminars in Spine Surgery, (2012)., 25-31.

[56] Delamarter, R, et al. Prospective, randomized, multicenter Food and Drug Administration investigational device exemption study of the ProDisc-L total disc replacement compared with circumferential arthrodesis for the treatment of two-level lumbar degenerative disc disease: results at twenty-four months. J Bone Joint Surg Am, (2011)., 705-715.

[57] Nechtow et al. Nechtow W, Hintner M, Bushelow M, Kaddick C (2006) Intervertebral disc replacement mechanical performance depends strongly on input parameters. 52nd Orthopaedic Research Society. Abstract 0118

[58] Grupp TM, Yue JJ, Garcia R Jr, Basson J, Schwiesau J, Fritz B, Blömer W (2009) Biotribological evaluation of artificial disc arthroplasty devices: influence of loading and kinematic patterns during in vitro wear simulation. Eur Spine J 18(1):98–108

[59] Ingham E, Fisher J (2000) Biological reactions to wear debris in total joint replacement. Proc Instn Mech Engrs 214:21–37

[60] Tropiano, P, et al. Lumbar disc replacement: preliminary results with ProDisc II after a minimum follow-up period of 1 year. J Spinal Disord Tech, (2003)., 362-368.

[61] McAfee PC, Cunningham B, Holsapple G, Adams K, Blumenthal S, Guyer RD, Dmietriev A, Maxwell JH, Regan JJ, Isaza J (2005) A prospective, randomized, multicenter Food and Drug Administration investigational device exemption study of lumbar total disc replacement with the CHARITE artificial disc versus lumbar fusion: part II: evaluation of radiographic outcomes and correlation of surgical technique accuracy with clinical outcomes. Spine (Phila Pa 1976) 30:1576–1583 (discussion E388–90)

[62] Chung, S. S, et al. The effect of lumbar total disc replacement on the spinopelvic alignment and range of motion of the lumbar spine. J Spinal Disord Tech, (2006)., 307-311.

[63] Le Huec J., et al.The effect of single-level, total disc arthroplasty on sagittal balance parameters: a prospective study. Eur Spine J, (2005)., 480-486.

[64] Huang, R. C, et al. Range of motion and adjacent level degeneration after lumbar total disc replacement. Spine J, (2006)., 242-247.

[65] Ensink, F. B, et al. Lumbar range of motion: influence of time of day and individual factors on measurements. Spine (Phila Pa 1976), (1996)., 1339-1343.

[66] Pearcy, M. J, & Bogduk, N. Instantaneous axes of rotation of the lumbar intervertebral joints. Spine (Phila Pa 1976), (1988)., 1033-1041.

Section 3

# Diagnostic Techniques

# Chapter 12

# X-Ray Digital Tomosynthesis Imaging: An Appropriate Reconstruction Algorithm for Arthroplasty

Tsutomu Gomi, Hiroshi Hirano and
Masahiro Nakajima

Additional information is available at the end of the chapter

## 1. Introduction

Digital tomosynthesis is a limited-angle method for image reconstruction. In this technique, a projection dataset of an object acquired at regular intervals during a single acquisition pass is used to reconstruct planar sections post priori. Tomosynthetic slices exhibit high resolution in planes that are parallel to the detector plane. Digital tomosynthesis enhances the existing advantages of conventional tomography, including low radiation dose, short examination time, and easy, low-cost availability of longitudinal tomographs, which do not include the partial volume effect. Furthermore, digital tomosynthesis provides the additional benefits of digital imaging (Ziedses et al 1971, Miller et al 1971, Grant et al 1972, Baily et al 1973, Kruger et al 1983, Sone et al 1991, Sone et al 1995) as well as the tomographic benefits of computed tomography (CT) at a decreased radiation dose and cost in an approach that is easily implemented in conjunction with chest radiography. This technique was developed by improving the old technique of geometric tomography, which is unpopular for chest imaging because of positioning difficulties, high radiation dose, and residual blur due to out-of-plane structures. Digital tomosynthesis overcomes these difficulties by enabling the reconstruction of numerous image slices from the data acquired from a single low-dose image. Digital tomosynthesis images are invariably affected by blurring because of objects lying outside the plane of interest and those superimposed on the focused image of the fulcrum plane by the limited acquisition angle. This results in poor object detectability in the in-focus plane. This technique has been investigated in angiography and the imaging of chest, hand joints, lungs, teeth and breasts (Stiel et al 1993, Duryea et al 2003, Sone et al 1995, Niklason et al 1997, Dobbins et al 2003).

Imaging by X-ray CT has improved over the past three decades and is now a powerful tool in medical diagnostics. It has become an essential, non-invasive imaging technique since the advent of spiral CT imaging in the 1990s, which led to shorter scan times and improved three-dimensional (3D) spatial resolution. CT provides a high resolution in the tomographic plane but limited resolution in the axial direction. However, the quality of images generated by a CT scanner can still be reduced by the presence of metal objects in the field-of-view. Imaging patients with metal implants such as marker pins, dental fillings or hip prostheses is susceptible to artifacts, generally in the form of bright and dark streaks, cupping, capping and so on. This artifact susceptibility is mostly due to quantum noise, scattered radiation and beam hardening (Hsieh 1995). Metal artifacts influence the image quality by reducing the contrast and obscuring details, thus hindering the ability to detect structures of interest and possibly leading to misdiagnosis. In addition, CT values are reduced, which can lead to errors while using these data e.g. for attenuation correction in positrin emission tomography (PET)/CT imaging (Kamel et al 2003). The metallic components of arthroplasty devices are high-contrast objects that generate artifacts when imaged using CT scans. These artifacts can make it extremely difficult or impossible to interpret images obtained by these devices. The presence of artifacts, along with the partial volume effect, severely limits the potential for the objective quantification of total joint replacement with CT.

Methods for reducing metal artifacts aim to improve the quality of images, affected by them. Recently, modified- iterative (Wang et al 1996, 1999, 2000, Man et al 2000) or wavelet-reconstruction techniques have produced promising results. However, these methods cannot be combined with the fast, robust filtered backprojection (FBP) algorithm, which is the standard reconstruction technique (Robertson et al 1997) implemented in modern CT scanners.

Digital tomosynthesis using the FBP algorithm shows satisfactory overall performance, but its effectiveness depends strongly on the region of the image. This type of digital tomosynthesis gives good results independent of the type of the metal present in the patient and effectively removes noise artifacts, especially at greater distances from the metal objects (Gomi et al 2008). In addition, flexibility in choosing digital tomosynthesis imaging parameters on the basis of the desired final images and generation of high-quality images may be beneficial.

In this study, we focus on the potential application of digital tomosynthesis using a different algorithm for an enhanced performance, which is used for imaging hip prosthesis phantoms (titanium) and human hip prostheses. The present study was performed to evaluate the clinical application of digital tomosynthesis in imaging these objects using the relatively commercial tomosynthesis method. Digital tomosynthesis was compared to the use of conventional reconstruction for tomosynthesis (FBP), metal-artifact-reduction processing reconstruction for tomosynthesis, iterative reconstruction for tomosynthesis [simultaneous iterative reconstruction technique; SIRT (Gordon et al 1970)], adaptive statistical iterative reconstruction CT and non-metal-artifact-reduction processing CT (conventional FBP reconstruction) scans of a hip prosthesis phantom and human hip prosthetic case.

## 2. Image reconstruction

### 2.1. Tomosynthesis

Existing tomosynthesis algorithms can be divided into three categories: (1) backprojection algorithms, (2) FBP algorithms, and (3) iterative algorithms. The backprojection algorithm is referred to as a shift-and-add (SAA) process, in which the projection images obtained at different angles are electronically shifted and added to generate an image plane, focused at a certain depth below the surface. The projection shift is adjusted such that the visibility of features in the selected plane is enhanced, whereas that in other planes is blurred. By using a digital detector, the image planes at all depths can be retrospectively reconstructed from one set of projections. The SAA algorithm is valid only if the motion of the X-ray focal spot is parallel to the detector (Gomi et al 2012).

In FBP algorithms, which are widely used in CT, many projections acquired at greater than 360º are used to reconstruct cross-sectional images. The number of projections typically ranges between a few hundred and approximately one thousand. The Fourier central slice theorem is fundamental to the FBP theory. In two-dimensional (2D) CT imaging, projecting an object corresponds to sampling it perpendicular to the X-ray beam in Fourier space (Kak et al 1988). For many projections, information of the object is well sampled, and the object can be restored by combining the information from all the projections. In 3D cone-beam imaging, the information of the object in Fourier space is related to the Radon transform of the object. The relationship between the Radon transform and cone-beam projections has been studied properly, and solutions to the cone-beam reconstruction have been provided (Smith 1985). The FBP algorithm generally provides highly precise 3D reconstruction images when an exact-type algorithm is employed (Feldkamp et al 1984). Therefore, this method has been adopted for the image reconstruction of 3D tomography and multi-detector cone-beam CT.

An iterative algorithm performs reconstruction recursively (Ruttimann et al 1984, Bleuet et al 2002), unlike the one-step operation in backprojection and FBP algorithms. During the iterative reconstruction, a 3-D object model is repeatedly updated until it converges to the solution, which optimizes an objective function. The objective function defines the criteria of the reconstruction solution. The objective function in SIRT are applied iteratively so that the projections of the reconstructed volume, computed from an image-formation model, resemble the experimental projections. A linear-projection model is a first-order approximation of the nonlinear image-formation process, occurring in tomosynthesis. Furthermore, although the noise is not white, the SIRT formula for white noise produces good estimates of the underlying structures.

Metal artifacts influence the image quality by reducing the contrast and obscuring the detail, thereby impairing the ability to detect structures of interest and making diagnosis impossible. Artifacts due to high-attenuation features in hip prostheses are observed in digital-tomosynthesis reconstruction because of the small number of projections and narrow angular range, typically employed in tomosynthesis imaging developed artifact-reduction methods on the basis of a modified Shepp–Logan reconstruction filter kernel by considering the additional weight of the direct current components in the frequency domain (Gomi et al 2009). Processing increases the ratio of low-frequency components in an image (Fig. 1). Artifact was reduced using basic and FBP algorithms. It provides a filtering method that can be used in combination with the backprojection algorithm to yield sliced images with the desired properties via tomosynthesis.

The tomosynthesis system (SonialVision Safire II, Shimadzu Co., Kyoto, Japan) comprised an X-ray tube with a 0.4-mm focal spot and a 362.88 × 362.88-mm digital flat-panel detector composed of amorphous selenium. Each detector element was 150 × 150 μm in size. Tomography was performed linearly with a total acquisition time of 6.4 s {80 kVp, 250 mA, 20 ms/view, effective dose: 1.33 mSv [International Commission on Radiological Protection (ICRP) 60], 0.69 mSv (ICRP 103)} and an acquisition angle of 40 degree. Projection images were sampled during a single tomographic pass (74 projections) using a matrix size of 1440 × 1440 with 12 bits per image and were used to reconstruct tomograms of a desired height. The reconstructed images (0.272 mm/pixel) were obtained with a 4-mm slice thickness at 1-mm reconstruction intervals. An antiscatter grid was used (focused type, grid ratio 12:1). The distance from the source to the isocentre was 980 mm and that from the isocentre to the detector was 1100 mm (3.0-mm aluminium equivalent filtration). The tomosynthesis images were reconstructed using FBP with the conventional Shepp–Logan filter kernel.

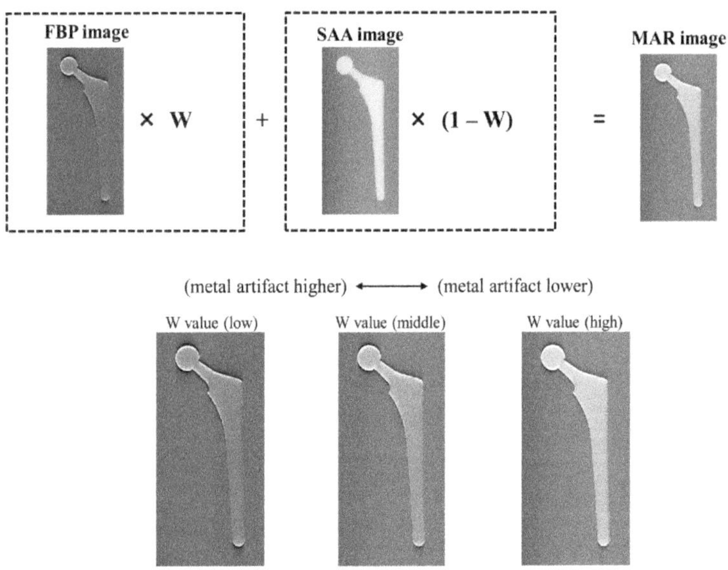


**Figure 1.** Concept of the metal-artifact-reduction processing method for tomosynthesis. The image is weighted by multiplying the different weight coefficients and adding them to the shift-added image and the conventional FBP image.

## 2.2. CT

The presence of metal artifacts has been a major problem in X-ray CT. Metal parts in the field-of-view attenuate most of the X-ray photons and generate dark and bright streaks after FBP, which is currently the selected reconstruction method for CT. These artifacts severely degrade the image quality, particularly near metal surfaces. Metal-artifact reduction has important applications in orthopaedic, oncologic, and dental imaging.

Iterative reconstruction algorithms, with and without the incorporation of a priori information, have been used to reconstruct incomplete projections. Although previous results using iterative reconstruction were unsatisfactory, a recently developed iterative-deblurring method has produced an image reconstruction of the incomplete data with few artifacts. Iterative reconstruction, which has recently become available on commercial CT scanners, enables metal-artifact-noise reduction without trade-off in spatial resolution (Main et al 2010). However, iterative reconstruction has unfavourable effects. Its use alters the texture of the image noise and can yield an unusually homogenous image. This may not be immediately appealing to most radiologists, who are usually accustomed to FBP images (Hara et al 2009). Moreover, an excessive degree of iterative reconstruction may obscure fine and subtle findings (Yanagawa et al 2010).

In computation with iterative reconstruction, the image has an initial condition of values, which are iteratively optimized according to the rules of the model. The FBP image is used for the initial condition in adaptive statistical iterative reconstruction (GE Healthcare Corp.; the initial value of each pixel) for the following reasons: it is presumably close to the final optimized solution (lessening the need for iterations), it is a valid indicator of specific-slice image noise and it can be obtained rapidly. For modelling and using iterative reconstruction, minimum convergence is achievable with adaptive statistical iterative reconstruction. However, a fully converged, 100% adaptive statistical iterative reconstruction image, has a noise-free appearance with an unusually homogeneous attenuation. Because some noise is inherent in CT, the use of 100% adaptive statistical iterative reconstruction may not be immediately appealing to most of the radiologists. However, blended images containing a linear mixture of the original FBP and this reconstruction can exhibit markedly decreased noise while retaining a more typical CT appearance. This blended image can be adjusted from 1% to 100% in adaptive statistical iterative reconstruction. The 40% level was chosen because 40% adaptive statistical iterative reconstruction should produce a diagnostically acceptable image with less noise than a full-dose FBP image. We selected the blending ratios of 20%, 40%, and 60% according to the results of a previous study (Hara et al 2009). In the conventional FBP reconstruction, standard reconstruction kernels were used.

CT scan was performed on a multi-slice CT scanner (64-slice Discovery CT 750HD scanner; GE Healthcare Corp., Milwaukee, WI) with 120 kVp, 150 mA, 0.625 mm × 64 collimation, and a 1-s gantry rotation time at a beam pitch of 0.984 [effective dose, 5.4 mSv (ICRP 60), 4.1 mSv (ICRP 103)]. The clinical task was to assess the hip prostheses. A 4-mm thick slice is generally used in clinical practice. In this study, we applied the slice thickness used during the screenings; therefore, the axial reconstructed images were obtained with a 4-mm slice thickness at 1-mm reconstruction intervals (512 × 512 pixels and 140-mm field-of-view).

# 3. Evaluation

In the study, the artifact-reduction performance was evaluated using the intensity profile, artifact spread function (ASF) and root-mean-square error (RMSE). The intensity profiles were compared using different reconstruction methods in the in-focus plane. Wu et al. proposed an ASF metric to quantify the artifacts observed in planes outside the focus image plane (Wu et al 2003). These artifacts are generated from real features located in the focus image plane and resemble the real feature. The artifacts exhibited in the image plane are defined by the ASF as $\frac{N_{artifact}(z)-N_{BG}(z)}{N_{artifact}(z_0)-N_{BG}(z_0)}$, where z to the base of 0 is the location of the in-focus plane of the real feature and z is the location of the off-focus plane. *N* to the base of artifact (z0) (*z*) and *NBG*(*z*0) are the average pixel intensities of the feature and the image background in the in-focus plane, respectively. *Nartifact*(*z*) and *NBG*(*z*) are the average pixel intensities of the artifact and the image background in the off-focus plane, respectively. Another important metric to be considered is RMSE, which can be computed by obtaining the root of the summation of the square of the standard deviation and the square of the bias. The errors in the image plane are defined in terms of RMSE as $RMSE = \sqrt{\sum_{i=1}^{n} (X - x_i)^2 / n}$, where $X$ is the observed image, $x_i$ is the referenced image, and $n$ is the number of compounds in the analysed set.

# 4. Results

## 4.1. Hip prosthesis phantoms (titanium)

A comparison of the intensity profiles and RMSEs of the tomosynthesis and CT images revealed that tomosynthesis (metal-artifact-reduction processing and the iterative algorithm) decreased the number of metal and beam hardening artifacts in the reconstructed images. Furthermore, this technique yielded a higher contrast detectability than the existing FBP algorithm. In the reconstructed images obtained from metal-artifact-reduction processing, the quantum noise structure decreased, and the noise structure was slightly smoother (Figs. 2–6).

The chart in Fig. 7 shows the ASF results for the prosthetic case. This chart shows ASF versus the distance from the in-focus slice in millimetres. There were nine reconstructed slices. The chart demonstrates that tomosynthesis with metal-artifact-reduction processing (*W* = high) removes the highest number of metal artifacts. Examining Fig. 7 through the entire thickness of the specimen shows that the order of ASF performance of the algorithm is as follows: (1) tomosynthesis (metal-artifact-reduction processing with FBP, *W* = high); (2) CT (20%, 40%, and 60% adaptive statistical iterative reconstruction and conventional FBP); (3) tomosynthesis (iterative algorithm, 100 iterations); and (4) tomosynthesis (conventional FBP).

### 4.2. Human hip prostheses

To demonstrate the potential benefits of digital tomosynthesis compared with CT in imaging hip prostheses, we used one clinical case, a 52-year-old female with total hip arthroplasty. The use of digital tomosynthesis improved the visualisation of the underlying tissue detail by blurring the overlying structures. CT provided information [multiplanar reformation (MPR) of images] on the hip prostheses, as shown in Fig. 8. MPR of CT images suffered from string artifacts in all regions. In addition, due to strong beam hardening and scattering, the femur region was poorly displayed. The artifacts in CT images, produced by FBP, were realistic and resembled actual patient images. The more metal was present in the field-of-view (metal-backed and bilateral prostheses), the more metal artifacts were produced. Reconstruction of the incomplete projection data by using iterative deblurring produced an essentially metal-artifact-free image for soft tissues and outperformed the FBP methods. The hip prostheses present on the digital tomosynthesis images could be removed effectively by blurring in the 74-projection digital tomosynthesis image. This allowed better visualisation of the tissue detail directly below the hip prostheses structures.

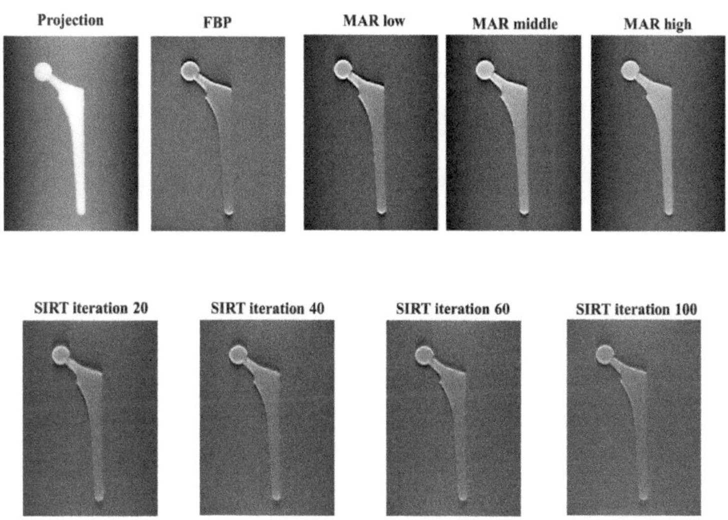


**Figure 2.** Comparison between tomosynthesis images and those obtained by metal-artifact-reduction processing, conventional FBP and SIRT imaging algorithms in the in-focus plane. (Reference is projection image.)

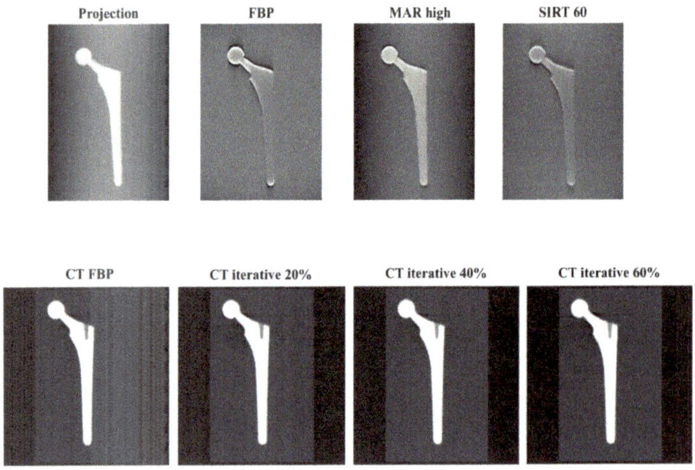


**Figure 3.** Comparison between excellent tomosynthesis images and those obtained by metal-artifact-reduction processing ($W$ = high), conventional FBP, SIRT imaging algorithms (60 iterations) in the in-focus plane and CT images (conventional FBP and iterative reconstruction). Metal-artifact-reduction processing provided a better visualisation of the hip prosthesis phantom by eliminating, blurring and reducing the artifacts, above, and the visualized planes, below.

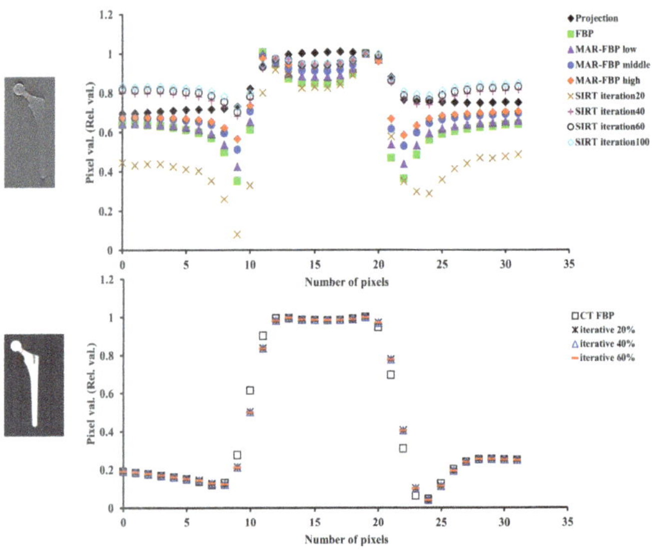


**Figure 4.** Comparison between intensity profiles using tomosynthesis and CT in the in-focus plane. Artifacts (part of undershooting) are reduced by metal-artifact-reduction processing and SIRT technique for tomosynthesis.

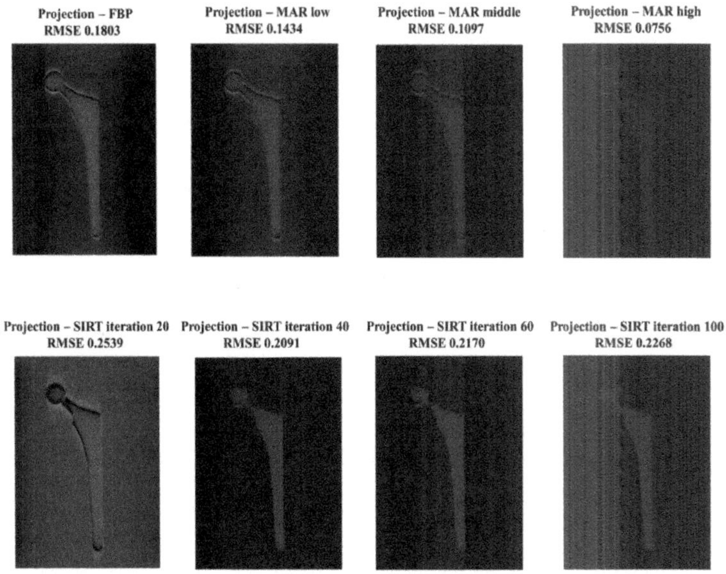


**Figure 5.** Comparison between tomosynthesis error images and RMSE of the images obtained by metal-artifact-reduction processing ($W$ = low, medium and high), conventional FBP and SIRT imaging algorithms in the in-focus plane. (Reference is the projected image.)

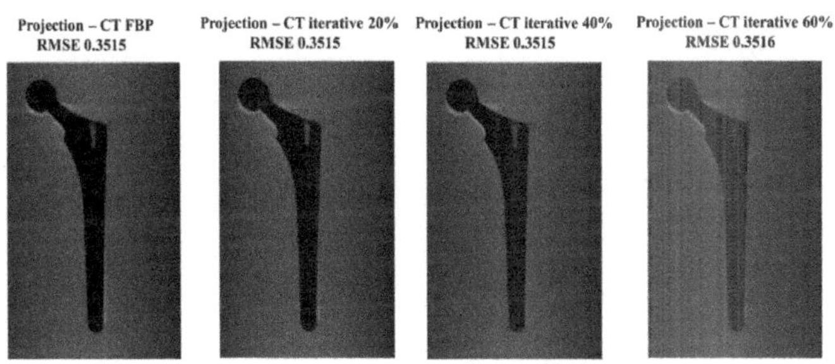


**Figure 6.** Comparison between CT error images and RMSE of images obtained from conventional FBP and iterative reconstruction algorithms in the in-focus plane. (Reference is the projected image.)

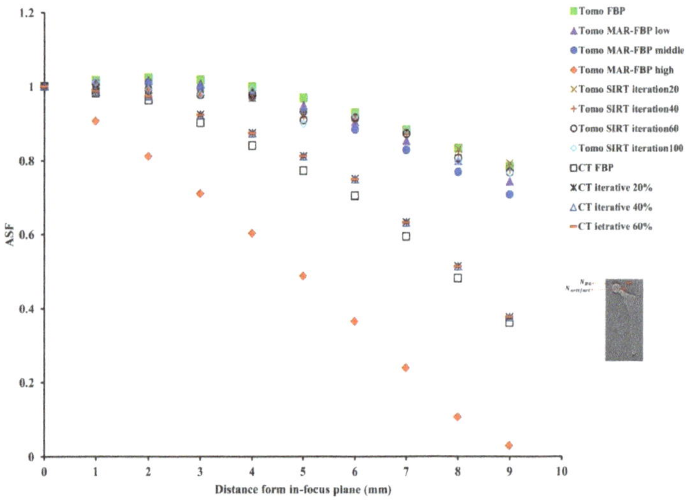


**Figure 7.** Comparison between ASF versus distance from the in-focus plane for tomosynthesis and CT. ASF chart demonstrates that tomosynthesis with metal-artifact-reduction processing results in the maximum removal of metal artifacts.

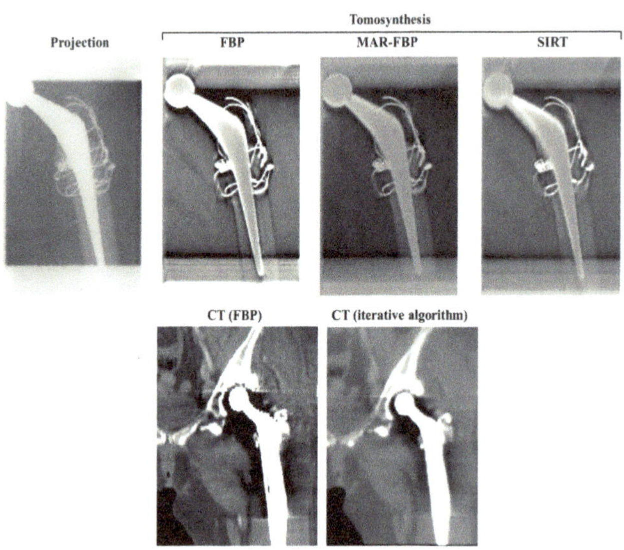


**Figure 8.** Case patient (52-year-old woman; coxarthrosis, after total hip arthroplasty). The use of metal-artifact-reduction processing tomosynthesis allowed a better visualisation of the left hip joint prosthesis by blurring the anatomic structures above and below the visualized planes. (MAR; metal-artifact-reduction)

## 5. Conclusion

Applicaton of metal-artifact-reduction processing digital tomosynthesis in imaging prostheses appears promising. The results of a prosthesis study suggest that digital tomosynthesis (metal-artifact-reduction processing and an iterative reconstruction algorithm) can produce improved image quality compared with that by conventional FBP tomosynthesis by removing the overlying structures and providing limited 3D information. In addition, the digital tomosynthesis method apparently facilitates the significant improvement of images corrupted by metal artifacts. Metal-artifact-reduction processing digital tomosynthesis provided higher quality images compared to those by CT. Metal-artifact-reduction processing digital tomosynthesis is the best solution when the high-attenuation feature causing the artifacts can be segmented accurately from the projection.

On the whole, metal-artifact-reduction processing performed satisfactorily, but its effectiveness depended strongly on the image region. Metal-artifact-reduction processing digital tomosynthesis images yielded good results, which were independent of the type of metal present in the phantom study or patient, and showed good removal of metal artifacts, particularly at greater distances from the metal objects. Flexibility in selecting the imaging parameters in metal-artifact-reduction processing digital tomosynthesis on the basis of the desired final images and realistic imaging conditions may be beneficial.

## Author details

Tsutomu Gomi[1], Hiroshi Hirano[2] and Masahiro Nakajima[3]

1 School of Allied Health Sciences, Kitasato University, Japan

2 Department of Radiology, Shinshu University Hospital, Japan

3 Department of Radiology, Dokkyo Medical University Hospital, Japan

## References

[1] Gordon R, Bender R, Hermen GT. (1970) Algebraic reconstruction techniques (ART) for three-dimensional electron microscopy and x-ray photography. Journal of theoretical biology, 29, pp.471-481 ISSN 0022-5193

[2] Ziedses des, Plante BG. (1932) Eine neue methode zur differenzierung in der roentgenographie (planigraphie). Acta radiologica, 13, pp.182-92, ISSN 0284-1851

[3] Miller ER, McCurry EM, Hruska B. (1971) An infinite number of laminagrams from a finite number of radiographs. Radiology, 98, pp.249-255, ISSN 0033-8419

[4] Grant DG. Tomosynthesis. (1972) A three-dimensional radiographic imaging technique. IEEE transactions on bio-medical engineering, 19, pp.20-8, ISSN 0018-9294

[5] Baily NA, Lasser EC, Crepeau RL. (1973) Electrofluoro-plangigraphy. Radiology, 107, pp.669-671 ISSN 0033-8419

[6] Kruger RA, Nelson JA, Ghosh-Roy et al. (1983) Dynamic tomographic digital subtraction angiography using temporal filteration. Radiology, pp.863-867, ISSN 0033-8419

[7] Sone S, Kasuga T, Sakai S et al. (1991) Development of a high-resolution digital tomosynthesis system and its clinical application. Radiographics, 11, pp.807-822, ISSN 0271-5333

[8] Stiel G, Stiel LG, Klotz E et al. (1993) Digital flashing tomosynthesis: A promising technique for angiographic screening. IEEE transactions on medical imaging, 12, pp. 314-21, ISSN 0278-0062

[9] Duryea J, Dobbins JT, Lynch JA. (2003) Digital tomosynthesis of hand joints for arthritis assessment. Medical Physics, 30, pp.325-33, ISSN 0094-2405

[10] Sone S, Kasuga T, Sakai F, et al. (1995) Image processing in the digital tomosynthesis for pulmonary imaging. European Radiology, 5, pp.96-101, ISSN 0938-7994

[11] Niklason LT, Christian BT, Niklason LE, et al. (1997) Digital tomosynthesis in breast imaging. Radiology, 205, pp.399-406, ISSN 0033-8419

[12] Dobbins JT III, Godfrey DJ. (2003) Digital x-ray tomosynthesis: curent state of the art and clinical potential. Physics in medicine and biology, 48, R65-106, ISSN 0031-9155

[13] Kak A, Slaney M. (1988) Principles of computerized tomographic imaging. IEEE, ISBN 0-89874-494-X, New York

[14] Smith DB. (1985) Image reconstruction from cone-beam projections: necessary and sufficient conditions and reconstruction methods. IEEE transactions on medical imaging, M1-4, pp.14-25, ISSN 0278-0062

[15] Feldkamp LA, Davis LC, Kress JW. (1984) Practical cone-beam algorithm. Journal of the Optical Society of America, A1, pp.612-619, ISSN 0030-3941

[16] Ruttimann U, Groenhuis R, Webber R. (1984) Restoration of digital multilane tomosynthesis by a constrained iteration method. IEEE transactions on medical imaging, MI-3, pp.141-8, ISSN 0278-0062

[17] Bleuet P, Guillemaud R, Magin I. Et al. (2002) An adapted fan volume sampling scheme for 3D algebraic reconstruction in linear tomosynthesis. IEEE transactions on nuclear science, 49, pp.2366-72, ISSN 0018-9499

[18] Hsieh J. (1995) computed tomography technology and applications; Image artifacts causes and correction, In: Medical CT and ultrasound, LW Goleman, JB Fowlkes, pp. 487-518, Advanced Medical Publishing ISBN 1-883526-03-5, Madison

[19] Kamel EM, Burger C, Buck A, et al. (2003) Impact of metallic dental implants on CT-based attenuation correction in a combined PET/CT scanner. European Radiology, 13, pp.724-8, ISSN 0938-7994

[20] Wang G, Snyder DL, O'Sullivan JA, et al. (1996) Iterative debluring for metal artifacts reduction. IEEE transactions on medical imaging, 15, pp.657-664, ISSN 0278-0062

[21] Wang G, Vannier MW, Cheng PC. (1999) X-ray cone-beam tomography for metal artifacts reduction and local region reconstruction. Microscopy and microanalysis, 5, pp.58-65, ISSN 1431-9276

[22] Wang G, Frei T, Vannier MW. (2000) A fast iterative algorithm for metal artifact reduction in x-ray CT. Academic Radiology, 7, pp.607-614, ISSN 1076-6332

[23] Man B De, Nuyts J, Dupont P, et al. (2000) Reduction of metal streak artifacts in x-ray computed tomography using a transmission maximum a posteriori algorithm. IEEE transactions on nuclear science, 47, pp.997-981, ISSN 0018-9499

[24] Robertson DD, Yuan J, Wang G, et al. (1997) Total hip prosthesis metal-artifact suppression using iterative deblurring reconstruction. Journal of computer assisted tomography, 21, pp.293-298, ISSN 0363-8715

[25] Wu T, Stewart A, Stanton M, McCauley T, et al. (2003) Tomographic mammography using a limited number of low-dose cone-beam projection images. Medical Physics, 30, pp.265-380, ISSN 0094-2405

[26] Gomi T, Hirano H. (2008) Clinical potential of digital linear tomosynthesis imaging of total joint arthroplasty. Journal of Digital Imaging, 21, pp.312-22, ISSN 0897-1889

[27] Gomi T, Hirano H, Umeda T. (2009) Evaluation of the X-ray digital linear tomosynthesis reconstruction processing method for metal artifact reduction. Computerized Medical Imaging and Graphics, 33, pp.257-274, ISSN 0895-6111

[28] Hara AK, Paden RG, Silva AC et al. (2009) Iterative reconstruction technique for reducing body radiation dose at CT. American Journal of Roentgenology, 193, pp. 764-771, ISSN 0361-803X

[29] Marin D, Nelson RC, Schindera ST et al. (2010) Low-tube-voltage, high-tube-current multidetector abdominal CT: improved image quality and decreased radiation dose with adaptive statistical iterative reconstruction algorithm-initial clinical experience. Radiology, 254, pp.145-153, ISSN 0033-8419

[30] Yanagawa M, Honda O, Yoshida S et al. (2010) Adaptive statistical iterative reconstruction technique for pulmonary CT: image quality of the cadaveric lung on standard- and reduced-dose CT. Academic Radiology, 17, pp.1259-1266, ISSN 1076-6332

[31] Gomi T, Hirano H, Nakajima M. (2012) Recent advance in arthroplasty "Chapter 6 x-ray digital linear tomosynthesis imaging of arhtoroplasty", pp.95-108, INTECH, ISSN 978-953-307-990-5, Croatia

Section 4

# Results of Arthroplasty by Etiology

Chapter 13

# Hip and Knee Arthroplasty in the Patient with Inflammatory Arthritis

Andrew Gordon, Hosam E. Matar and
J. Mark Wilkinson

Additional information is available at the end of the chapter

## 1. Introduction

The term inflammatory arthritis refers to an inflammatory arthropathy in patients suffering from one of a number of chronic inflammatory conditions including rheumatoid arthritis (RA), and the seronegative spondyloarthropathies of ankylosing spondylitis (AS), psoriatic arthritis (PsA), spondyloarthritis associated with inflammatory bowel disease and undifferentiated spondyloarthritis. This chapter will focus on a review of the surgical management of patients with RA, AS, and PsA, as these represent the most common of the inflammatory arthropathies.

Knowledge of the inflammatory arthritidies is important for lower limb arthroplasty surgeons as awareness of both the local changes within the affected joints and how extra-articular manifestations can adversely affect anaesthesia, surgery and rehabilitation is necessary to ensure good surgical outcomes. In addition to the local and systemic manifestations of the inflammatory diseases, patients may be prescribed multiple medications, including disease modifying anti-rheumatic drugs (DMARDs) or biological therapies that may affect the local surgical site or affect the patient systemically and have an impact on rehabilitation and patient outcome. In addition, quality of life and functional outcome of patients with chronic inflammatory arthropathies may also be reduced compared to simple osteoarthritis because of the chronicity and systemic nature of the inflammatory disease. Finally, the choice of implant and the method of fixation may affect implant survival and revision burden.

The term inflammatory arthropathy covers a wide spectrum of diseases which ultimately manifest themselves with joint destruction, systemic features and disability. In the following section the pathophysiology, presentation, diagnosis and medical treatments for the inflammatory conditions will be considered separately to the treatment of hip and knee 'inflammatory arthritis'.

## 2. Rheumatoid arthritis

### 2.1. Epidemiology and pathophysiology

Rheumatoid arthritis (RA) is the most common chronic inflammatory condition and affects 3% of women and 1% of men, and has its peak age of onset between 35 and 45 years. The aetiology of RA remains unclear but involves environmental and heritable factors. Several susceptibility loci reside in the HLA region on chromosome 6 and within this region, normal genetic variation may increase a patient's susceptibility to or severity of rheumatoid disease. Although many genetic variants have been identified [1-4], the impact of individual variants on the risk of developing RA is low. Research into the functional mechanisms by which these genetic variants confer disease susceptibility is on-going, with the ultimate goal of identifying discrete biological pathways which pathologically induce chronic inflammation. From this research, medical therapies to specifically target RA may be further developed. Environmental triggers which may increase the risk of RA include smoking, high alcohol intake, coffee, vitamin D levels and low socio-economic group [5-10].

The underlying pathophysiology of RA is of over-activation of intra and extra-cellular inflammatory cascades including over the expression of tumour necrosis factor and other inflammatory cytokines including interleukin (IL) 6 and IL-1 [11-14]. The cells that drive the inflammatory response include B and T lymphocytes, macrophages and synovial cells [15]. The activation of inflammatory pathways result in persistent synovial inflammation with subsequent joint and periarticular bone destruction.

### 2.2. Presentation

#### *2.2.1. Joint features*

Patients with RA typically present with a persistent symmetrical polyarthritis. The small joints of the hand and foot are most commonly affected, although any synovial joint may be involved. The natural history of the affected joint is one of low grade chronic inflammation with periods of intense pain and stiffness during a 'flare.' Between flares, joint stiffness is usually worst in the morning or after a period of rest.

#### *2.2.2. Systemic features*

Extra articular manifestations (EAM) of RA affect many organ systems and can be classified by the Malmö criteria [16] into severe and non-severe (Table 1). EAM may be present in up to 41% of patients with RhA and up to 22% of patients may develop the severe EAMs [17]. These EAMs must be considered in any patient presenting to the orthopaedic surgeon and investigated further in conjunction with rheumatology and anaesthetic specialists prior to any surgery. In addition, patients with RA may suffer from general malaise, anorexia, anaemia, weight loss and depression.

| Affected tissue or organ | EAM | | Co-morbidities |
|---|---|---|---|
| | Not severe | Severe | |
| Skin | Nodules<br>Raynaud's phenomenon | Petechiae, purpura, ulcers, gangrene | Cancer |
| Pulmonary system | Bronchiolitis obliterans<br>Organizing pneumonia | Pleuritis<br>Interstitial lung disease | Lung carcinoma |
| Heart | Valvular heart disease<br>Myocarditis<br>Arrhythmias | Pericarditis<br>Coronary vasculitis and aortitis | Hypertension<br>Heart failure<br>Ischaemic heart disease |
| Nervous system | Non identified | Mono/polyneuritis multiplex<br>Central nervous system vasculitis | Depressive syndrome<br>Cervical myelopathy |
| Eyes | Secondary Sjögren's syndrome<br>Sicca syndrome | Episcleritis or scleritis<br>Retinal vasculitides | None identified |
| Haematological system | None identified | Felty's syndrome | Non-Hodgkin lymphoma<br>Lymphadenopathy<br>Splenomegaly |
| Kidneys | None identified | Glomerulonephritis<br>Interstitial nephritis<br>Amyloid deposition | None identified |
| Bone | None identified | None identified | Osteoporosis |

**Table 1.** Extra-articular manifestations (EAM) in rheumatoid arthritis (RA). (Reproduced with permission from Prete M *et al* [17]).

### 2.3. Diagnosis

Diagnostic criteria have been designed to differentiate RA from other joint diseases. In 1987 the American College of Rheumatology (ACR) published seven diagnostic criteria to aid the diagnosis [18]. For a patient to be diagnosed with RA, four of the seven criteria have to be present and morning stiffness, arthritis in three or more joints, symmetrical arthritis and hand arthritis had to be present for at least 6 weeks (Table 2).

| | ACR Criteria for Rheumatoid Arthritis |
|---|---|
| 1 | Morning stiffness (present for at least 1 hour) |
| 2 | Arthritis of 3 or more joints. |
| 3 | Arthritis of hand joints (>1 swollen joint) |
| 4 | Symmetrical arthritis |
| 5 | Rheumatoid Nodules |
| 6 | Serum Rheumatoid factor |
| 7 | Radiographic changes |

**Table 2.** The American College of Rheumatology diagnostic criteria for Rheumatoid Arthritis [18].

However, the ACR classification has been criticised for its low sensitivity and specificity for early RA [19], a time which is critical since early pharmacological intervention increases remission rate. Further, early treatment can limit the severity of the disease and prevent bony destruction [9]. This has led to the development of another classification system by the ACR and the European League Against Rheumatism (ELAR) (Table 3) [20]. This more recent classification system assesses joint involvement, and duration of symptoms along with serological markers including acute-phase reactants and detection of antibodies against citrullinated peptides (ACPA). The detection of ACPA antibodies increases the sensitivity of the serological tests greater than the detection of rheumatoid factor. The common radiographic features of RA are shown in Table 4.

| | ACR/EULAR 2010 criteria |
|---|---|
| 1 | Joint involvement (0-5)<br>One medium to large joint (0)<br>Two to ten medium to large joints (1)<br>One to three small joints (large joints not counted( (2)<br>Four to ten small joints (large joints not counted) (3)<br>More than ten joints (at least one small joint) (5) |
| 2 | Serology (0-3)<br>Negative RF and negative ACPA (0)<br>Low positive RF and low positive ACPA (2)<br>High positive RF or high positive ACPA (3) |
| 3 | Acute-phase reactants (0-1)<br>Normal CRP and normal ESR (0)<br>Abnormal CRP or abnormal ESR (1) |
| 4 | Duration of symptoms (0-1)<br>Less than 6 weeks (0)<br>Greater than 6 weeks (1) |

**Table 3.** The 2010 American College of Rheumatology &European League Against Rheumatism classification criteria for Rheumatoid Arthritis [20].

| Soft tissue overlying the joint |
| --- |
| Swelling |
| Effusion |
| Rheumatoid nodules |
| **Intra-articular changes** |
| Global joint space narrowing |
| Marginal erosions |
| Secondary osteoarthritic change (osteophytes, sclerosis, cysts) |
| **Peri-articular changes** |
| Juxta-articular osteoporosis |
| Metaphyseal cysts (geodes) |
| Periostitis (common at the digits, rare at large joints) |
| Joint mal-alignment (alignment abnormalities due to ligament incompetence, joint subluxation, joint dislocation) |

**Table 4.** Common radiographic features in rheumatoid arthritis [48]

## 2.4. Medical management

The classes of medication therapies used in rheumatoid and in other inflammatory arthropathies include simple analgesics non-steroidal anti-inflammatories (NSAIDs), disease modifying anti-rheumatic drugs (DMARDs), glucocorticosteroids and biological agents.

In RA, reduction of pain and stiffness may be achieved with the use of simple analgesics and NSAIDs. However, the long-term use of NSAIDs is limited by their cardiac and renal toxic effects and their lack of impact on disease progression [9]. DMARDs are the first line of treatment for rheumatoid disease. Although they are a heterogeneous group of drugs, they all decrease pain and stiffness, improve function, and may limit disease progression and induce disease remission. The most frequent DMARD used in RA remains methotrexate. Others include sulfasalazine, leflunomide, hydroxychloroquine, and gold. Serious adverse effects are associated with these potential agents and require careful monitoring. Hepatotoxicity, pancreatitis, interstitial lung disease, blood dyscrasias, marrow aplasia, induction of autoimmune diseases and acute kidney injury are all adverse effects of DMARDs. In particular, methotrexate can induce bone marrow suppression, induction of liver enzymes and folic acid depletion, necessitating concurrent folic acid supplementation.

Glucocorticosteroids may be used as an effective local treatment when given intra-articularly. They may also be administered systemically for controlling acute flares, as they reduce synovitis, however with longer term use the adverse effects of osteoporosis, increased risk of infection and chronic adrenal suppression limit their use.

To date, five anti-tumour necrosis factor (anti-TNF) antibodies have been licenced as biological therapy for RA. They act in one of two ways, Enterocept blocks the effect of TNF by acting as a soluble TNF receptor whereas Infliximab, Golimumab, Adalimumab and Certolizumab are monoclonal antibodies which bind and block TNF. A recent meta-analysis of the efficacy of the TNF blocking agents concluded that TNF blockers as a monotherapy were efficacious but only as much as the DMARD methotrexate [21]. Combination therapy of methotrexate and an anti-TNF were more efficacious than either of the treatments in isolation. Adverse reactions and complications of anti-TNF treatment has been widely reported and includes local injection site reactions, infusion reactions, reactivation of latent infections, especially tuberculosis and an increased risk of sepsis, both local and systemic. Other biological approaches to disease modification include depletion in B cell numbers that drive inflammation using Rituximab, a monoclonal antibody to a protein found of the surface of B cells.

## 3. Ankylosing spondylitis

### 3.1. Epidemiology and pathophysiology

Ankylosing spondylitis (AS) is a chronic seronegative autoimmune arthropathy and is the most common of the spondyloarthritis subtypes. It predominantly affects the axial skeleton especially the sacroiliac joints and the spine, however the lower limb joints, the entheses and peripheral joints may be affected. AS typically starts in the third decade of life, has a prevalence of up to 1.2% and is 2.5 times more common in men than women [22, 23]. All of the spondyloarthropathies have a strong heritable component to susceptibility, most strongly with the HLAB27 variant on chromosome 6. 90-95% of patients with ankylosing spondylitis are positive for HLAB27. However, only 5% of subjects carrying this variant develop a spondyloarthropathy.

### 3.2. Bony features

Bony changes in AS commonly include new bone formation which arises from the cortical surfaces. Bony spurs from the vertebral bodies (syndesmophytes) extend vertically and may bridge across the intervertebral disc ultimately leading to a rigid 'bamboo' spine appearance. Entheses are also affected by new bone formation and patients may develop bony spurs in the Achilles tendon or plantar fascia. In addition, patients with AS have an increased risk of osteoporosis which can lead to devastating spinal fractures and cord compromise. The hip joint is more commonly affected than the knee joint in AS, 20% of patients who develop AS during adolescence go onto total hip arthroplasty (THA) [24].

### 3.3. Systemic features

AS is a systemic disease and extra-articular features (EAMs) are present in up to 40% of patients [25]. The most common EAMs include anterior uveitis, inflammatory bowel disease, lung disease, cardiac abnormalities (including conduction defects, valvular disease and cardiomyopathy) and renal disease secondary to deposition of IgA and renal amyloid [25].

### 3.4. Diagnosis

The main clinical manifestations of AS are pain and stiffness within the axial skeleton. A number of radiographic grading systems have been developed in AS, however magnetic resonance imaging (MRI) is more sensitive and can detect inflammation within the sacroiliac joints before radiographic changes are apparent [26, 27]. The clinical diagnosis of AS can approach a sensitivity of 70% and a specificity of 81% if two of the four criteria developed by Rudwaleit *et al* are present [28] (Table 5). Other investigations that aid the diagnosis include typing for HLAB27 and C-reactive protein however this may be elevated in only 50% of cases [27]. Serum alkaline phosphatase is elevated in severe disease.

In established disease, lumbar spine and pelvis plain radiographs may show squaring of the lumbar vertebrae (a consequence of inflammatory bone remodelling), syndesmoses and structural changes within the sacroiliac joint. MR imaging reveals bony oedema, inflammation and bony erosions within the sacroiliac joints before radiographic changes are apparent.

| New criteria for inflammatory back pain in young to middle-aged adults (<50 yrs) with chronic back pain |
|---|
| Morning stiffness >30 minutes |
| Improvement in back pain with exercise but not with rest |
| Awakening because of back pain during the second half of the night only |
| Alternating buttock pain |
| The criteria are fulfilled at least two of four of the parameters are present (sensitivity 70.3%, specificity 81.2%). |

**Table 5.** Clinical criteria for the diagnosis of Ankylosing Spondylitis [25].

### 3.5. Medical management

Simple NSAIDs and cyclooxygenase-2 inhibitors are used to control pain and stiffness. In addition NSAIDs may limit the osteoprolific component of the disease as they block the osteoblastic effects of prostaglandin E2. Again the adverse effects of long term NSAIDs however limit protracted use. Intense physiotherapy may assist individual patients but its role has not been proven to be of benefit when evaluated in Cochrane systematic reviews [29].

As with RA, AS is a systemic disease and the DMARDs methotrexate, sulphasalazine and leflunomide have been used to treat symptoms and prevent or slow disease progression. Clinical results and results from RCTs unfortunately have been disappointing. Methotrexate may be effective at treating the peripheral joint disease but its use for axial disease has not been proven. Similar results are seen with other DMARs as well perhaps reflecting a different pathophysiology in AS compared to RhA.

The recent introduction of anti-TNF biological agents has greatly aided the medical management of AS. RCTs have shown that these agents control symptoms, improve function and limit or halt disease progression. The adverse reactions of these drugs have been previously documented but in selected patients therapy is well tolerated both in the short term and up to 6 years [30, 31].

## 4. Psoriatic arthritis

### 4.1. Epidemiology and pathophysiology

Psoriatic arthritis (PsA) is usually a seronegative spondyloarthropathy associated with psoriasis. Five subsets were described by Moll and Wright in 1973 [32] and are widely used in clinical practise, these include; distal interphalangeal arthritis, asymmetrical oligoarthritits, symmetrical arthritis, spondylitis and arthritis mutilans. The prevalence of psoriasis in Western Europe is 2-3% and up to 30% of patients with psoriasis develop an arthritis [33]. However this prevalence varies considerably due to geographic variation and variation in diagnostic criteria.

PsA has a strong genetic component to susceptibility, and has been linked to the MHC region and HLA-B28, HLA-B39 and HLA-B27. This latter association is much weaker in PsA than ankylosing spondylitis [34, 35]. As with the other major spondyloarthropathies, upregulation of the T-cells and increased expression of inflammatory cytokines are features of the disease. A bacterial or traumatic environmental trigger has been proposed with PsA, however no conclusive evidence for this has been found to date [36, 37].

### 4.2. Presentation

PsA differs from RA in that fewer joints are affected, and the pattern of joint involvement is commonly asymmetric, and involves the distal interphalangeal joints and nail lesions [38]. Dactylitis, spondylitis and sacroiliitis are common features of PsA, the involved joints are tighter, contain less fluid and are less tender than those in RA [38]. The systemic features of PsA are less significant than RhA but patients may still suffer from EAMs of anterior uveitis and a disease pattern similar to SAPHO (synovitis, acnes, pustulosis, hyperostosis and oseitis). The incidence of and mortality from cardiovascular complications is increased in patients with PsA which is thought to be secondary to an increase in atherosclerosis [39, 40].

### 4.3. Diagnosis

Many diagnostic criteria have been used to detect psoriatic arthropathy, the most recent in 2006 by the Classification Criteria for Psoriatic Arthritis (CASPAR) group [41] (Table 6). The sensitivity and specificity for psoriatic arthritis may reach 98.7 and 91.4 respectively [42]. No single laboratory finding in PsA is diagnostic however acute phase reactants are elevated in approximately 50% of cases [43].

### 4.4. Medical management

Methotrexate, retinoids and psoralen combined with ultraviolet A (PUVA) treatment appear to be most effective at treating skin and joints together [43]. The role of biological agents remains unclear with limited data evaluating their use in PsA [33].

| Category | Point |
|---|---|
| Current psoriasis | 2 |
| Personal history of psoriasis | 1 |
| Family history of psoriasis | 1 |
| Typical psoriatic nail dystrophy (onycholysis, pitting, hyperkeratosis) | 1 |
| Negative rheumatoid factor | 1 |
| Current dactylitis or history of dactylitis (recorded by a rheumatologist) | 1 |
| Hand or foot plain radiography: evidence of juxta-articular new bone formation, appearing as ill-defied ossification near joint margin (excluding osteophytes) | 1 |

**Table 6.** Caspar Classification of Psoriatic Arthritis [41]

## 5. Surgical interventions for inflammatory arthritis

Optimal management of the patient with inflammatory arthropathy requires a multidisciplinary approach both in primary and secondary care. The hospital management of the inflammatory arthropathies is predominantly led by the rheumatologist with support from physiotherapy, occupational therapy, the surgeon, dieticians, social workers, orthotists and chiropodists. Community care is also paramount to maintain and optimise pain control and function. The multidisciplinary approach comprises general practitioners, district nursing, occupational therapy and social workers. Patients also often require support through housing agencies for home adaptation, community care workers and employment services [44].

In the lower limb, patients with inflammatory arthritis can present with a combination of progressive pain, restricted movement, instability particularly in the knee joint and progressive loss of function. Arthroplasty should be considered when optimal medical and non-drug supportive therapies have failed.

### 5.1. Pre-operative assessment

The systemic features of RA and the spondyloarthropathies need to be thoroughly identified through a detailed history, examination and appropriate investigations (Table 7). Abnormalities which may affect fitness for surgery or rehabilitation need to be discussed with the anaesthetist, rheumatologist and where necessary other relevant medical and allied professionals. Cardiovascular pathology maybe silent because of low physical demand. The incidence of silent myocardial infarction is six times that of the general population and is responsible for much of the 10 year reduced life expectancy in the rheumatoid population versus the background population [45]. Any abnormalities within the history in a patient with inflammatory arthritis therefore need to be investigated further.

| | |
|---|---|
| History | Disease onset<br>Pattern and temporal sequence of joints involved<br>Presence and persistence of joint swelling<br>Pain: site, severity and radiation<br>Morning stiffness and duration<br>Functional difficulties<br>Presence of non-articular features (e.g. nodules)<br>Systemic features (e.g. anorexia, fatigue, weight loss)<br>Psychological effects<br>Full review of systems<br>Previous anaesthetic and surgical history<br>Drugs and allergies |
| Examination | Complete medical<br>Evidence of joint inflammation<br>Joint damage, range of motion, and previous surgical scars<br>Tendon and ligamentous damage<br>Presence of extra-articular features (e.g. plenomegaly, leg ulcers, vasculitis)<br>Grip strength<br>General health, anaemia, muscle atrophy<br>Dental inspection, assessment of mouth opening ability, dysphonia<br>Neurological assessment for cervical myelopathy and peripheral neuropathy |
| Investigations | Full blood count, urea, creatinine, electrolytes, and liver function tests<br>Chest radiograph, lateral cervical spine flexion and extension radiographs<br>Electrocardiogram<br>Urine dipstick; culture to exclude occult infection<br>Pulmonary function tests in patients with limiting lung disease<br>Echocardiogram in patients with limiting cardiac involvement |

**Table 7.** Preoperative assessment of the Rheumatoid Patient, Wilkinson *et al* [48]

Airway management in the rheumatoid patient may also present difficulties because of laryngomalacia and atlanto-axial subluxation (AAS). AAS may be anterior, posterior, vertical, lateral/rotatory and sub-axial. The less common posterior and lateral subluxations place the spinal cord in jeopardy during extension of the neck. Cervical pathology is common. In a review of rheumatoid patients awaiting orthopaedic surgery, Neva *et al* found that 44% of patients had cervical spine subluxation or previous fusion [46]. Interestingly, they found no difference in neck pain, headaches or upper limb radiculopathy between patients with or without cervical spine instability. Flexion and extension views of the cervical spine or computed tomography (CT) scanning may aid AAS diagnosis and although this diagnosis may not change anaesthetic practise it will ensure that neck handling is kept to a minimal and ensure that staff with adequate training are present for anaesthesia [45]. Further cervical spine difficulties are encountered in the AS patient who may have fixed spinal deformities. These fixed deformities in the presence of osteoporosis place patients at high risk of fracture and subsequent neurological deficit. The anaesthetist needs to be made aware of these issues before surgery. Cervical spine involvement is not common in psoriatic arthritis and the most common clinical feature is a decrease in range of movement secondary to apophysial joint ankylosis [47]. Radiographically, the prevalence of anterior atlanto-axial instability is less than 10%. Published data with regards to the incidence of cervical spine involvement with spondyloarthritis secondary to inflammatory bowel disease is extremely limited.

Finally, patients with chronic inflammatory disease often have anaemia both as a result of their disease or secondary to medication. Optimising pre-operative haemoglobin levels, intraoperative cell salvage and reinfusion post-operative drains should be planned before surgery is undertaken.

### 5.2. The order of surgery

Patients with inflammatory arthritis often present with many symptomatic joints of both the upper and lower limbs. Careful consideration to the order of surgical intervention requires assessment on an individual level. Surgical priority should be given to structures that are at high risk of failure (for example symptomatic cervical spine instability or imminent tendon rupture). In general, lower limb surgical procedures precede those of the upper limb as post-operative rehabilitation using crutches can compromise upper limb reconstructive surgery. Within the lower limb, total knee arthroplasty implant positioning and rotational alignment is simpler once femoral length and rotation have been restored with a total hip arthroplasty [48], however generally the order of surgery should be dictated by managing the most painful and functionally limiting joints first. In patients with severe forefoot disease, consideration should be given to undertaking forefoot arthroplasty prior to hip or knee joint replacement (Figure 1).

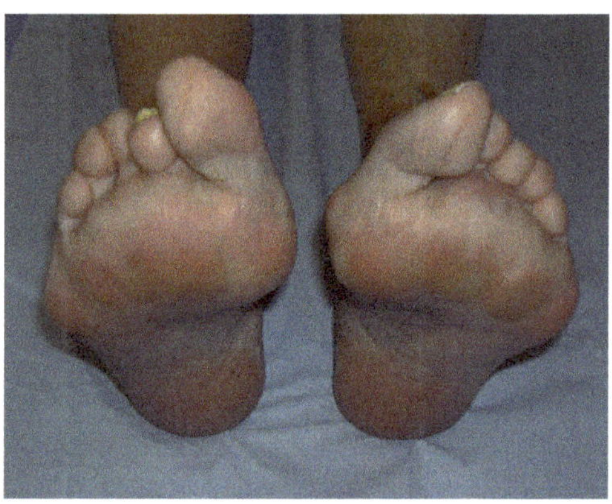

**Figure 1.** Soles of the feet in a patient with rheumatoid arthritis. There is distal subluxation of the forefoot fad pad 1
with exposure of subluxed metatarsal heads and resultant callosity formation.

### 5.3. The perioperative management of medical therapies

The adverse effect profile of many of the medications used to control symptoms and influence disease progression in inflammatory arthropathy may affect a wide variety of organ systems and an awareness of these and of their potential drug interactions is required.

NSAIDs increase the risk of gastric ulceration and patients may benefit from perioperative gastric protection with proton pump inhibitors. Long term use may also impair renal function increasing the risk of acute kidney injury secondary to post-operative dehydration.

The risk of an Addisonian crisis, an insufficient adrenal response to stress, is increased in patients with long term glucocorticosteroid use. Exognous steroid use results in adrenal atrophy secondary to suppression of corticotropin-releasing hormone and adrenocorticotropic hormone (ACTH). Patients in Addisonian crisis may present with symptoms ranging from lethargy, abdominal pain and syncope to coma. Biochemically, hypoglycaemia, hyponatraemia, hyperkalaemia and hypercalcaemia may be present. Local practice governs the regimen of hydrocortisone supplementation in the perioperative period, however typical dosing includes 100mg of intravenous hydrocortisone at induction of anaesthesia and 100mg 6 or 8 hourly for 3 days. Lower dosing regimens with a total of 150mg per day are also used [48].

While the effects of NSAIDs and glucocorticoids are well understood, there is no consensus on the perioperative management of the DMARDs. A randomised controlled trial in RA patients revealed that the infection rate was lower in patients continuing methotrexate versus those who stopped methotrexate prior to surgery (2% versus 15% respectively) [49]. A recent systematic review of the use of methotrexate in RA patients undergoing elective orthopaedic surgery found that continuing methotrexate was not associated with increasing risk of surgery complications, and led to fewer disease flares in the perioperative period [50]. Disease activity is also better controlled when methotrexate weekly administration remains un-interrupted [51]. Also, a study examining late infection rates with uninterrupted methotrexate use found no evidence of increased risk of late deep infection in 65 patients undergoing elective orthopaedic surgery over 10 years of follow up [52].

There is, to date, no clear evidence on the perioperative risk of orthopaedic infections in patients receiving biological agents, such as anti-TNF therapy [53]. A review of the limited published data in this area reveals much heterogeneity. RA patients have shown no increase in superficial wound infection rates following arthroplasty surgery with the continued use of biological agents [54, 55]. Conversely other studies have shown an increased rate of post-operative infection [56]. In a retrospective review of 81 total hip arthroplasties (THA) and 339 total knee arthroplasties (TKA), there was an increased odds ratio for superficial skin infection of up to 9.8 with continued use of anti-TNF therapy [57]. In a much larger Japanese study [58], 1626 patients treated with biological agents versus 29,903 patients not on a biological agent, reported an odds ratio for superficial infection of 2.1 with the use of biological agents even when these were stopped prior to surgery. The general recommendations of the American College of Rheumatology (ACR) guidelines in 2008 [59] and its update in 2012 [60] on the perioperative management of DMARDs are as follows:

i. Methotrexate: continue perioperatively for all procedures.

ii. Sulfasalazine: discontinue 1 day before surgery, resume 3 days after surgery.

iii. Leflunomide: discontinue 2 days before surgery, resume 2 weeks after surgery.

iv. Hydroxychloroquine: continue perioperatively for all procedures.

v. Biological agents (eg. Anti-TNF- $\alpha$): discontinue 1 week before surgery, resume 2 weeks after surgery. The ACR guidelines also recommend that the time period for cessation of biological agents is dependent upon the half-life of the biological agent used. Gilson et al. [110] recommends that the cessation of anti-TNF therapy should allow levels to fall by 5 half-lives prior to surgery in order to ensure that the drug has been eliminated.

## 6. Surgical challenges and choice of implant in inflammatory arthritis

Patients with inflammatory arthritis may be regular attenders to primary and secondary care. A good rapport and doctor-patient relationship is essential to gain trust and understanding and help to manage patients expectations. Some orthopaedic challenges stem from the general chronicity of the inflammatory disease or from the medications used to treat it. Others are joint-specific.

### 6.1. General features

Many patients will have had previous hip or knee procedures or had surgery at other sites. The overall function of these sites, as well as the presenting joint, must be assessed as they may affect rehabilitation and outcome. Soft tissue pathology may manifest as joint contracture, tendon attenuation or rupture, ligamentous instability, skin loss, chronic ulceration, vascular or neurological insufficiency, or a combination of these features (Figure 2). Previous surgical scars, especially around the knee, may affect planning, exposure and outcome after surgery. Bony disease can result in extensive bone loss secondary to erosive disease, avascular necrosis, or osteoporosis with increased fracture risk and deformity and challenges in establishing primary implant fixation.

### 6.2. Surgical challenges for hip arthroplasty

Surgical challenges at the hip include acetabular protrusio, focal bone loss and osteoporosis. Flexion contractures may be present in patients who have been chair-bound for a considerable time prior to seeking treatment for their joint disease.

Protrusio may be primary, or secondary, and can occur with or without medial wall defects and is common in all inflammatory arthritidies (Figure 3). Protrusio was first recognised by Otto in 1816 [61] and it was 1935 when Overgaard [62] presented the first useful classification into primary and secondary, since modified by Gilmour [63]. Other classifications have also emerged e.g. Charnley [64] and Hirst [65].

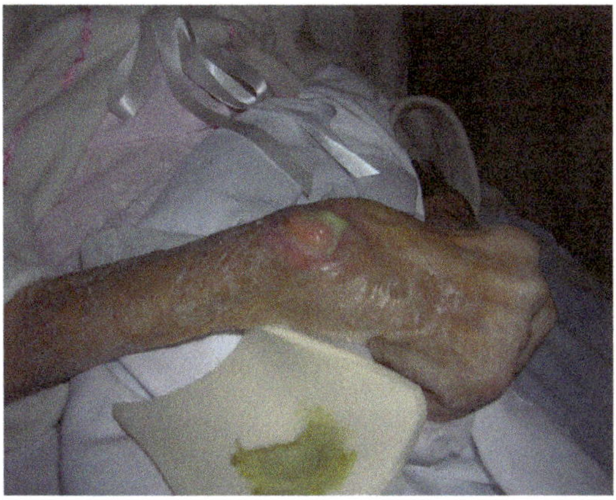

**Figure 2.** Thin skin, ligamentous damage, infection, and soft tissue loss at the wrist in a patient with rheumatoid arthritis. Similar problems at the foot are common, and may impact on hip and knee reconstructive options.

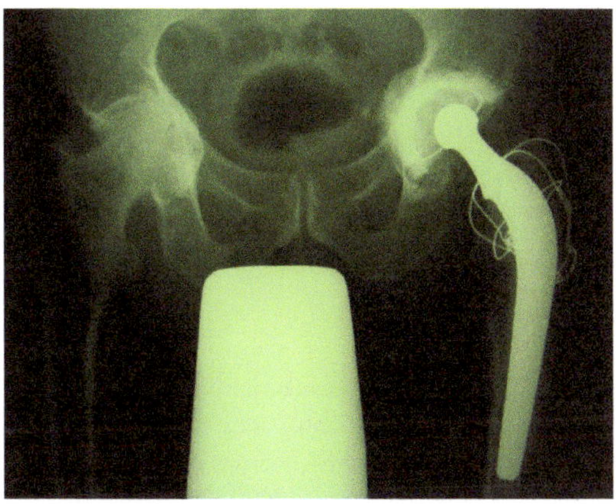

**Figure 3.** Plain radiograph of the pelvis in a patient with rheumatoid arthritis. On the right side there is protrusio acetabuli, on the left this has been treated with cemented total hip arthroplasty plus impaction of morsellised allograft to the protrusio defect.

Charnley graded protrusio acetabuli by measuring the distance between the medial wall of the acetabulum and the iliopectineal line. In Grade I protrusio the medial acetabular wall is medial to the line by 1-5mm, Grade II 6-15mm and Grade III greater than 15mm. Edstein and Murphy recognised that using the ilioischial line as a reference point that there was sex specific variation of the medial wall of the acetabulum, in males the medial wall was 2mm lateral to the line and females were 1mm medial [66]. Hirst graded the protrusio taking into account this sex related variation [65](Table 8).

| Grade | Men | Women |
|---|---|---|
| I | 3-8 mm | 6-11 mm |
| II | 8-13 mm | 12-17 mm |
| III | >13 mm | >17 mm with fragmentation |

**Table 8.** Protrusio acetabuli classification by Hirst [65]

In Grade III cases dislocation of the femoral head may be difficult and the surgeon should be confident with his/her ability to divide the femoral neck in situ and remove the femoral head as a secondary procedure. The normal anatomy of the sciatic nerve may also be altered and it should be actively sought for in posterior approaches to the hip. Anatomical restoration of the centre of hip rotation lateral to Kohler's line is essential. Anatomical restoration optimises hip biomechanics and prevents impingement; therefore further deepening of the acetabulum should be avoided. Medial wall supplementation and anatomical restoration can be achieved with the use of bone grafting or metal augmentation. Hirst [65] initially described the use of 2mm thick femoral head slices impacted into the medial acetabular wall and Rosenburg *et al* have reported a 90% survival rate at 12 years using morsellised impaction bone grafting [67]. Larger defects require medial wall supplementation. The clinical results of support with metal mesh in these large defects is poor [68] and therefore cage supplementation prior to impaction bone grafting is needed. These systems report good outcomes, up to 95% survival at 9 year follow-up [69], in revision surgery for large defects. However there are few long term studies assessing the clinical and radiographic outcomes of primary hip arthroplasty in Grade III protrusio defects in inflammatory arthritis. Studies utilising trabecular metal supplementation are awaited.

### 6.3. Choice of implant for hip arthroplasty

Cemented or cementless THA components may be used in patients with RA. A study from the Finish Arthroplasty register found comparable long-term results between cemented and cementless components in 4,019 patients who were over 55 years when revision for any reason was used as an end point [70]. Similarly, in a study of 2,557 patients under the age of 55 years there were no significant differences in overall survival between different components [71]. The 15-year survival rate for cementless proximally circumferentially porous-coated stems was 87% and for cemented stems was 81%. However, the 15-year survivorship for cementless cups was poorer than cemented cups, 67% versus 80%, respectively.

In another study from the Danish Hip Arthroplasty registry [72], 1,395 (1,661 primary hips) patients with RA were followed for up to 14 years and results were compared with 64,858 patients with osteoarthritis (RA: cemented cups 47%, cemented stems 73%, OA: cemented cups 43%, cemented stems 68%). There was no difference in survival of cups between primary THAs in rheumatoid versus osteoarthritis patients. In contrast, there was better overall survival of stems in rheumatoid versus osteoarthritis patients, both for revision due to aseptic loosening (adjusted relative risk = 0.58; 95% CI: 0.34-0.99) and for any reason (adjusted relative risk = 0.63; 95% CI: 0.45-0.88).

In a 10-year follow up study of 75 patients with RA (106 hips) who received a cemented THA, stem survival was 98% and cup survival was 92% [73]. In cemented Charnley THA in young patients with rheumatoid arthritis (63 patients, 100 hips) versus osteoarthritis (54 patients, 66 hips), 25-year survivorship of the femoral component was 85% in patients with rheumatoid arthritis versus 74% in patients with osteoarthritis, and of the acetabular component was 79% versus 59%, respectively [74]. Finally, in a recent systematic review of 23 small case series and 5 national implant registers of THA in rheumatoid patients there was no evidence in favour of cemented components over cementless ones [75].

The role of resurfacing arthroplasty in RA remains unclear. In a recent international register study, 47 rheumatoid patients (54 hips) were gender and age matched with 131 osteoarthritis patients (138 hips) and all had uncemented acetabular and cemented femoral hip resurfacing with Birmingham Hip Resurfacing implant. At 8-year average follow up, the survival rate was 96.3% in the RA group and 97.8% in OA group [76]. In another small series of 10 patients (13 hips) who had metal-on-metal resurfacing, no failures were reported at short term 3-year follow up [77]. However, recent data on the survival of resurfacing prostheses in general suggests avoiding this type of prosthesis in women, and in smaller men, phenotypic characteristics that are common in the rheumatoid population.

### 6.4. Surgical challenges for Total Knee Arthroplasty (TKA)

Soft tissue destruction leading to ligamentous instability, focal bone loss particularly of the femoral condylar bone leading to loss of height within the lateral compartment and fixed valgus deformity (Figure 4a and b), and periarticular osteoporosis are common features in the rheumatoid knee [48]. Valgus deformities with a variable degree of hyperextension rather than fixed flexion are commonly seen. Varus deformities are often secondary to osteoarthritic changes with a degree of fixed flexion [78]. The surgical challenge is to ensure correct soft tissue balance to avoid unequal loading and asymmetric stresses on the implant and eventual loosening. A stepwise approach to the release of contracted tissue is required [79-81]. A medial parapatellar or a lateral approach is used and structural bone grafting or prosthetic augmentation blocks may be required to restore large bone defects [48, 82]. Soft tissue insufficiency and ligamentous imbalance often favours the use of a cruciate sacrificing, rather than a posterior cruciate-retaining prosthesis. The survivorship of cruciate retaining prostheses is reported as poor in some series [83][84]. In cases of ligamentous incompetence a fully constrained prosthesis may be required [85]. The role of patella resurfacing in the rheumatoid patient is unclear. In a randomised controlled trial of 26 patients with RA who had bilateral TKA and patellar replacement performed in one randomly selected knee in each patient demonstrated improved pain and function in the patella resurfacing group [86].

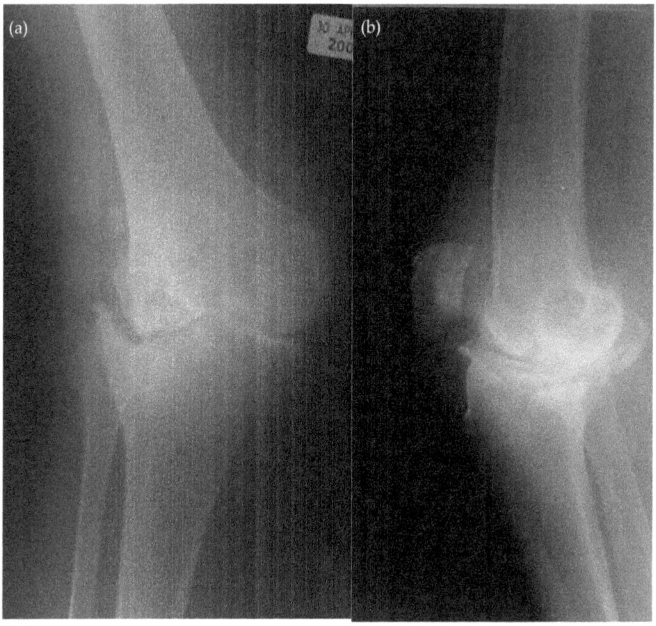


**Figure 4.** Plain anteroposterior (a) and lateral (b) radiographs of the knee in a patient with rheumatoid arthritis. Degenerative changes are present in all 3 joint compartments. There is collapse of the lateral compartment with resultant valgus deformity. Erosion of the anterior aspect of the distal femoral metaphysis due to pannus is also seen.

### 6.5. Choice of implant for knee arthroplasty

Cemented TKA has been considered the gold standard prosthesis for the rheumatoid patient. The 10-year revision rate of cemented TKA between 2001 and 2010 in rheumatoid patients reported to the Swedish Knee Arthroplasty register was 4% [87]. Fifteen-year survival rate of cemented Kinematic TKA was 93.7% in 25 rheumatoid patients (36 knees) [88]. However, recent survivorship data on cementless TKA also show good results, with a survival rate of 96.8 % at 10 years in a cohort of 112 patients (179 knees) [89]. The cementless Hi-Tech Knee II cruciate-retaining prosthesis was evaluated in 31 Japanese patients with RA with an average 8-year follow up and a reported survival rate 96.9% [90]. Similarly, 16-year survival rate of cementless low contact stress TKA in 47 patients was 94% [91]. Unicompartmental prostheses are not appropriate for RA patients as the degenerative changes are pan-articular, and their use is associated with high failure rates [92].

# 7. Complications of hip and knee arthroplasty in inflammatory arthritis

When compared to the general arthroplasty population, patients with inflammatory arthritis have more comorbidities and are taking more prescription medication. This is reflected by the higher risk of systemic and surgery specific complications. Mortality rates in rheumatoid patients are 1.5-1.6 fold higher than in the general population [93]. In a ten-year survivorship analysis from the Scottish register, greater mortality rate was associated with rheumatoid disease. Cardiovascular disease is the most commonly attributed cause of death, although other complications, such as infection, pulmonary and renal disease, are also more prevalent in the rheumatoid population [94].

In a population based study on risk of revision for infection in THA and TKA from the Norwegian Arthroplasty register, data from 6,629 (2,462 TKA, 4,167 THA) patients with RA were compared with 102,157 osteoarthritis patients (21,832 TKA, 80,325 THA). On an average 8-9 year follow up, rheumatoid patients with TKA had a 1.6 times higher risk of revision for infection than osteoarthritis patients, whereas there was no difference in the THAs [95]. In a population based study from Mayo clinic, 462 patients with RA (657 total joint replacements) the prosthetic infection rate at 4 years follow up was 3.7% [96]. Da Cunha *et al* [97] found no significant difference in infectious complications when compared perioperative infections in 49 rheumatoid patients (28 TKA, 47 THA) with 75 gender and age matched osteoarthritis patients (56 TKA, 75 THA).

A retrospective review of nearly 5 million patients demonstrated that RA was an independent risk factor for pulmonary embolism and deep vein thrombosis (DVT) in hospital patients, with a relative risk of 2.25 and 1.9 respectively [98]. In a recent comparative study, the risk of DVT was compared in 199 patients (238 knees) with RA and 156 patients (169 knees) with osteoarthritis and was found to be higher in the osteoarthritis group [99]. Earlier studies have also demonstrated lower risk in rheumatoid patients, which has been attributed to the use of NSAIDs [100]. The use of NSAIDs is also believed to cause lower incidence of heterotopic ossification in the rheumatoid patient as compared with those with osteoarthritis [101].

The risk of dislocation is also reported as higher in RA patients in a recent population based study from the Scottish National arthroplasty register, 62,175 total hip arthroplasties performed from April 1989 to March 2004 [102]. This is supported by the results of a prospective study assessing dislocation 2-years following THA in inflammatory arthritis patients [103]. Finally, periprosthetic fractures are reported more common in RA patients compared to OA, this can be explained by the poor bone quality and comorbidities [104, 105]

### 7.1. Functional outcomes

Successful functional outcome requires realistic understanding of goals and expectations of surgery with active inclusion of the patient in the decision making process [109]. In measuring the success of lower limb arthroplasty in patients with inflammatory arthritis, condition specific outcome measures should be used. Scoring systems have been developed to measure disease activity and functional deficit. The American College of Rheumatology has developed the "ACR20 response score" [106], this was modified and adapted by the European League Against Rheumatism "EULAR score"[107]. The ACR score is considered the gold standard and it is based on seven clinical end points: swollen joint count, tender joint count, the physician's assessment of disease activity, the patient's assessment of disease activity, pain, and physical function, and levels of an acute-phase reactant (either the C - reactive protein levels or the erythrocyte sedimentation rate). The "ACR20 response'' [106], defined as at least 20% improvement in in both the tender joint count and the swollen joint count and at least 20% improvement in 3 of the 5 other core set measures listed above. ACR20 aims to provide an objective assessment of disease status and is used in longitudinal studies to measure the effectiveness of medical and surgical interventions. The use of these scores helped to provide objective assessment of patients outcomes, better preoperative scores are associated with better surgical outcome [108].

The outcome of surgery is influenced by the local pathology, nature of the procedure and the severity of the disease [53, 88, 110]. In a systematic review of patients characteristics affecting the surgical outcome of total joint arthroplasty, older age was related to worse function particularly among women, whilst age and sex did not influence the outcome of pain [111]. There is good evidence that an increase in joint damage is associated with an increase in functional disability [112] and joint surgery has improved the function and quality of life of patients with RA [113].

However, when compared to patients with osteoarthritis, those with inflammatory arthritis have a slower, more gradual functional improvement in clinical outcomes scores [114]. Functional outcomes following THA are poorer in rheumatoid compared with non-inflammatory arthritis [73], this is perhaps explained by the multiple joints involvement in this group and its effects on functional outcomes [115]. Nevertheless, following THA in 50 rheumatoid patients, Harris hip score improved from 22 to 82 at 9 years mean follow up [116], and from 25 to 89 at 11 years follow up in another cohort of 20 patients [117].

Studies on TKA in rheumatoid patients have also reported good long term functional outcomes. When using the knee society score, 46 patients (71 knees) achieved 77% 'Good' or 'Excellent' at 10 years follow up [118]. In another study, 25 patients (36 knees) achieved 78% 'Good' or 'Excellent' at 15 year follow up [88]. However, when compared with osteoarthritis patients who had TKA, 207 rheumatoid patients younger than 55 years achieved less postoperative improvement [119]. On the other hand, when assessing patient satisfaction following TKA, there was a significantly better subjective outcome in rheumatoid versus osteoarthritis patients [120].

## 8. Conclusions

Hip and knee reconstruction are important surgical interventions in the management of the patient with inflammatory arthritis. Evidence to date suggests that both cemented and cemented prosthesis give good long term results. The functional benefit achieved in an individual patient will be affected by the systemic nature of the disease, and other joint involvement. Because inflammatory arthropathy involves the whole joint, partial and uni-compartmental joint replacement should be avoided. The perioperative management of the patient with inflammatory arthropathy requires multidisciplinary input, and recognition and appropriate management of comorbidities that are common in this patient group. Finally, an awareness of the pharmaceutical and biological agents taken by the patient, and their appropriate peri-operative management is important to minimise the risk of iatrogenic complications.

## Author details

Andrew Gordon[1], Hosam E. Matar[1] and J. Mark Wilkinson[2]

*Address all correspondence to: a.gordon@sheffield.ac.uk

*Address all correspondence to: hematar@doctors.org.uk

*Address all correspondence to: j.m.wilkinson@sheffield.ac.uk

1 Department of Orthopaedics The Northern General Hospital, Sheffield, United Kingdom

2 Academic Unit of Bone Metabolism, University of Sheffield, Sheffield, United Kingdom

## References

[1] Ceccarelli F, D'Alfonso S, Perricone C, Carlomagno Y, Alessandri C, Croia C, et al. The role of eight polymorphisms in three candidate genes in determining the susceptibility, phenotype, and response to anti-TNF therapy in patients with rheumatoid arthritis. Clinical and Experimental Rheumatology 2012;Epub ahead of print

[2] de Rooy DP, Yeremenko NG, Wilson AG, Knevel R, Lindqvist E, Saxne T, et al. Genetic studies on components of the Wnt signalling pathway and the severity of joint destruction in rheumatoid arthritis. Annals of Rheumatic Diseases 2012;Epub ahead of print.

[3] Han SW, Sa KH, Kim SI, Lee SI, Park YW, Lee SS, et al. CCR5 gene polymorphism is a genetic risk factor for radiographic severity of rheumatoid arthritis. Tissue Antigens 2012;80:416-23.

[4] Orozco G, Goh CL, Al Olama AA, Benlloch-Garcia S, Govindasami K, Guy M, et al. Common genetic variants associated with disease from genome-wide association studies are mutually exclusive in prostate cancer and rheumatoid arthritis. British Journal of Urology International 2012.

[5] Bergstrom U, Jacobsson LT, Nilsson JA, Berglund G, and Turesson C. Pulmonary dysfunction, smoking, socioeconomic status and the risk of developing rheumatoid arthritis. Rheumatology (Oxford) 2011;50:2005-13.

[6] Lundberg K, Bengtsson C, Kharlamova N, Reed E, Jiang X, Kallberg H, et al. Genetic and environmental determinants for disease risk in subsets of rheumatoid arthritis defined by the anticitrullinated protein/peptide antibody fine specificity profile. Annals of Rheumatic Diseases 2012.

[7] Mikuls TR, Cerhan JR, Criswell LA, Merlino L, Mudano AS, Burma M, et al. Coffee, tea, and caffeine consumption and risk of rheumatoid arthritis: results from the Iowa Women's Health Study. Arthritis & Rheumatism 2002;46:83-91.

[8] Ruiz-Esquide V and Sanmarti R. Tobacco and other environmental risk factors in rheumatoid arthritis. Reumatologia Clinica 2012.

[9] Scott IC, Steer S, Lewis CM, and Cope AP. Precipitating and perpetuating factors of rheumatoid arthritis immunopathology: linking the triad of genetic predisposition, environmental risk factors and autoimmunity to disease pathogenesis. Best Practice & Research Clinical Rheumatology 2011;25:447-68.

[10] Song GG, Bae SC, and Lee YH. Association between vitamin D intake and the risk of rheumatoid arthritis: a meta-analysis. Clinical Rheumatology 2012.

[11] Bhardwaj N, Santhanam U, Lau LL, Tatter SB, Ghrayeb J, Rivelis M, et al. IL-6/IFN-beta 2 in synovial effusions of patients with rheumatoid arthritis and other arthritides. Identification of several isoforms and studies of cellular sources. Journal of Immunology 1989;143:2153-9.

[12] Cope AP, Aderka D, Doherty M, Engelmann H, Gibbons D, Jones AC, et al. Increased levels of soluble tumor necrosis factor receptors in the sera and synovial fluid of patients with rheumatic diseases. Arthritis & Rheumatism 1992;35:1160-9.

[13] Houssiau FA, Devogelaer JP, Van DJ, de Deuxchaisnes CN, and Van SJ. Interleukin-6 in synovial fluid and serum of patients with rheumatoid arthritis and other inflammatory arthritides. Arthritis & Rheumatism 1988;31:784-8.

[14] Waage A, Kaufmann C, Espevik T, and Husby G. Interleukin-6 in synovial fluid from patients with arthritis. Clinical Immunology and Immunopathology 1989;50:394-8.

[15] Brennan FM, Foey AD, and Feldmann M. The importance of T cell interactions with macrophages in rheumatoid cytokine production. Current Topics in Microbiology and Immunology 2006;305:177-94.

[16] Turesson C, Jacobsson L, and Bergstrom U. Extra-articular rheumatoid arthritis: prevalence and mortality. Rheumatology (Oxford) 1999;38:668-74.

[17] Prete M, Racanelli V, Digiglio L, Vacca A, Dammacco F, and Perosa F. Extra-articular manifestations of rheumatoid arthritis: An update. Autoimmunity Reviews 2011;11:123-31.

[18] Arnett FC, Edworthy SM, Bloch DA, McShane DJ, Fries JF, Cooper NS, et al. The American Rheumatism Association 1987 revised criteria for the classification of rheumatoid arthritis. Arthritis & Rheumatism 1988;31:315-24.

[19] Banal F, Dougados M, Combescure C, and Gossec L. Sensitivity and specificity of the American College of Rheumatology 1987 criteria for the diagnosis of rheumatoid arthritis according to disease duration: a systematic literature review and meta-analysis. Annals of Rheumatic Diseases 2009;68:1184-91.

[20] Funovits J, Aletaha D, Bykerk V, Combe B, Dougados M, Emery P, et al. The 2010 American College of Rheumatology/European League Against Rheumatism classification criteria for rheumatoid arthritis: methodological report phase I. Annals of Rheumatic Diseases 2010;69:1589-95.

[21] Aaltonen KJ, Virkki LM, Malmivaara A, Konttinen YT, Nordstrom DC, and Blom M. Systematic review and meta-analysis of the efficacy and safety of existing TNF blocking agents in treatment of rheumatoid arthritis. PLoS One 2012;7:e30275.

[22] Braun J, Bollow M, Remlinger G, Eggens U, Rudwaleit M, Distler A, et al. Prevalence of spondylarthropathies in HLA-B27 positive and negative blood donors. Arthritis & Rheumatism 1998;41:58-67.

[23] Feldtkeller E, Khan MA, van der Heijde D, van der Linden S, and Braun J. Age at disease onset and diagnosis delay in HLA-B27 negative vs. positive patients with ankylosing spondylitis. Rheumatology International 2003;23:61-6.

[24] Braun J and Sieper J. Ankylosing spondylitis. Lancet 2007;369:1379-90.

[25] El Maghraoui A. Extra-articular manifestations of ankylosing spondylitis: prevalence, characteristics and therapeutic implications. European Journal of Internal Medicine 2011;22:554-60.

[26] Hermann KG, Landewe RB, Braun J, and van der Heijde DM. Magnetic resonance imaging of inflammatory lesions in the spine in ankylosing spondylitis clinical trials: is paramagnetic contrast medium necessary? The Journal of Rheumatology 2005;32:2056-60.

[27] Oostveen J, Prevo R, den BJ, and van de Laar M. Early detection of sacroiliitis on magnetic resonance imaging and subsequent development of sacroiliitis on plain radiography. A prospective, longitudinal study. The Journal of Rheumatology 1999;26:1953-8.

[28] Rudwaleit M, Metter A, Listing J, Sieper J, and Braun J. Inflammatory back pain in ankylosing spondylitis: a reassessment of the clinical history for application as classificatoin and diagnositc criteria. Arthritis & Rheumatism 2006;54:569-78.

[29] Dagfinrud H, Kvien TK, and Hagen KB. The Cochrane review of physiotherapy interventions for ankylosing spondylitis. The Journal of Rheumatology 2005;32:1899-906.

[30] Saougou I, Markatseli TE, Voulgari PV, and Drosos AA. Maintained clinical response of infliximab treatment in ankylosing spondylitis: a 6-year long-term study. Joint Bone Spine 2010;77:325-9.

[31] Woodward LJ and Kam PC. Ankylosing spondylitis: recent developments and anaesthetic implications. Anaesthesia 2009;64:540-8.

[32] Moll JM and Wright V. Psoriatic arthritis. Seminars in Arthritis and Rheumatism 1973;3:55-78.

[33] Woolacott N, Bravo Vergel Y, Hawkins N, Kainth A, Khadjesari Z, Misso K, et al. Etanercept and infliximab for the treatment of psoriatic arthritis: a systematic review and economic evaluation. Health Technology Assessment 2006;10:1-239.

[34] Khan MA. Update on spondyloarthropathies. Annals of Internal Medicine 2002;136:896-907.

[35] Winchester R, Minevich G, Steshenko V, Kirby B, Kane D, Greenberg DA, et al. HLA associations reveal genetic heterogeneity in psoriatic arthritis and in the psoriasis phenotype. Arthritis & Rheumatism 2012;64:1134-44.

[36] Scarpa R, Del PA, di GC, della VG, Lubrano E, and Oriente P. Interplay between environmental factors, articular involvement, and HLA-B27 in patients with psoriatic arthritis. Annals of Rheumatic Diseases 1992;51:78-9.

[37] Wang Q, Vasey FB, Mahfood JP, Valeriano J, Kanik KS, Anderson BE, et al. V2 regions of 16S ribosomal RNA used as a molecular marker for the species identification of streptococci in peripheral blood and synovial fluid from patients with psoriatic arthritis. Arthritis & Rheumatism 1999;42:2055-9.

[38] Gladman DD, Stafford-Brady F, Chang CH, Lewandowski K, and Russell ML. Longitudinal study of clinical and radiological progression in psoriatic arthritis. Journal of Rheumatology 1990;17:809-12.

[39] Eder L, Zisman D, Barzilai M, Laor A, Rahat M, Rozenbaum M, et al. Subclinical atherosclerosis in psoriatic arthritis: a case-control study. The Journal of Rheumatology 2008;35:877-82.

[40] Tam LS, Tomlinson B, Chu TT, Li M, Leung YY, Kwok LW, et al. Cardiovascular risk profile of patients with psoriatic arthritis compared to controls--the role of inflammation. Rheumatology (Oxford) 2008;47:718-23.

[41] Taylor W, Gladman D, Helliwell P, Marchesoni A, Mease P, and Mielants H. Classification criteria for psoriatic arthritis: development of new criteria from a large international study. Arthritis & Rheumatism 2006;54:2665-73.

[42] Chandran V, Schentag CT, and Gladman DD. Sensitivity of the classification of psoriatic arthritis criteria in early psoriatic arthritis. Arthritis & Rheumatism 2007;57:1560-3.

[43] Cantini F, Niccoli L, Nannini C, Kaloudi O, Bertoni M, and Cassara E. Psoriatic arthritis: a systematic review. International Journal of Rheumatic Diseases 2010;13:300-17.

[44] Sandles L. An holistic approach to the management of rheumatoid disease. Occupatonal Therapy in Rheumatology. London: Chapman and Hall; 1990, p. 41-50.

[45] Samanta R, Shoukrey K, and Griffiths R. Rheumatoid arthritis and anaesthesia. Anaesthesia 2011;66:1146-59.

[46] Neva MH, Hakkinen A, Makinen H, Hannonen P, Kauppi M, and Sokka T. High prevalence of asymptomatic cervical spine subluxation in patients with rheumatoid arthritis waiting for orthopaedic surgery. Annals of Rheumatic Diseases 2006;65:884-8.

[47] Shen FH, Samartzis D, Jenis LG, and An HS. Rheumatoid arthritis: evaluation and surgical management of the cervical spine. Spine Journal 2004;4:689-700.

[48] Wilkinson JM, Haslam P, and Getty CJM. (ii) Hip and knee reconstruction in the rheumatoid patient. Current Orthopaedics 2007;21:330–9.

[49] Grennan DM, Gray J, Loudon J, and Fear S. Methotrexate and early postoperative complications in patients with rheumatoid arthritis undergoing elective orthopaedic surgery. Annals of Rheumatic Diseases 2001;60:214-7.

[50] Loza E, Martinez-Lopez JA, and Carmona L. A systematic review on the optimum management of the use of methotrexate in rheumatoid arthritis patients in the perioperative period to minimize perioperative morbidity and maintain disease control. Clinical and Experimental Rheumatology 2009;27:856-62.

[51] Heldmann F and Braun J. Perioperative use of methotrexate. Clinical and Experimental Rheumatology 2010;28:S110-3.

[52] Sreekumar R, Gray J, Kay P, and Grennan DM. Methotrexate and post operative complications in patients with rheumatoid arthritis undergoing elective orthopaedic surgery-a ten year follow-up. Acta Orthopaedica Belgica 2011;77:823-6.

[53] da Cunha BM, Maria Henrique da Mota L, and Dos Santos-Neto LL. Risk of orthopedic surgical site infections in patients with rheumatoid arthritis treated with antitumor necrosis factor alfa therapy. International Journal of Rheumatology 2012;2012:369565.

[54] Talwalkar SC, Grennan DM, Gray J, Johnson P, and Hayton MJ. Tumour necrosis factor alpha antagonists and early postoperative complications in patients with inflammatory joint disease undergoing elective orthopaedic surgery. Annals of Rheumatic Diseases 2005;64:650-1.

[55] Wendling D, Balblanc JC, Brousse A, Lohse A, Lehuede G, Garbuio P, et al. Surgery in patients receiving anti-tumour necrosis factor alpha treatment in rheumatoid arthritis: an observational study on 50 surgical procedures. Annals of Rheumatic Diseases 2005;64:1378-9.

[56] Giles JT, Bartlett SJ, Gelber AC, Nanda S, Fontaine K, Ruffing V, et al. Tumor necrosis factor inhibitor therapy and risk of serious postoperative orthopedic infection in rheumatoid arthritis. Arthritis & Rheumatism 2006;55:333-7.

[57] Momohara S, Kawakami K, Iwamoto T, Yano K, Sakuma Y, Hiroshima R, et al. Prosthetic joint infection after total hip or knee arthroplasty in rheumatoid arthritis patients treated with nonbiologic and biologic disease-modifying antirheumatic drugs. Modern Rheumatology 2011;21:469-75.

[58] Suzuki M, Nishida K, Soen S, Oda H, Inoue H, Kaneko A, et al. Risk of postoperative complications in rheumatoid arthritis relevant to treatment with biologic agents: a report from the Committee on Arthritis of the Japanese Orthopaedic Association. Journal of Orthopaedic Science 2011;16:778-84.

[59] Saag KG, Teng GG, Patkar NM, Anuntiyo J, Finney C, Curtis JR, et al. American College of Rheumatology 2008 recommendations for the use of nonbiologic and biologic disease-modifying antirheumatic drugs in rheumatoid arthritis. Arthritis & Rheumatism 2008;59:762-84.

[60] Singh JA, Furst DE, Bharat A, Curtis JR, Kavanaugh AF, Kremer JM, et al. 2012 update of the 2008 American College of Rheumatology recommendations for the use of disease-modifying antirheumatic drugs and biologic agents in the treatment of rheumatoid arthritis. Arthritis Care & Research (Hoboken) 2012;64:625-39.

[61] Otto AW. Ein Becken, mit kugelformig augedehnten Pfannen. In: E Heft editor. Seltene Beobachtungen zur Anatomie, Physiologie und Pathologie gehorig. Breslau: Verlag Willibald August Holaufer; 1816, p. 19–20.

[62] Overgaard K. Otto's disease and other forms of protrusio acetauli. Acta Radiologica 1935;16 390-419.

[63] Gilmour J. Adolescent deformities of the acetabulum: an investigation into the nature of protrusio acetabuli. British Journal of Surgery 1939;26:670-99.

[64] Sotelo-Garza A and Charnley J. The results of Charnley arthroplasty of hip performed for protrusio acetabuli. Clinical Orthopaedics and Related Research 1978:12-8.

[65] Hirst P, Esser M, Murphy JC, and Hardinge K. Bone grafting for protrusio acetabuli during total hip replacement. A review of the Wrightington method in 61 hips. Journal of Bone and Joint Surgery (Br) 1987;69:229-33.

[66] Edelstein G and Murphy WA. Protrusio acetabuli: radiographic appearance in arthritis and other conditions. Arthritis & Rheumatism 1983;26:1511-6.

[67] Rosenberg WW, Schreurs BW, de Waal Malefijt MC, Veth RP, and Slooff TJ. Impacted morsellized bone grafting and cemented primary total hip arthroplasty for acetabular protrusion in patients with rheumatoid arthritis: an 8- to 18-year follow-up study of 36 hips. Acta Orthopaedica Scandinavica 2000;71:143-6.

[68] Buttaro MA, Comba F, Pusso R, and Piccaluga F. Acetabular revision with metal mesh, impaction bone grafting, and a cemented cup. Clinical Orthopaedics and Related Research 2008;466:2482-90.

[69] Jones L, Grammatopoulos G, and Singer G. The Burch-Schneider cage: 9-year survival in Paprosky type 3 acetabular defects. Clinical and radiological follow-up. Hip International 2012;22:28-34.

[70] Mäkelä KT, Eskelinen A, Pulkkinen P, Virolainen P, Paavolainen P, and Remes V. Cemented versus cementless total hip replacements in patients fifty-five years of age or older with rheumatoid arthritis. Journal of Bone and Joint Surgery (Am) 2011;93:178-86.

[71] Eskelinen A, Paavolainen P, Helenius I, Pulkkinen P, and Remes V. Total hip arthroplasty for rheumatoid arthritis in younger patients: 2,557 replacements in the Finnish Arthroplasty Register followed for 0-24 years. Acta Orthopaedica Scandinavica 2006;77:853-65.

[72] Rud-Sørensen C, Pedersen AB, Johnsen SP, Riis AH, and Overgaard S. Survival of primary total hip arthroplasty in rheumatoid arthritis patients. Acta Orthopaedica Scandinavica 2010;81:60-5.

[73] Creighton MG, Callaghan JJ, Olejniczak JP, and Johnston RC. Total hip arthroplasty with cement in patients who have rheumatoid arthritis. A minimum ten-year follow-up study. Journal of Bone and Joint Surgery (Am) 1998;80:1439-46.

[74] Sochart DH and Porter ML. The long-term results of Charnley low-friction arthroplasty in young patients who have congenital dislocation, degenerative osteoarthrosis, or rheumatoid arthritis Journal of Bone and Joint Surgery (Am) 1997;79:1599–617.

[75] Zwartelé RE, Witjes S, Doets HC, Stijnen T, and Pöll RG. Cementless total hip arthroplasty in rheumatoid arthritis: a systematic review of the literature. Archives of Orthopaedic and Trauma Surgery 2012;132:535-46.

[76] Aulakh TS, Kuiper JH, Dixey J, and Richardson JB. Hip resurfacing for rheumatoid arthritis: independent assessment of 11-year results from an international register. International Orthopaedics 2011;35:803-8.

[77] Wisk LE and Amstutz HC. Metal-on-metal hip resurfacing in rheumatoid patients. A report on thirteen hips with minimum 3 year follow-up. Hip International 2011;21:59-65.

[78] Mihalko WM, Saleh KJ, Krackow KA, and Whiteside LA. Soft-tissue balancing during total knee arthroplasty in the varus knee. Journal of the American Academy of Orthopaedic Surgeons 2009;17:766-74.

[79] Kanamiya T, Whiteside LA, Nakamura T, Mihalko WM, Steiger J, and Naito M. Ranawat Award paper. Effect of selective lateral ligament release on stability in knee arthroplasty. Clinical Orthopaedics 2002;404:24-31.

[80] Peters CL, Mohr RA, and Bachus KN. Primary total knee arthroplasty in the valgus knee: creating a balanced soft tissue envelope. Journal of Arthoplasty 2001;16:721-9.

[81] Wang W and Niu D. Balancing of soft tissues in total knee arthroplasty for patients with rheumatoid arthritis with kneeflexion contracture. Zhongguo Xiu Fu Chong Jian Wai Ke Za Zhi 2008;22:1173-6.

[82] Clarke HD, Fuchs R, Scuderi GR, Scott WN, and Insall JN. Clinical results in valgus total knee arthroplasty with the "pie crust" technique of lateral soft tissue releases. Journal of Arthoplasty 2005;20:1010-4.

[83] Archibeck MJ, Berger RA, Barden RM, Jacobs JJ, Sheinkop MB, Rosenberg AG, et al. Posterior cruciate ligament-retaining total knee arthroplasty in patients with rheumatoid arthritis. Journal of Bone and Joint Surgery (Am) 2001;83:1231-6.

[84] Miller MD, Brown NM, Della Valle CJ, Rosenberg AG, and Galante JO. Posterior cruciate ligament-retaining total knee arthroplasty in patients with rheumatoid arthritis: a concise follow-up of a previous report. Journal of Bone and Joint Surgery (Am) 2011;93:e130(1-6).

[85] Morgan H, Battista V, and Leopold SS. Constraint in primary total knee arthroplasty. Journal of the American Academy of Orthopaedic Surgeons 2005;13:515-24.

[86] Kajino A, Yoshino S, Kameyama S, Kohda M, and Nagashima S. Comparison of the results of bilateral total knee arthroplasty with and without patellar replacement for rheumatoid arthritis. A follow-up note. Journal of Bone and Joint Surgery (Am) 1997;79:570-4.

[87] Swedish knee arthroplasty register annual report 2011 (www.ort.lu.se/kneeS). 2011.

[88] Ito J, Koshino T, Okamoto R, and Saito T. 15-year follow-up study of total knee arthroplasty in patients with rheumatoid arthritis. Journal of Arthoplasty 2003;18:984-92.

[89] Woo YK, Kim KW, Chung JW, and Lee HS. Average 10.1-year follow-up of cementless total knee arthroplasty in patients with rheumatoid arthritis. Canadian Journal of Surgery 2011;54:179–84.

[90] Yamanaka H, Goto K, and Suzuki M. Clinical results of Hi-tech Knee II total knee arthroplasty in patients with rheumatoid athritis: 5- to 12-year follow-up. Journal of Orthopaedic Surgery and Research 2012;22:9.

[91] Sharma S, Nicol F, Hullin MG, and McCreath SW. Long-term results of the uncemented low contact stress total knee replacement in patients with rheumatoid arthritis. Journal of Bone and Joint Surgery (Br) 2005;87:1077–80.

[92] Robertsson O, Knutson K, Lewold S, Goodman S, and Lidgren L. Knee arthroplasty in rheumatoid arthritis. A report from the Swedish Knee Arthroplasty Register on 4,381 primary operations 1985–1995. Acta Orthopaedica Scandinavica 1997;68:545-53.

[93] Sokka T, Abelson B, and Pincus T. Mortality in rheumatoid arthritis: 2008 update. Clinical and Experimental Rheumatology 2008;26:S35-61.

[94] Clement ND, Jenkins PJ, Brenkel IJ, and Walmsley P. Predictors of mortality after total knee replacement: a ten-year survivorship analysis. Journal of Bone and Joint Surgery (Br) 2012;94:200-4.

[95] Schrama JC, Espehaug B, Hallan G, Engesaeter LB, Furnes O, Havelin LI, et al. Risk of revision for infection in primary total hip and knee arthroplasty in patients with rheumatoid arthritis compared with osteoarthritis: a prospective, population-based study on 108,786 hip and knee joint arthroplasties from the Norwegian Arthroplasty Register. Arthritis Care & Research (Hoboken) 2010;62:473-9.

[96] Bongartz T, Halligan CS, Osmon DR, Reinalda MS, Bamlet WR, Crowson CS, et al. Incidence and risk factors of prosthetic joint infection after total hip or knee replacement in patients with rheumatoid arthritis. Arthritis & Rheumatism 2008;59:1713-20.

[97] da Cunha BM, de Oliveira SB, and Santos-Neto L. Incidence of infectious complications in hip and knee arthroplasties in rheumatoid arthritis and osteoarthritis patients. Revista Brasileira de Reumatologia 2011;51:609-15.

[98] Matta F, Singala R, Yaekoub AY, Najjar R, and Stein PD. Risk of venous thromboembolism with rheumatoid arthritis. Journal of Thrombosis and Haemostasis 2009;101:134-8.

[99] Niki Y, Matsumoto H, Hakozaki A, Mochizuki T, and Momohara S. Rheumatoid arthritis: a risk factor for deep venous thrombosis after total knee arthroplasty? Comparative study with osteoarthritis. Journal of Orthopaedic Science 2010;15:57-63.

[100] Buchanan RR and Kraag G. Is there a lower incidence of deep venous thrombosis after joint replacement in rheumatoid arthritis? The Journal of Rheumatology 1980;7:551-4.

[101] Eggli S and Woo A. Risk factors for heterotopic ossification in total hip arthroplasty. Archives of Orthopaedic and Trauma Surgery 2001;121:531-5.

[102] Meek RM, Allan DB, McPhillips G, Kerr L, and Howie CR. Late Dislocation after Total Hip Arthroplasty. Clinical Medicine & Research 2008;6:17-23.

[103] Zwartelé RE, Brand R, and Doets HC. Increased risk of dislocation after primary total hip arthroplasty in inflammatory arthritis: a prospective observational study of 410 hips. Acta Orthopaedica Scandinavica 2004;75:684-90.

[104] Lindahl H, Malchau H, Oden A, and Garellick G. Risk factors for failure after treatment of a periprosthetic fracture of the femur. Journal of Bone and Joint Surgery (Am) 2006;88:26-30.

[105] Pap G and Neumann HW. Periprosthetic fractures in patients with rheumatoid arthritis. Zeitschrift fur Rheumatologie 2007;66:22-7.

[106] Felson DT, Anderson JJ, Boers M, Bombardier C, Furst D, Goldsmith C, et al. American College of Rheumatology: preliminary definition of improvement in rheumatoid arthritis. Arthritis & Rheumatism 1995;38:727–35.

[107] van Gestel AM, Prevoo ML, van 't Hof MA, van Rijswijk MH, van de Putte LB, and van Riel PL. Development and validation of the European League Against Rheumatism response criteria for rheumatoid arthritis. Comparison with the preliminary American College of Rheumatology and the World Health Organization/International League Against Rheumatism Criteria. Arthritis & Rheumtism 1996;39:34-40.

[108] Fortin PR, Penrod JR, Clarke AE, St-Pierre Y, Joseph L, Bélisle P, et al. Timing of total joint replacement affects clinical outcomes among patients with osteoarthritis of the hip or knee. Arthritis & Rheumatism 2002;46:3327-30.

[109] Sledge CB. Introduction to surgical management of patients with arthritis. In: S Ruddy, ED Harris, and CB Sledge editors. Kelley's textbook of rheumatology. Philadelphia: W.B.Saunders, p. 1691–8.

[110] Gilson M, Gossec L, Mariette X, Gherissi D, Guyot MH, Berthelot JM, et al. Risk factors for total joint arthroplasty infection in patients receiving tumor necrosis factor alpha-blockers: a case-control study. *Arthritis Research & Therapy* 2010;12:R145.

[111] Santaguida PL, Hawker GA, Hudak PL, Glazier R, Mahomed NN, Kreder HJ, et al. Patient characteristics affecting the prognosis of total hip and knee joint arthroplasty: a systematic review. Canadian Journal of Surgery 2008;51:428-36.

[112] Bombardier C, Barbieri M, Parthan A, Zack DJ, Walker V, Macarios D, et al. The relationship between joint damage and functional disability in rheumatoid arthritis: a systematic review. Annals of Rheumtic Diseases 2012;71:836-44.

[113] Benoni AC, Bremander A, and Nilsdotter A. Patient-reported outcome after rheumatoid arthritis-related surgery in the lower extremities: a report from the Swedish National Register of Rheuma Surgery (RAKIR). Acta Orthopaedica 2012;83:179-84.

[114] Nguyen-Oghalai TU, Ottenbacher KJ, Caban M, Granger CV, Grecula M, and Goodwin JS. The impact of rheumatoid arthritis on rehabilitation outcomes after lower extremity arthroplasty. Journal of Clinical Rheumatology 2007;13:247-50.

[115] Bischoff-Ferrari HA, Lingard EA, Losina E, Baron JA, Roos EM, Phillips CB, et al. Psychosocial and geriatric correlates of functional status after total hip replacement. Arthritis & Rheumatisim 2004;51:829-35.

[116] Katsimihas M, Taylor AH, Lee MB, Sarangi PP, and Learmonth ID. Cementless acetabular replacement in patients with rheumatoid arthritis: a 6- to 14-year prospective study. Journal of Arthroplasty 2003;18:16–22.

[117] Tang WM and Chiu KY. Primary total hip arthroplasty in patients with rheumatoid arthritis. International Journal of Orthopaedics 2001;25:13-6.

[118] Kristensen O, Nafei A, Kjaersgaard-Andersen P, Hvid I, and Jensen J. Long-term results of total condylar knee arthroplasty in rheumatoid arthritis. Journal of Bone and Joint Surgery (Br) 1992;74:803-6.

[119] Ritter MA, Lutgring JD, Davis KE, Faris PM, and Berend ME. Total knee arthroplasty effectiveness in patients 55 years old and younger: osteoarthritis vs. rheumatoid arthritis. Knee 2007;14:9-11.

[120] Bullens PH, van Loon CJ, de Waal Malefijt MC, Laan RF, and Veth RP. Patient satisfaction after total knee arthroplasty: a comparison between subjective and objective outcome assessments. Journal of Arthroplasty 2001;16:740-7.

Chapter 14

# Revision Hip Arthroplasty: Management of Bone Loss

Plamen Kinov and Peter Tivchev

Additional information is available at the end of the chapter

## 1. Introduction

Total hip arthroplasty (THA) is one of the most successful surgical procedures with well documented survivorship at up to 25 years. With ageing of the population and higher arthritis prevalence in older adults, the demand for the procedure increases worldwide [89]. In addition, over the last two decades the age range has been broadened to include younger patients. Over 270 000 hip replacements are performed annually in the US alone, and the annual volume of hip joint replacement is projected to double by the year 2030 [89]. Although very successful procedure, significant percentage of patients undergoing total hip arthroplasty require revision within 10 to 15 years after the surgery. Aseptic loosening and the associated osteolysis have been recognized as the main reason for implant failure in 71% of cases [66]. Other indications for revision include periprosthetic fracture, dislocation, and infection. New technologies in implant design and advances in surgical technique have improved the outcomes after primary total hip arthroplasty and decreased the rate of complications. However, as a consequence of increased rate of primary THA's the prevalence of revision hip surgery is increasing proportionally. The increased rate and costs of revision procedures impose high demands on both surgeon and healthcare system. Moreover, the cost of hip replacement is exponentially increasing [82].

Bone loss is the major challenge in revision setting. In 2009, Bozic et al. reviewed the most common causes for revision hip arthroplasty [8]. Aseptic loosening, instability, and infection were reported as the main reasons for revision surgery. This study underlined the need for a complex approach to evaluation and management of patients with implant failure after hip replacement. Such approach will guarantee precise diagnosis, proper selection of revision implant and surgical approach, uncomplicated surgery, and optimal clinical result.

This chapter provides an overview of aseptic loosening of revision hip arthroplasty and outlines the management strategies in the clinical scenario of a failed hip prosthesis.

## 2. Patient evaluation

Various signs and symptoms can occur in the clinical setting of a failed hip prosthesis. Painful hip arthroplasty is the most common complication after total hip arthroplasty reaching 18% of patients in some series [6]. Most of these painful hips will require revision. Groin pain can be referred to implant failure easily whereas occasional hip pain, pain in the buttock, knee pain or migrating pain can have different etiology. Other diseases and conditions such as disk disease, radiculopathy, inguinal or femoral hernia, pelvic infections, tumors, and trauma may have manifestations similar to that of a failed prosthesis.

The differential diagnosis of hip pain requires a careful history and examination. In simple cases, the reason could be identified with clinical examinations and standard radiographs only. Thorough examination elicits the underlying cause of hip complains such as infection, neurological injury, referred pain, wear, aseptic loosening or instability. In many cases, the diagnosis is a challenge to the surgeon. In addition to clinical history and physical examination, radiographic examination and advanced imaging techniques could help establish exact localization of pain, and its possible connection with the implant. Additional radiographic examinations as well as an algorithmic approach with special diagnostic imaging and tests help establishing precise diagnosis. Computed tomography and 3-D computed tomography is often helpful in establishing periprosthetic osteolysis and its severity. In addition to plain radiographs arthrography with contrast medium could be considered in certain cases.

Once extrinsic and periarticular diseases have been excluded as a reason for the hip pain, septic loosening should be excluded. Laboratory investigations are the initial tests that help differentiate septic from aseptic loosening. A standard set includes WBC, Erythrocyte sedimentation rate (ESR), C-reactive protein (CRP), complete chemistries and urinalysis. In addition to plain radiographs and laboratory tests joint aspiration is considered the most important diagnostic tool in ruling out periprosthetic infection. The aspirate should be sent for cell count and anaerobic and aerobic cultures. Recently, local markers such as interleukin-6 (IL-6) and other cytokines [34], synovial CRP, and leukocyte esterase (LE) [118] from joint aspirate have been proposed. All of these local markers have shown accuracy of more than 90% in predicting periprosthetic infection. Nuclear medicine scans with technetium-99m-HDP, gallium citrate, and labeled WBC have been used to diagnose the presence of infection. However, because of poor sensitivity, specificity, and accuracy, it is cost-prohibitive and remains a tertiary tool. Nuclear medicine is used only if infection could not be proven otherwise. Intraoperatively, diagnostic evaluations such as Gram stains and frozen sections have been proposed.

Guidelines and algorithms for evaluation of painful hip arthroplasty have been published in the literature and implemented in practice [119]. Such approach helps eliminate infection of the failed hip that would change treatment approach and could exclude one-stage revision.

## 3. Classification systems for bone defects

It is important to have a practical, relatively simple classification system for assessment of bone defects associated with loose hip implants. The use of a radiographic classification system helps to establish the severity and localization of bone defects, and to guide treatment decisions. It should allow the surgeon to be prepared for the possible intraoperative findings and to plan adequate treatment approach. Numerous classification systems have been described in the literature [17,23,25,32,40,58,60,99,116,137,158].

### 3.1. AAOS classification

The American Academy of Orthopedic Surgeons (AAOS) classification system of bone defects, described by D'Antonio et al. identifies the pattern and localization of osteolysis but does not quantify the bone loss [23-25]. It is one of the most widely used classification system in the literature.

### 3.2. Paprosky classification

Perhaps the most widely used classification system, the Paprosky Classification [32,116,158] (Tables 1, 2) was developed to establish bone defect type, size, and localization in order to allow selection of appropriate cementless reconstructive option for a given bone loss pattern. We base our clinical decisions on this classification system.

The key advantage of this classification is the assessment of the host bone ability to provide initial stability of a cementless implant until bone ingrowth occurs. The bone defects are usually classified on the basis of plain radiographs. However, final assessment is made intraoperatively, after removal of the failed implant and thorough debridement of the host bone. Intraoperative assessment of implant stability is made with help of trial components. The remaining host bone determines the stability of the implant and the type of the defect.

| Type | Radiographic and intraoperative findings |
|---|---|
| 1 | Minimal metaphyseal bone loss |
| 2 | Extensive metaphyseal bone loss and an intact diaphysis |
| 3A | Extensive metadiaphyseal bone loss and a minimum of 4 cm of intact cortical bone in the diaphysis |
| 3B | Extensive metadiaphyseal bone loss and <4 cm of intact cortical bone in the diaphysis |
| 4 | Extensive metadiaphyseal bone loss and a nonsupportive diaphysis |

**Table 1.** Paprosky classification systems for femoral defects.

| Type | Radiographic and intraoperative findings |
|---|---|
| 1 | Acetabular rim, anterior-posterior column intact |
| 2 | Less than 3 cm superior migration<br>Distorted acetabular rim. Intact anterior and posterior columns<br>Adequate stability with Trial. Greater than 50% contact surface |
| 2A | Superior and medial cavitation defect. Intact rim |
| 2B | Segmental supero-lateral defect (less than 1/3 of circumference) |
| 2C | Medial defect with cup medial to Kohler's line (Protrusio) |
| 3 | Greater than 3 cm superior migration<br>Non-supportive acetabular rim for biological fixation |
| 3A | Lateral to Kohler's line. Intact medial support<br>Moderate ischial lysis (<15 mm below superior obturator line)<br>Medial limb of teardrop is intact<br>Superior and lateral migration "up and out"<br>Contact of trial with bone over 40-60% |
| 3B | Broken Kohler's line. No medial or superior support<br>Extensive ischial osteolysis (>15 mm below superior obturator line)<br>Complete destruction of tear drop<br>Superior and medial migration "up and in"<br>Under 40% contact surface. High risk of occult pelvic discontinuity |

**Table 2.** Paprosky classification system for acetabular defects.

## 4. Preoperative planning

Careful preoperative planning is a prerequisite for successful revision surgery. The principle aims in revision hip arthroplasty are to achieve supportive host bone, secure implant fixation and to restore hip center and joint kinematics. The type and severity of host bone loss determine the method of reconstruction. Careful preoperative planning improves effectiveness during surgery, and helps distinguish more complex alternatives for reconstruction if needed.

Thorough clinical and radiographic examination is essential for determining the extent and severity of bone loss, quality of the host bone, exclusion of infection, additional deformities, and potentially confounding factors. Computed tomography may be needed in the presence of massive bone loss. In case of medial migration of the failed components angiography with contrast medium should be considered. Manual or digital templating helps for adequate selection (size, diameter, length) of revision implant and reduce the operative room inventory. Templating also helps determine whether stable initial fixation could be obtained and the need for additional procedures. Preoperative planning is critical for the assessment of the need of graft, tools for implant removal, and selection of proper components available at the time of surgery. Appropriate surgical exposure should be planned with an extensile approach often necessary. Classification system of bone defects based on radiographs that assesses the severity of bone loss according to the type of fixation for a given bone loss pattern is beneficial. In our practice, we find the Paprosky classification system a useful tool for guidance of clinical decisions. Any attempt should be made to identify the failed implant. The implant manufacturer should be contacted for implant-specific extraction devices if available. In case of isolated partial revision, it is advisable to have an option for partial (liner or head) exchange.

## 5. Surgical approaches in revision arthroplasty

The aims of revision surgery are to extract the failed prosthesis with minimal soft tissue and bone damage, to restore bone loss, and to implant prosthesis with stable and durable fixation. Ultimate goals are long-lasting and painless joint function. To obtain these goals arthroplasty surgeons may require a variety of approaches for adequate exposure of the femur and acetabulum in different revision settings. Usually arthroplasty surgeons are familiar and most comfortable with a certain approach and use it in most surgeries. However, in order to obtain reproducible results after revision of most difficult cases, surgeons should be familiar with all approaches to the hip joint. Next to standard approaches used in primary total hip arthroplasty, extensile approaches were developed in order to minimize damage to the host bone, safely remove the loose implant and provide good visualization for correct insertion of the revision components. Contained defects can be reconstructed through any conventional approach. For uncontained defects, we prefer to have wide access and, therefore, we use transtrochanteric approach or trochanteric slide osteotomy with preserved insertion of vastus lateralis. If greater exposure is needed extended trochanteric osteotomy is advisable.

### 5.1. Extended trochanteric osteotomy

The extended trochanteric osteotomy (ETO) is one of the significant achievements in revision surgery [9] (Figure 1).

It is safe and straightforward, saving time and minimizing risk of fracture during cement and failed implant removal. However, it limits femoral component options to those that rely on distal fixation. Advantages of the technique are: predictable healing of the osteotomy, decrease in intraoperative fractures and femoral perforations, direct access to the distal canal for cement removal and neutral reaming, and decreased surgical time [9,104]. Favorable clinical results after use of ETO have been published in the literature [9,104].

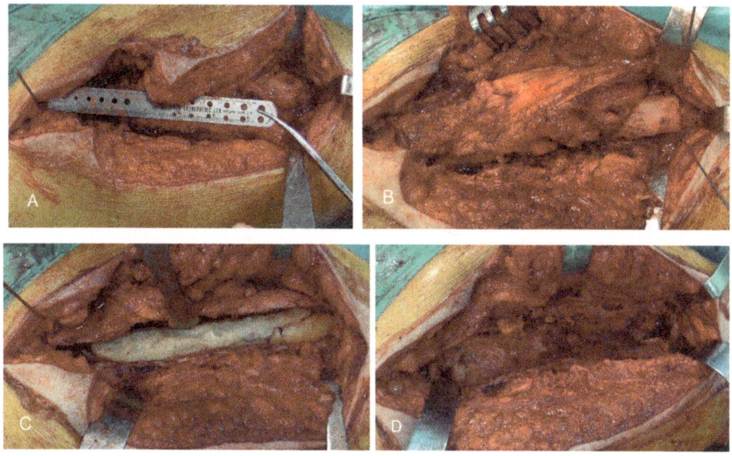


**Figure 1.** (A) The Extended trochanteric osteotomy is performed by cutting from the greater trochanter distally along the long axis of the femur. (B) The bone is cut with a saw. (C) The flap with the attached muscles is elevated. (D) Exposed femoral bone bed.

## 6. Surgical revision options

Majority of hip revisions could be performed using cementing technique. However, patients with severe bone loss and poor bone quality require complex alternatives for revision.

### 6.1. Options for Femoral revision

#### *6.1.1. Cemented fixation of the femoral component*

Various studies publish the outcomes after cemented femoral revision [2,13,122]. Use of the early cementing technique produced disappointing results [2,69]. Gaining more extensive experience resulted in acceptable short- to mid-term results [13,81,122]. Re-revision rates ranging from 4.3% to 6.0% and radiographic loosening ranging from 12% to 44% after mid-term follow-up of 3.4 to 4.5 years were reported (Table 3). However, long-term studies showed suboptimal outcomes after revision with an early cementing technique. At 8.1-year follow-up of the initial group of cemented revisions, Pellicci et al. found more than doubled incidence of re-revision and radiographic loosening ranging from 5.4% to 19% and from 13.6% to 29%, respectively [121]. Similar results were published by Kavanagh et al. in a 10-year follow-up study [79]. Sixty-four per cent of the stems had been revised or were radiographically loose. The incidence of revision had more than doubled from 18% at 3 years to 39% at final follow-up.

| Authors | Year | Hips (No) | Follow-up (yrs) | Re-revision rate (%) | Radiographic loosening (%) |
|---|---|---|---|---|---|
| | | **Early technique** | | | |
| Amstutz et al. [2] | 1982 | 66 | 2.1 | 9.0 | 29.9 |
| Pellicci et al. [122] | 1982 | 110 | 3.4 | 5.4 | 13.6 |
| Pellicci et al. [121] | 1985 | 99 | 8.1 | 19.0 | 29.0 |
| Kavanagh et al. [81] | 1985 | 166 | 4.5 | 6.0 | 44.0 |
| Engelbrecht et al. [39] | 1990 | 138 | 7.4 | 8.8 | 38.0 |
| | | **Improved technique** | | | |
| Rubash and Harris [134] | 1988 | 43 | 6.2 | 2.0 | 11.0 |
| Katz et al. [78] | 1997 | 79 | 11.9 | 5.4 | 16.0 |
| Callaghan et al. [13] | 1985 | 139 | 3.6 | 4.3 | 12.0 |
| Estok and Harris [43] | 1994 | 38 | 11.7 | 10.5 | 10.5 |
| Mulroy and Harris [109] | 1996 | 43 | 15.1 | 20.0 | 6.0 |

**Table 3.** Results of cemented femoral revision.

The main reason for suboptimal results with early cemented revisions was difficulty in obtaining stable and long-lasting fixation in compromised host bone stock where the rate of re-revision was very high [83]. In early studies, the reactive sclerotic bone between the fibrous membrane and the native cancellous bone was not removed [12]. Poor fixation of the revision femoral component compared to that in the primary setting may be due to inadequate excision of residual fibrous membrane, incomplete drying of bone, suboptimal cement filling technique, or insufficient cement-bone interlock on the smooth sclerotic bone surface. In such setting, even long cemented stems, are generally difficult to be inserted with adequate primary and long lasting stability. Femoral revision using so-called modern cementing techniques may yield promising results (Figure 2).

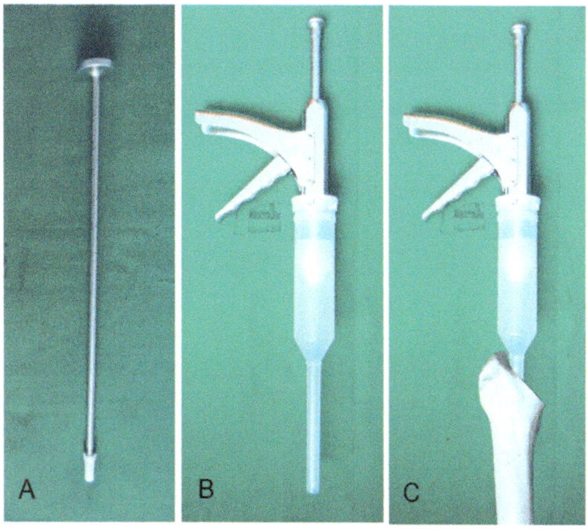


**Figure 2.** Modern cementing technique. (A) Distal cement plug. (B) Cement injector. (C) Delivery and pressurization of cement using cement injector.

Different studies have demonstrated that modern cementing techniques have improved implant survival and clinical outcome compared with the mid-term results after revision with use of so-called first-generation technique [71,85,109,128,134] (Figure 3).

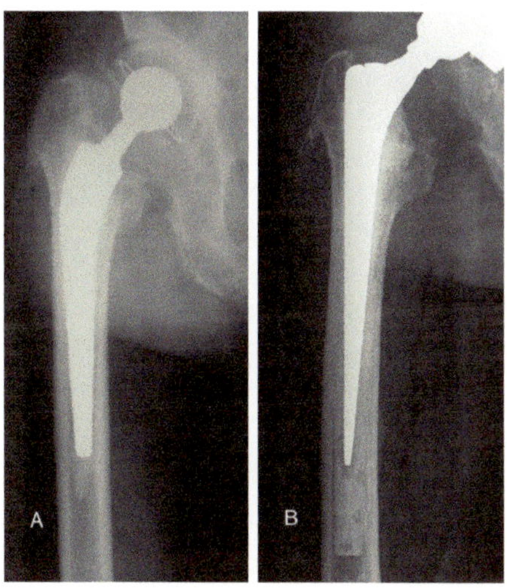


**Figure 3.** (A) Preoperative radiograph of a failed cemented prosthesis. (B) Grade A cemented fixation achieved with modern cementing technique.

Cemented femoral revision has several advantages in elderly patients. It allows early mobilization, a shorter operating time, and possibly less risk of a peroperative fracture. Use of modern cementing techniques seems to improve fixation of the femoral components and clinical outcomes and justifies its use. Whenever possible the failed arthroplasty should be revised before occurrence of severe bone loss and femoral enlargement.

*6.1.1.1. Cement-within-cement fixation of the femoral component*

Removal of the well-fixed cement mantle around the stem can be extremely difficult, time consuming, and risky procedure. A solution to the problem, cement-within-cement revision was first proposed by Eftekhar who advised on preserving the existing well cemented mantle and re-cementing the new stem into it [36]. In a biomechanical study, Greenwald et al. demonstrated that the separation strength was 94% that of a single block when the existing cement mantle was adequately prepared [56]. The technique requires that the old cement surface be dried and roughened in order to provide contact area for fixation of the new cement. The cement should be injected in the early liquid phase in order to prevent lamination and to promote polymerization within the existing cement mantle.

This technique has been questioned by other authors [96], but subsequent biomechanical and clinical studies have favored its use in properly selected cases [35,67,97]. In a cadaver study, Rosenstein et al. demonstrated that cut strength at the cement-cement interface was greater than the strength at the cement bone interface [133]. However, the cut strength of the cement bone interface was 30% weaker when cement was placed against a revised bone surface.

*6.1.2. Impaction grafting technique for femoral revision*

Femoral impaction grafting with a cemented stem was first performed in Exeter in 1987 [67] (Figure 4). The rationale behind this simple concept is to rebuild femoral bone stock and to provide secure fixation to the femoral stem. The biologic approach of bone restoration during revision hip arthroplasty is a highly appealing solution for restoring host bone stock a difficult procedure with usually deficient femurs.

Following the initial report of Gie and coworkers of highly successful results after 56 revisions with follow-up of 18-49 months [53] the technique received wide attention and spread rapidly [64,114,141,161]. Further studies confirmed the favorable outcomes, and it became evident that the technique resulted in restoration of femoral bone loss as the impacted allograft was incorporated and remodeled [67,161].

The technique of impaction grafting appeared to be reliable, reproducible, can be learned rapidly, and produced predictably favorable outcomes. In a series of 226 revisions, Halliday et al. reported the Exeter initial experience with femoral impaction grafting [64]. The overall rate of mechanical failure was 7% (16/221) at a minimum follow-up of five years. Ten to 11-year survivorship with removal of the stem for any reason as the end point was 90.5% and survivorship with revision for aseptic loosening as the end point was 99.1% [64]. In 2006, Schreurs et al. published their results with the technique using a cemented polished tapered stem at an average 10.4-year follow-up [140]. The average subsidence of the stem within the cement mantle was 3 mm, and seven stems migrated 5 mm. [140]. No stem was revised for aseptic loosening. Three periprosthetic fractures at the sults of 1305 femoral revisions with impaction grafting from the Swedish arthroplasty registry [114]. Survivorship at 15 years for aseptic loosening was 99.1%, for infection 98.6%, for subsidence 99.0%, and for fracture 98.7%.

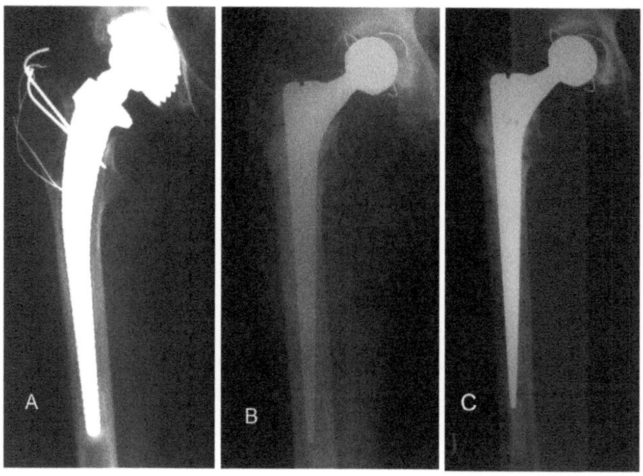


**Figure 4.** Femoral impaction grafting. (A) Preoperative radiograph. B) Immediate postoperative and, (C) at 8 years after revision.

However, other authors reported higher percentage of intraoperative complications, mainly femoral fractures and suboptimal cementing technique [84,86,101,123]. A high incidence of up to 12% intraoperative femoral fractures have been reported [64,140,103]. Stem subsidence of greater than 5 mm is a typical complication with this technique with a prevalence of up to 38% in some series [38,49,86,101]. Impaction grafting has certain disadvantages: it is prone to femoral fractures [103]; has a steep learning curve; and shows highly variable outcomes, probably related to the surgical technique. The causes of early subsidence of the stem might be insufficient impaction of the allograft, suboptimal cement penetration and interdigitation, use of synthetic graft substitutes, or other graft additives, loss of primary fixation of the allograft-cement composite due to soft-tissue infiltration and substitution of the allograft in the process of remodeling and revascularization, unrecognized femoral fracture, or fracture of the cement-allograft composite. However, in a study on saw femurs, Flannery et al. and Cummins et al. were unable to find a correlation between threshold force needed to achieve stable construct in impaction bone grafting without fracture and bone mineral density, canal-cortex ratio, or cortical thickness [22,48]. According to Gokhale et al. four variables (age, intramedullary canal diameter, stem design, and density of the graft at the tip of the stem) affected the subsidence of the stem [54].

The original technique of impaction grafting utilized the Exeter stem [53]. The impacted graft is subjected to continuous loading and deformation. Thus, the use of double-tapered polished stem appears suitable option as the stem could achieve secondary stability after subsidence. Arguing that the technique is more important than the type of prosthesis other authors have used different implant designs from those of Exeter wedge shaped prosthesis [49,77, 124]. Uncemented technique was also used with an equally good outcome at mid-term follow-up [100].

Femoral impaction bone grafting is a suitable indication for cases with severe bone deficiency. The technique is expensive, prone to complications, hast steep learning curve, and results depend on surgical skills. It may be a viable revision option for young patients with severe bone loss.

*6.1.3. Proximal femoral allografts in revision surgery*

Severe bone loss in femoral revision is increasing problem as the number of patients with multiple previous revision increases. These complex cases are further increasing as the age of patients undergoing hip replacement is diminishing.

A stable initial fixation is hardly obtainable in complex cases with circumferential proximal bone loss >5 cm in length. Severe bone loss makes femoral revision using conventional techniques difficult. Alternatives include distal fixation of the stem or use of a proximal femoral allograft. Distal fixation requires the use of a proximally femoral replacement prosthesis or megaprosthesis. This has some disadvantages such as: instability due to poor soft-tissue attachment [62,120], early loosening of the distally fixed stem [47], stress shielding [10,46,110], intraoperative fractures [110] or difficulty with fixation in an ectatic femur. Various studies of revisions using megaprosthesis reported survival rate within the range 58% to 84% at five to ten year follow-up [98,120,164].

The viable revision technique using proximal femoral allograft consists of a long-stem prosthesis cemented to the allograft but not to the host bone [59] (Figure 5). Uncemented fixation of the allograft prosthesis construct would not result in long lasting stability of the prosthesis as neither in-growth nor on-growth could be expected at the allograft-implant interface. The importance of the allograft-host bone contact is a key factor for achieving stability of the construct and ensuring long-term stability of the implant [136].

Individual studies published encouraging results after use of proximal femoral allograft-prosthesis construct in large segmental defects of the proximal femur. In a series of 44 revisions with a mean follow-up of 7.2 years Vastel et al. observed two deep infections, two aseptic loosening and two fractures bellow the tip of the prosthesis [155]. The final prosthesis survivorship rate with revision as the end point was 82.4% at 14 years of follow-up. The nonunion of the greater trochanter was considered major complication and was observed in 25 cases. In another series of 30 hips who underwent revision total hip replacement with an allograft prosthetic composite Sternheim et al. observed favorable long-term outcome [149]. The survivorship at 10, 15 and 20 years was 93%, 75.5% and 75.5%, respectively. Encouraging results were published by Blackley et al. with 78% successful results for an average of eleven-year follow-up [7]. The allograft-prosthesis construct survivorship at five years was 90% and at 10 years was 86%. A recent systematic review of 498 hips with a mean follow-up of 8.1 years reported survival rate of 82% [131]. The major complications were aseptic loosening observed in 13.7% of patients followed by dislocation in 12.8%.

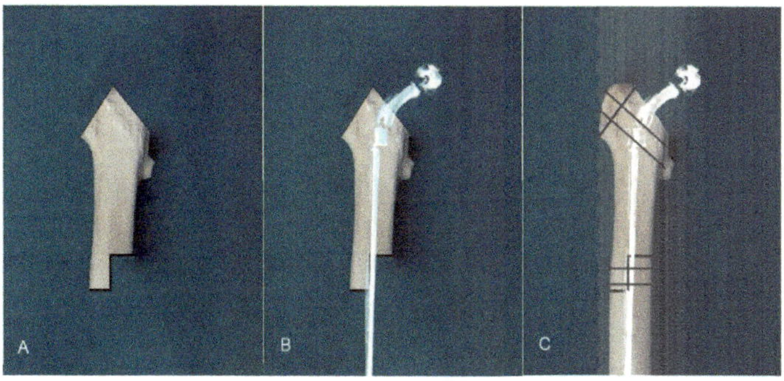


**Figure 5.** The technique of bone reconstruction with use of a proximal femoral allograft-prosthesis construct as described by Gross et al. [59]. (A) The proximal allograft is shaped from a proximal femoral allograft according to the preoperative planning. It should accommodate the selected stem and the step cut of approximately 2 by 2 cm of the host bone. (B) The stem is cemented in the femoral allograft. The contact surface of the allograft to the host bone should be free of cement. (C) The proximal femur-allograft construct is stabilized to the host bone by the stem of the implant. The step cut is reinforced by cerclage wires. Usually, the construct is reinforced with cortical struts prepared from the remnants of the allograft or from bone-bank allografts.

The use of a proximal femoral allograft-prosthesis construct has some inherited disadvantages characteristic for complex surgery. Allograft resorption eventually leading to failure of the revision is of major concern with longer follow-up [61]. Usually, it was observed after several years of follow-up but did not progress [7,155]. Authors that utilize uncemented distal fixation support the concept of direct loading of the host-allograft junction and argue that it minimizes allograft resorption [7,59]. On the other hand, cementing the prosthesis to the distal femur and thus stress shielding the allograft may explain the high rate of allograft resorption [61]. Nonunion of the allograft-host junction [7] or the greater trochanter [61,155] are of major concern with this technique. A step-cut osteotomy may provide rotational stability while an oblique osteotomy may provide greater surface area for bone healing compared to a transverse osteotomy. Dislocation is a frequent complication after revision with proximal femoral allograft with incidence ranging from to 7.3% to 16.7% [15, 61,131,155]. As with other cases, the high risk of dislocation may be lowered by optimal reconstruction of length, adequate version and high offset of the prosthesis-allograft construct and by maintaining the soft tissue tension and its attachment to the host femur [131]. The infection rates after revision with allograft-prosthesis construct are higher than that reported after primary hip arthroplasty. Rates of infection ranging from 0 to 10.9% were reported [15,94,132,136,155]. However, considering the high complexity of the technique these levels of infection are not unacceptable.

Femoral revision using proximal femoral allograft cemented to a long-stem prosthesis is appealing option for revision. The current data from the literature support the use of the technique as a durable solution, with available evidence reporting a long-term survivorship up to 86%. It is of a particular interest in the young patients because of its potential to improve bone stock and provide a substrate for subsequent revision. The development and refinement of this technique should be encouraged.

*6.1.4. Cementless fixation of the femoral component*

Obtaining stable and long lasting fixation in femoral revision in patients with severe bone deficiency is a difficult task. Long-term results after cemented revision have not been optimal [81,83,121]. High failure rates ranging between 12% to 44% at mid-term follow-up have been reported [2,81,83,121]. The main reason was difficulty in obtaining stable and long-lasting fixation in severe bone loss. Cementless fixation proved a promising alternative and was soon introduced in practice. However, for fears of stress shielding the ingrowth surface of first-generation designs was confined to the proximal part of the stem. Although highly successful in primary arthroplasty, the limited amount of porous coating with proximal fixation led to less favorable results in revision surgery (Table 4). Failure rates of 4% to 10% were reported at short- to mid-term follow-up. These results were slightly better than those obtained with an early cementing technique. The technique yielded acceptable results in less severe deformities [71]. Retrieval studies have demonstrated that less bone ingrowth occurs in revision stems compared to primary stems [21]. Porous surface extending to the diaphysis is needed to ensure stable primary fixation. In support of this, various authors have reported promising long-term results after revision with use of extensively coated uncemented stems [1,41,88,115].

Proximal femoral deficiency results from osteolysis, infection, fracture or bone damage during implant extraction. In such cases with severe bone loss, distal fixation with cylindrical, tapered or fluted stem designs is a viable option [4,14,41]. The technique requires accurate preparation of 4 cm to 7 cm of diaphyseal bone [41,92,102]. It is adaptable and can be used in situations with different severity of bone loss. Moreover, it can be used in periprosthetic fractures and is adjustable with extended trochanteric osteotomy. Distal stem fixation is the most successful strategy in terms of primary and secondary mechanical stability, bone osteointegration, and most importantly clinical results [4]. The main reason for its success is the fact that the implant is in contact with viable bone. Success rates of 90% to 95% have been reported with extensively coated monoblock stems over 10-year follow-up [105,115,158]. However, issues, such as thigh pain and proximal stress shielding, were reported frequently.

The principles of the Wagner stem are utilized in the tapered stems [156]. The cone prosthesis achieves good contact between the supportive distal diaphysis and the middle or distal third of the stem (Figure 6). The conical shape and the longitudinal splines promotes primary axial and rotational stability, which are prerequisites for osteointegration and long-lasting endurance of the cementless implant. The concept of modularity was introduced in the tapered stems with the advantages of versatile proximal fill and distal fit [76]. By modularity the sizes and shapes of the prosthesis can be increased by varying the diameter and shape of the proximal and distal part of the stem and locking them in different way. Modularity offers certain advantages such as correction and restoration of leg length, correction of offset and version, selection of optimal proximal fill, as well as compatibility with extended trochanteric osteotomy [4,92]. The potential problem of thigh pain was not associated with tapered stem design [156]. Disadvantages of modular taper stem designs include complexity, risk of stem fracture, fretting and corrosion of the junction, increased inventory, and higher cost.

| Authors | Year | Hips (No) | Follow-up (yrs) | Re-revision rate (%) | Radiographic loosening (%) |
|---|---|---|---|---|---|
| Lawrence et al. [95] | 1993 | 174 | 7.4 | 5.7 | 1.1 |
| Engh et al. [42] | 1988 | 127 | 4.4 | 1.6 | 2.4 |
| Kang et al. [76] | 2008 | 39 | 2 (minimum) | 2.6 | 0 |
| Krishnamurthy el al. [88] | 1997 | 297 | 8.3 | 1.7 | 0.7 |
| Harris et al. [65] | 1988 | 23 | 2 (minimum) | 0 | 4.3 |
| Moreland and Bernstein [106] | 1995 | 175 | 5.0 | 1.1 | 4.2* |
| Moreland and Moreno [105] | 2001 | 137 | 9.3 | 4 | - |

* Mechanical failure

**Table 4.** Results of cementless femoral revision.

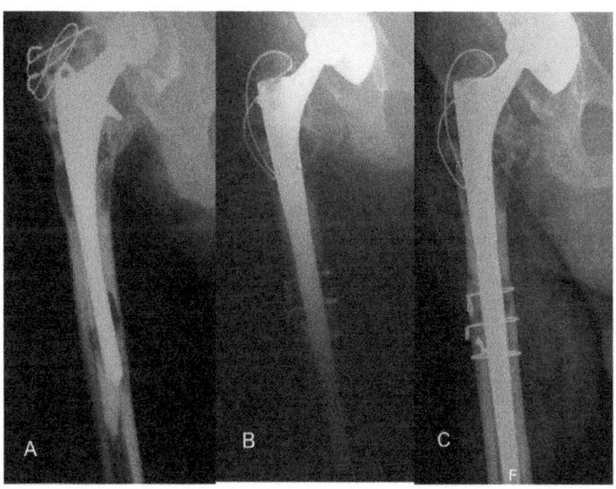


**Figure 6.** Cementless revision of Paprosky type 3A defect with a modular tapered stem (A) resulting in good initial (B) and mid-term stability at 2 years (C).

Various studies have reported favorable outcomes of various uncemented tapered distal fixation stems with high survival of more than 95% at 5 to 10-year follow-up [41,88,102]. The technique of cementless revision with distal fixation of the stem has been shown to be a reliable and straightforward. It ads no additional risks or complications. It can be used in all but the most severe segmental defects [4,14,41,102]. When the simple principles of the method are followed it provides stable and durable fixation of the revision implant. However, distal fixation does not restores host bone, thus making further revision surgery more difficult.

### 6.2. Options for acetabular revision

The goals of revision arthroplasty are to relieve pain and to improve function. In order to obtain these goals stable and durable fixation of the revision components must be achieved with restoration of hip center. Acetabular revision is the most difficult part of hip revision. Unfortunately, there is no single surgical technique to solve the problem of fixation. The achievement of stable initial and long-lasting fixation is challenged by the severity of different acetabular defects and soft tissue damage. The main acetabular reconstruction option is cementless pres-fit fixation of the cup with or without allograft [19,73]. When severe combined segmental and cavitary bone deficiencies, poor bone quality and viability or pelvic discontinuity are identified, other more complex options for acetabular reconstruction are required. These include trabecular metal (TM) cups, modular metallic augments, reconstruction cages, reinforcement rings, cup-cages, and structural or morsellized allografts that can be used to support the reconstruction.

#### *6.2.1. Cemented fixation of the acetabular component*

In cases with no or moderate bone loss revision could be performed with simple cemented exchange of the implant. Historically, early revisions were performed with the same technique that had been used for primary arthroplasty. However, difficulties in achieving consistent long-term results had prevented use of this technique. Failure to achieve adequate cement interdigitation explained poor results reported with early cementing techniques. Key factors for good cementing technique are optimal exposure of cancellous bone, adequate containment of the cup, and a clean and dry socket [130]. Sutherland and colleagues demonstrated that preservation of the subchondral bone can increase stiffness and stress concentration at the bone-cement junction [150]. Callaghan et al [13] reported 4.3% revisions and 34% radiographic loosening at 3.6-year follow-up of cemented revisions. Similar high rates of loosening were reported by Pellicci et al at 3.4-year follow-up [122]. The long-term results after cemented revision were considerably worse [121]. Even with improvement of the cementing technology, the cemented acetabular fixation has not improved (Table 5).

At longer follow-up, using modern cementing techniques failure rates ranging from 35% to 65% were reported [78,112]. Ten-year survivorship of the acetabular component with radiographical loosening as the endpoint event was 72% [78]. Consequently, cement fixation of the acetabular component has become less popular among orthopedic surgeons. In contrast, hemispherous porous-coated cups with bone ingrowth potential were developed and demonstrated consistently better results.

| Authors | Year | Hips (No) | Follow-up (yrs) | Re-revision rate (%) | Radiographic loosening (%) |
|---|---|---|---|---|---|
| Raut et al. [127] | 1995 | 387 | 5.5 | 6.2 | 18.8 |
| Estok and Harris [43] | 1994 | 32 | 11.7 | 22.0 | 19.0 |
| Mulroy and Harris [109] | 1996 | 29 | 15.1 | 38.0 | 44.0 |
| Katz et al. [78] | 1997 | 79 | 11.9 | 16.0 | 23.5 |
| Eisler et al. [38]* | 2000 | 83 | 3.6 | 8.0 | 22.0 |
| Huo and Salvati [70] | 1993 | 113 | 4.1 | 1.0 | 5.0 |

* Third generation cementing technique

**Table 5.** Results of acetabular revision using modern cementing technique.

### *6.2.2. Cementless fixation of the acetabular component*

The approach to each individual case depends upon the severity and localization of host bone loss. Results after cementless revision of the acetabular component have outperformed cemented fixation [30,31,44]. With supportive and viable host bone and a reliable ingrowth surface a hemispheric metal shell supported with screws is a straightforward solution for acetabular reconstruction (Table 6). The success of the technique has been so dramatic that it is currently considered the gold standard by most arthroplasty surgeons in the USA.

| Authors | Hips (No) | Follow-up (yrs) | Re-revision rate (%) | Radiographic loosening (%) |
|---|---|---|---|---|
| Della Valle CJ et al. [30] | 138 | 15.0 (minimum) | 4.5* | 1.5 |
| Park et al. [117] | 138 | 20.0 (minimum) | 8.0* | 5.0 |
| Wysocki et al. [162] | 187 | 5.0 (minimum) | 2.0 | 5.0 |
| Lachiewicz and Hussamy [91] | 60 | 5.0 | 0 | 0 |
| Tanzer et al. [152] | 140 | 3.4 | 0.7 | 4.3 |
| Silverton et al. [145] | 109 | 8.3 | 0 | 5.0 |
| Templeton et al. [153] | 61 | 12.9 | 0 | 3.0 |

*Combined wear and loosening

**Table 6.** Results of cementless cup revision.

In minor or contained defects, hemispherical cup with/without grafting produced excellent results [30,31,44]. Cementless fixation is suitable for patients with Paprosky types 1, 2A and 2B defects: without hip center migration or pelvic discontinuity. As a general rule, at least 50% of the host bone is needed to be in contact with the implant in order to support a hemispherical cup. Transfixational screws are usually used to support ingrowth of the press-fit cup. Morcellized allografts could be used to fill the cavitary defects. In a deficient acetabulum with major bone loss such as Paprosky type 3 defects a hemispherical cup could be placed against the intact supportive roof ("high hip center"). Sometimes extra large (jumbo cup) or oblong cups can bypass severe bone defects and provide stable initial fixation for bone ingrowth. Cementless fixation results in a anatomical hip center or in a high hip center [26].

*6.2.2.1. High hip center*

The failed acetabular components migrate in the direction of joint reaction forces creating a deficient acetabular bed with greater superoinferior dimension compared to the antero-posterior dimension. In such revision setting implantation of the cementless hemispheric press-fit cup in the anatomical hip center is not possible. A straightforward decision for treatment of such defects is to place a small hemispherical press-fit cup against the supportive bone at the roof of the acetabular defect - the so-called high hip center (Figure 7). Most authors consider arbitrary the hip center high if it is proximally greater than 35 mm to the inter-teardrop line [27].

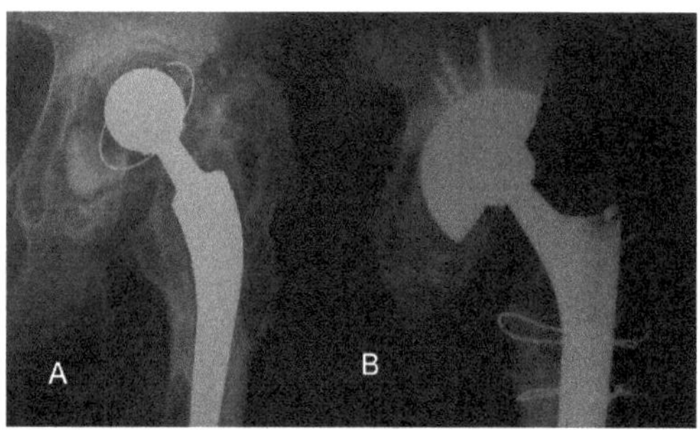


**Figure 7.** Type 3A defect of the acetabulum (A) resulting in high placement of the cup (B).

Results after cementless press-fit fixation of the acetabular component inserted with screws outperformed cemented revision. With use of this approach, despite extensive acetabular bone loss excellent implant fixation was consistently reported. The durability of cementless acetabular fixation was proven in long-term studies, too. In the study of Templeton et al., none of the cementless cups have been revised for aseptic loosening at 12.9-year follow-up and only 3 cups have migrated [153]. In a study with minimum follow-up of 20 years, Park et al. demonstrated 95% survivorship with revision of the cup for aseptic loosening or radiographic signs for loosening as the end point [117]. However, with longer follow-up, the problem of polyethylene wear and osteolysis emerged. In their series, re-revisions for wear and osteolysis were first performed at approximately twelve years postoperatively [117]. At last follow-up 20 years after revision, the incidence of reoperations for polyethylene wear and/or osteolysis continued to increase.

The technique saves costs, time, and eliminates the use of structural allografts or cement. However, high rate of complications was reported [27,74]. This might reflect the complexity of the procedure. Certain disadvantage of the technique is restoration of limb-length discrepancy on the femoral side whereas the defect is on the acetabular side. This would result in abnormal hip biomechanics. Increased hip joint reactive forces with high hip center and impingement might partially explain the relatively higher rate of dislocation with this technique [117,162].

Considering the excellent results reported with porous coated press-fit acetabular components in terms of implant fixation, we believe that the use of press-fit cups should be considered in every revision setting if there is sufficient host bone stock to support the cup.

*6.2.2.2. Jumbo cups*

Extra-large cups offer certain advantages in maximizing the contact area between the cup and host bone when revising deficient acetabulum. There is no universally-accepted definition of the jumbo cup. Extra-large cups are arbitrary defined compared to the size of the pelvis, the hip joint, and the previous implant. Whaley and coworkers defined jumbo cups as having a minimum outside diameter of 66 mm (men) or 62 mm (women) [159]. This was based upon the fact that the revision cups used at their institution were 10 mm larger than the mean implant diameters used for primary hip arthroplasty.

The method has certain advantages [126]: the acetabulum is prepared straightforward by reaming to a large hemispere; the large implant fills in the deficiencies and bone grafting is usually unnecessary; the center of rotation is transferred inferiorly and to some extent laterally restoring hip biomechanics (Figure 8); the large implant provides greater contact area and greater lever arm. Disadvantage of the technique are the limitations in restoring bone stock. Moreover, most of the defects are oblong with a greater superoinferior dimension than anteroposterior dimension. Converting an oblong defect to a hemispherical with extensive reaming may disrupt posterior wall or column which is critical for cup stability [159]. This risk of host bone compromise may result in high implantation of the socket.

Whaley et al. reported on 89 acetabular revisions using extra-large hemispherical components from the Mayo clinic [159]. The probability of survivorship of the cup at eight years was 93% with removal for any reason as the end point, and 95% with radiographical loosening or revision for aseptic loosening as the end point [159]. Wedemeyer et al., Obenaus et al., and Dearborn and Harris published similar results with cup survivorship with an end point aseptic loosening higher than 94% at mid-term follow-up [26,113,157].

The technique saves costs, time, and eliminates the use of structural allografts or cement. However, the rate of complications reported was rather high. In the series of Park et al., the most common reason for revision in 11.6% of 138 hips was infection and dislocation [117]. Similar high rates of revision were reported by Dearborn and Harris [26] and Della Valle et al. [30]. This might reflect the complexity of the procedures.

Extra large cups are a reasonable alternative in patients with moderate defects (Paprosky type 2).

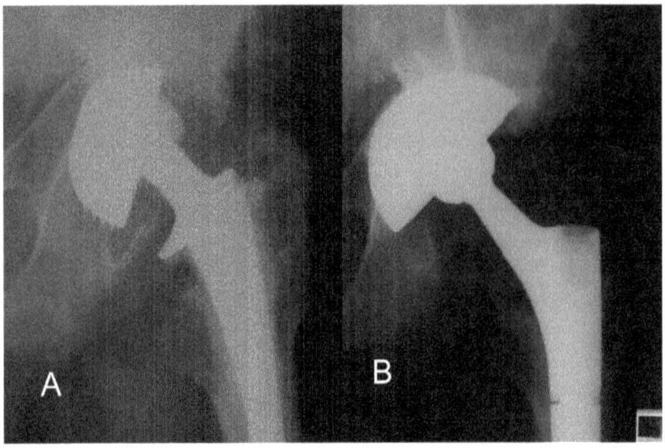


**Figure 8.** Correction of the center of rotation with a large oversized cup.

### 6.2.2.3. *Oblong cups*

As described earlier, large oval contained defects cannot be filled-in superoinferiorly without excessive reaming of the anterior or posterior column of the acetabulum to produce hemisphere. Another option is high placement of the cup. Attractive alternative in such cases is oblong cup. Oblong cup has smaller anteroposterior and mediolateral dimensions compared to the superiorinferior dimension. By accommodating the implant to the defect oblong cups can restore hip center and increase implant contact with host bone. Advantages of the technique are: lack of increased reaming of the anterior or posterior columns or metallization of the cup; increased contact between the device and the host bone; restoration of hip center [19,73]; and avoidance of structural allografts [5]. Disadvantages include higher cost, difficulties in cases with insufficient contact [16], possible component malpositioning, failure to restore bone [5], and excessive bone removal in order to achieve press-fit [126].

In a multicenter study on 38 hips revised with oblong press-fit cups, Berry et al. published good results at mean 3 years after surgery [5]. There was only one failure for acetabular loosening that required re-revision. Mean Harris Hip Score (HHS) increased from 50 points preoperatively to 90 points after revision. The hip center was 37 mm above the inter-teardrop line before the operation and was corrected to 25 mm above the inter-teardrop line. Civinini et al. published good mid-term results after revising with oblong cup Paprosky type 2 and 3 acetabular defects [19]. In a series of 55 hips followed-up for an average of 7.2 years only one cup was revised for loosening. Similar good results were reported by DeBoer and Christie on 18 hips revised with oblong press-fit cups [28]. At the latest follow-up, 4.5 years after revision no component was loose and the mean HHS increased from 41 points preoperatively to 91 points after revision. The authors reported near anatomic restoration of the hip center to 17 mm above the inter-teardrop line after revision. Chen and Engh reported less favorable results in 37 revisions (29 with massive type 3 defects) followed-up for an average of 41 months [16]. Eight percent of the hips were probably loose and 16% were unstable. Eight of the 14 hips that had more than two centimeters of superior migration of the component and disruption of Koehler's line on preoperative radiographs failed [16]. The authors found a correlation between loosening and average distance from the inferior edge of the cup and the interteardrop line. Five of the six unstable components initially had not reached to the level of the radiographic teardrop or distal to it [16]. In their early series, Sutherland [151] reported a 50% failure rate (3 of 6) after revision with an oblong cup of type 3 defects. Discouraging mid-term results were published by Babis et al. using a cementless oblong cup for revision of Paprosky 3A defects [3]. After a mean follow-up of 60.5 months 18 hips (29.0%) were revised and a further four hips (6.4%) were loose and awaited revision. Further analyses proved that careful patient selection is critical for the success of this revision technique.

Acetabular revision with an oblong cup is an attractive alternative, especially when the surgeon plans correction of an elevated hip center [16,108]. The technique is suitable for Paprosky type 2A, 2B and 3A defects where the acetabular defect is oval. Obtaining initial stability and supplementary fixation by screws are mandatory for the stability of the implant and are key factors for long-term success of the reconstruction. However, the medial wall should be intact and the failed component should not have migrated more than two centimeters. Pelvic discontinuity is also a contraindication for this technique. Alternative techniques such as structural allograft or cage should be considered in such revision settings.

### *6.2.3. Impaction grafting technique for acetabullar revision*

Cemented acetabular revision yielded unacceptably high rate of loosening [13,80,81]. Possible reason is the deficient, weaken and sclerotic acetabular bone frequently found at revision. An attractive alternative for cup fixation in massive contained defects is impaction grafting where the cup is cemented on a premoulded bed of impacted morsellized cancellous bone. In such revision setting the contact with host bone is very limited if not absent. The morsellized bone has osteoinductive and osteocunductive properties and is used as a filler scaffold of contained defects. The technique of impaction bone grafting and cemented fixation of the cup was first described in 1984 by Slooff and coworkers [146], and later standardized by the same authors with minor modifications and technique-specific instrumentation [11,142]. Morsellized graft could be used with a cementless hemispherous cup if more than 50% of the cup is in contact with viable host bone [57]. Transfixing screws should be used for additional stabilization of the cup. In cases with less than 50% contact between the cup and viable host bone the cemented cup into impacted cancellous bone should be used [146].

The technique can provide stable and durable reconstruction of the hip joint. However, initial mechanical stability of the morsellized allograft-cemented cup composite is a prerequisite for a successful biological reconstruction. Subsequent remodeling and incorporation of grafts, provides long-term stability. In contrast to cementless revision, this technique could restore bone loss. The modern evolved technique consists of reconstruction of segmental and rim defects with use of a metal mesh or a solid graft. The sclerotic areas are perforated with multiple 2-mm drill-holes, and fresh-frozen morsellized bone chips are impacted layer by layer into the acetabulum. The clinical success of the of impaction grafting depends on the surgical technique and on the biological and mechanical properties of the morsellized bone graft. Various factors connected with the graft such as graft type (cancellous, cortical-cancellous, chemical composites, synthetic additives), graft processing (fresh frozen, freeze-dried, irradiated), graft particle size and grade influence the clinical result. The originators of the technique use fresh frozen allografts [11,142,143].

The technique of acetabular impaction grafting is well-established and various authors demonstrated reproducible results [20,51,143,154]. Schreurs et al. reported good results after acetabular revision with impaction allografting at 15 to 20-year follow-up [142]. With revision for aseptic loosening as the endpoint, cup survivorship was 84% at 15 years [142]. In a 20 to 28-year follow-up study, Busch et al. from the same study group evaluated 42 patients with impaction grafting younger than 50 years [11]. With revision for aseptic loosening as the end point, survivorship was 85% after twenty years and 77% after twenty-five years [11]. With end point event signs of loosening on radiographs, survival was 71% at twenty years and 62% at twenty-five years. Results declined over time, but the authors concluded that the technique is useful in younger patients with major bone defects [11].

Acetabular revision using impaction grafting is a reliable alternative for biologic restoration of hip joint mechanics. The procedure is technically demanding and exacting. Results comparable to those after revision with cementless hemispheric cups were obtained after use of correct surgical technique.

### *6.2.4. Reconstruction cages*

Reconstruction cages and antiprotrusio rings are an established method of treatment for severe acetabular bone loss if contact with 50% host bone could not be established [57]. They have the advantage of fixation into viable host bone of the ileum and ischium with flanges while protecting allograft (Figure 9). Failure rates higher than 60% at an average of 2.9 years have been reported in cases with massive allografts not supported by cages [116]. Because of the poor results following use of unsupported structural allograft use of reconstruction cages has been advised [148]. Reinforcement rings or reconstruction cages can provide adequate support for the reconstruction with massive allografts in Paprosky type 2C and type 3 defects. Favorable results were reported after use of reconstruction cages by different authors [50,68,107,125]. Recently, this treatment approach has been questioned as TM implants provide more favorable conditions for graft incorporation and bone ingrowth [148].

The reconstruction cages and antiprotrusio rings have definite advantages: the cage and ring allow for restoration of hip center; they provide uniform load to the allograft stimulating bone remodeling and incorporation into host bone [72]; cementing allows use of local antibiotic protection; allow correct placement of the cemented cup independent of the cage or ring. The cage protects either the morsellized or structural allograft while it remodels, and if the cage fails cementless revision can be done [55,57].

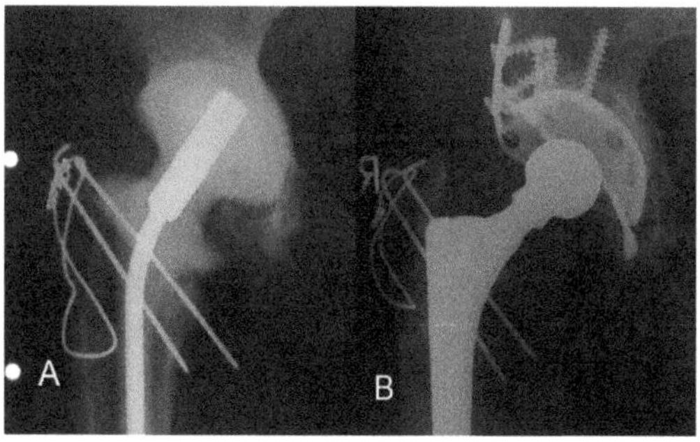


**Figure 9.** Reconstruction of a Paprosky type 2C defect (A) with a cage (B). Remodeling of the allograft at 2 years.

Disadvantages include higher cost, need for wide surgical exposure of the superolateral part of the ileum. The later may risk injury of the superior gluteal nerve and limping. The major concern with standard nonporous cages and rings is that they do not allow bone ingrowth. Finally, they loosen and break. However, this inability of bone ingrowth is compensated by the mechanical stability and incorporation of the graft reducing the risk of fatigue fracture of the cage. Close fit between the cage and the allograft as well as adequate fixation of the cage are a prerequisite for successful reconstruction. Cement augmentation of screws is recommended in cases with severe osteolysis or osteoporosis.

The limits of using antiprotrusio rings were demonstrated by Haentjens and coworkers and Zehntner and Ganz [63,163]. High rate of migration up to 44% (12/27) at mid-term follow-up of 7.2 years was reported [163]. Previous designs of reconstruction cages did not allow bone ingrowth and a failure rate of 16.4% due to loosening was reported on average 4.6 years after surgery [55]. Sporer et al. reported a 2- to 8-year follow-up of 45 hips where a cage was used for a type 3 defects [148]. Nine hips were revised for aseptic loosening, and an additional nine hips were radiographically loose.

In contrast, Winter et reported no loosening or revision in 38 hips followed-up at mean 7.3 years after revision with cage [160]. In a long-term study, 18 acetabular revisions for pelvic discontinuity have been reported on average 13.5 years after surgery [129]. Two cages were revised for aseptic loosening, and another two allografts showed signs of severe osteolysis. Survivorship of the acetabular component at 16.6 years with end points revision for any reason, loosening or nonunion of the allograft was 72%. The increased rate of loosening and revision is probably multifactorial and reflexes the increased case load. Frequent indication for use of reconstruction cages is pelvic discontinuity. However, designs without bone ingrowth do not have potential for biologic fixation and rely solely on mechanical fixation.

Antiprotrusio cages and rings are an effective technique for treatment of severe bone defects. However, in recent years, newer implant designs have gained popularity. In cases with more than 50% host bone support cementless cup transfixed with screws is the treatment method of choice. Trabecular metal implants, porous augments, and triflanged acetabular components are an attractive alternative for complex acetabular reconstructions,

[33,57,148]. TM cups have been proposed if contact with viable host bone is 30% to 50%. If contact with viable host bone is less than 30% a cup-cage construct was suggested [57]. Longer follow-up studies are needed to support the clinical use of these new implants.

*6.2.5. Structural acetabular allografts*

One of the most difficult scenarios in revision surgery is a reconstruction of a massive acetabular bone loss. Structural acetabullar allografts are a suitable revision option for uncontained bone defects (Paprosky type 2B, 3A and 3B). The size of the allograft may range from a femoral head in superolateral uncontained defects to total acetabular allograft when severe uncontained defects or pelvic discontinuity are present.

Advantages of the technique include restoration of hip center and restoration of bone stock for future revisions [50,68,90,125]. However, actual restoration of viable and mechanically competent bone is questionable. Moreover, results are unpredictable. The technique is demanding and associated with various complications.

Results after revision with structural allografts have been largely controversial. Harris initially reported successful results after reconstruction of severe acetabular defects with structural allografts [135]. However, the encouraging period of initial good functioning for 5 to 10 years was followed by later failures. In 1993, Kwong et al. reported 47% failures in 30 hips with a mean follow-up period of 10 years [90]. In 1997, the senior author reported total rate of revision or loosening 60% at an average of 16.5 years [144]. High hip center for placement of the cup was suggested in cases with severe acetabular bone loss [135].

In a series of 33 hips followed-up on average 7 years after revision with a structural allograft, Garbuz et al. reported 55% success rate [50]. Fifteen hips were revised: seven hips because of failure of the prosthesis and eight hips because of failure of both the allograft and the prosthesis. Gross et al. reported on 107 hips reconstructed with bulk allograft [58]. Thirty hips (28%) were revised and in 15.9% of cases (17 hips) the indication was aseptic loosening. The authors reported 76% successful results in the 33 hips with minimum duration of follow-up of 5 years (average, 7.1 years) after the revision. However, eight hips needed additional reoperation because of failure of the graft and another six hips were revised for loosening. Hooten et al. reported on a series of 31 revisions with structural allograft and cementless cup followed-up on average 46 months after surgery [68]. Twelve (44%) cups were radiographically loose and five of these hips were revised. In contrast, Paprosky et al. reported a failure rate of 19 per cent (6/31) at an average follow-up of 5.7 years after revision with use of a structural allograft [116]. The only failures in that series were in hips in which the allograft supported more than 50 per cent of the cup. In another study, Morsi et al. found a success rate of 86% (25/29) at mean follow-up of 7.1 years [107]. They used a minor bulk allograft that supported less than 50% of the cup.

Although results after revision with structural allograft are controversial, most authors agree that the rate of success increases if more than 50% of the cup is in contact with viable host bone [50,68,116]. According to Morsi et al. [107] and Pollock and Whiteside [125] a repeat revision does not mean failure of the reconstruction. This complex reconstruction can be considered successful if bone stock is restored for future revisions.

Revision with structural allograft is a suitable option for restoration of hip center. The role of the allograft is to support the cementless cup with partial stability until adequate ingrowth occurs. The success after the procedure is technically-related. In order to optimize result after revision with structural allograft a number of principles should be followed. Structural allografts combined with antiprotrusio cages, and a cemented cup should be considered only in cases with insufficient host bone to provide a stable fixation for a press-fit cup [26].

For an optimal result, an appropriate allograft must be selected to match the mechanical requirements of the desired reconstruction. The method of processing of the bone allografts is important for the clinical result. Greater success rate with fresh frozen bone allografts was obtained compared to freeze-dried allografts [58]. The trabecullae of the allograft should be in the direction of load for optimal stress transfer. After trimming of the allograft in order to obtain maximal contact with the host bone the allograft is fixed with 6.5 mm parallel screws in the direction of load. In case of pelvic discontinuity, the column should be fixed with a plate before fixating the allograft. Use of reinforcement cages improves results after reconstruction with structural allograft [50,138].

*6.2.6. Custom triflanged implants*

Custom triflanged prostheses have been proposed for treatment of massive acetabular defects and pelvic discontinuity, but the experience is limited and the rate of complications is high [75]. The implant is manufactured from 3-D CT data reconstruction of the degree and localization of bone loss as well as its spatial orientation.

In 2007, DeBoer et al. evaluated the outcome of revision with a custom-designed porous-coated triflanged acetabular implant in 20 hips at an average 10-year follow-up [28]. A definite healing of the pelvic discontinuity was found in 18 hips (90%). The remaining two implants were radiographically stable and did not migrate even when discontinuity persisted. However, the overall dislocation rate in the series was 25%. Christie et al. followed-up retrospectively 67 complex revisions with custom-made triflanged implant [18]. Two discontinuities persisted, but both were asymptomatic and no implant was revised. Six (7.8%) hips were revised for recurrent dislocation. Using custom triflanged acetabular components Dennis reported three failures in 24 revisions with mid-term follow-up of 4 years [33]. He questions the value of the technique in pelvic discontinuity unless supplemented with additional column plating.

The technique has high cost, it is time consuming, requires extensile exposure, and lacks modularity. It could not be used in urgent clinical situation where it is not possible to wait for manufacturing the product. With complex implant and technically challenging surgery custom-designed triflanged prosthesis should be reserved for cases where less costly and less technically demanding options could not be used. Many surgeons consider it a salvage procedure for cases where the bone loss is catastrophic.

### 6.2.7. Trabecular metal cups

Trabecular metal cups can be used in massive contained or uncontained defects. As tantalum provides favorable environment for biological fixation, TM cups have been suggested for revision of Paprosky type 3 defects [57,148] instead of an allograft-cage construct.

Early results with use of TM implants have been encouraging [111]. TM has decreased the need for at least 50% contact of the implant with viable host bone. In Paprosky 3A an 3B defects, because cages do not provide biologic fixation, Gross suggested use of a cup and cage construct (the so-called cup-cage technique) when less than 30% contact can be made with viable host bone [57]. The rationale behind the technique is that load will be taken off the cage, once bone ingrowth occurs into the trabecular metal cup. So early and mid-term failures of the cages will be prevented.

Sporer et al. reported on 13 hips with pelvic discontinuity revised with tantalum cups with or without augments [147]. At mean 2.6 years after revision 12 of the 13 cups were radiographically stable. Lakstein et al. reported on 53 revisions of contained defects with 50% or less contact with host bone using TM cups [93]. Two cups (4%) were revised, and two additional cups (4%) had radiographical evidence of probable loosening at a mean 45-month follow-up. The fact that some of the TM cups lacked contact with a viable host bone is impressive. Four hips (8%) dislocated and one (2%) sciatic nerve palsy was observed. In a large multicenter study, 263 revisions with tantalum TM cups were followed-up at an average 7 years after surgery. At the most recent follow-up, all cups were radiographically stable and no revision for loosening was reported. Eight dislocations (3%) in the series were successfully treated with closed reduction, and one sciatic palsy partially resolved at last follow-up. Kosashvili et al. reported on 26 revisions of pelvic discontinuities using cages combined with trabecular metal components and morsellized bone (cup-cage technique) [87]. At mean follow-up of 45 months 23 hips (88.5%) were radiographically stable.

Promising midterm results have been demonstrated after revision with use of these new techniques. Currently, the preference is to biological fixation whenever possible, and to alternative options when initial stability could not be obtained.

### 6.2.8. Modular components (metal augments)

Modular metal augments of various sizes and shape are used to decrease defect size and to restore bone defect to contained one capable of supporting a revision cup (Figure 10).

The size and placement of augments is highly dependable on the bone loss pattern. Augments are secured with multiple screws to host bone and remaining defects are filled in with morsellized bone. The hemispherical cup is impacted into the defect with the interface between the shell and the metal augment cemented.

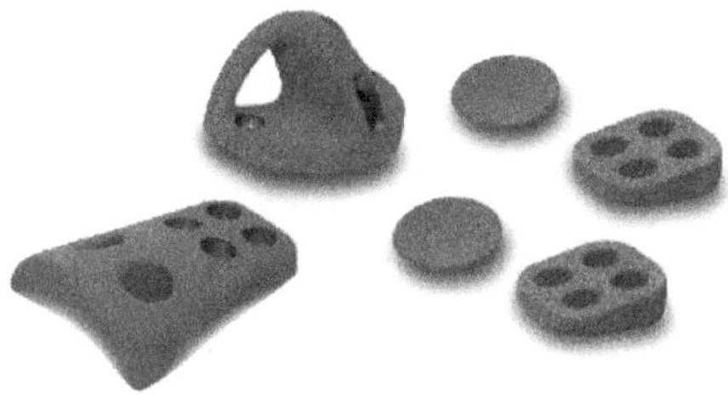

**Figure 10.** TM modular augments (courtesy of Zimmer, Warsaw, IN, USA).

## 7. Conclusion

During the last two decades, revision hip arthroplasty is constantly in the focus of orthopedic surgeons as the numbers of these difficult and risky surgeries are increasing. Up to date, he paradigms of revision surgery has been evolving constantly. From polyethylene wear, osteolysis and loosening, to complexities such as pelvic discontinuity, there is a wide range of surgical options for successful reconstruction. Analysis of clinical results from various studies outlines the preference for biological fixation of the revision implant whenever possible. It is vital for the surgeon to be familiar with different treatment approaches and to anticipate various intraoperative scenarios. Systematic approach with considerable preoperative evaluation and planning will achieve a good result. Prerequisite for a successful and durable revision include viable host bone, adequate surgical technique, and stable and endurable implant. Current improvements in surgical techniques, implant designs, as well as biomaterials and bearing surfaces are a significant contribution for obtaining favorable outcome after revision hip arthroplasty. However, we do not have complex solution. The optimal surgical approach for revision THA varies considerably among different settings. On the other hand, the economic burden of total joint replacement is increasing at a steep rate. This necessitates improved methods for evaluation of existing technology and particularly patient-derived outcomes assessment instruments. Further research and well-designed clinical studies are needed in order to provide optimal treatment to the increasing number of patients requiring revision surgery in the future.

## Author details

Plamen Kinov and Peter Tivchev

Queen Giovanna – ISUL University Hospital, Department of Orthopedics and Traumatology, Medical University of Sofia, Bulgaria

## References


[1] Amanatullah DF, Meehan JP, Cullen AB, Kim SH, Jamali AA. Intermediate-term radiographic and patient outcomes in revision hip arthroplasty with a modular calcar design and porous plasma coating. J Arthroplasty 2011; 26(8):1451-4.

[2] Amstutz HC, Ma SM, Jinnah RH, Mai L. Revision of aseptic loose total hip arthroplasties. Clin Orthop Relat Res 1982; 170:21-33.

[3] Babis GC, Sakellariou VI, Chatziantoniou AN, Soucacos PN, Megas P. High complication rate in reconstruction of Paprosky type IIIa acetabular defects using an oblong implant with modular side plates and a hook. J Bone Joint Surg Br 2011; 93(12): 1592-6.

[4] Barrack RL. Orthopaedic crossfire - Stem modularity is unnecessary in revision total hip arthroplasty: in the affirmative. J Arthroplasty 2003; 18(3 Suppl 1):98-100.

[5] Berry DJ, Sutherland CJ, Trousdale RT, Colwell CW Jr, Chandler HP, Ayres D, Yashar AA. Bilobed oblong porous coated acetabular components in revision total hip arthroplasty. Clin Orthop Relat Res 2000; 371:154-60.

[6] Bin Nasser A, Beaulé PE, O'Neill M, Kim PR, Fazekas A. Incidence of groin pain after metal-on-metal hip resurfacing. Clin Orthop Relat Res 2010; 468(2):392-9.

[7] Blackley HR, Davis AM, Hutchison CR, Gross AE. Proximal femoral allografts for reconstruction of bone stock in revision arthroplasty of the hip. A nine to fifteen-year follow-up. J Bone Joint Surg Am 2001; 83(3):346-54.

[8] Bozic KJ, Kurtz SM, Lau E, Ong K, Vail TP, Berry DJ. The epidemiology of revision total hip arthroplasty in the United States. J Bone Joint Surg Am 2009; 91:128-33.

[9] Bradford MS, Jablonsky WS, Paprosky WG, Younger TI. Revision of the difficult femur using the extended proximal femoral osteotomy. AAOS 1999; 48:19.

[10] Bruns J, Delling G, Gruber H, Lohmann CH, Habermann CR. Cementless fixation of megaprostheses using a conical fluted stem in the treatment of bone tumours. J Bone Joint Surg Br 2007; 89(8):1084-7.

[11] Busch VJ, Gardeniers JW, Verdonschot N, Slooff TJ, Schreurs BW. Acetabular reconstruction with impaction bone-grafting and a cemented cup in patients younger than fifty years old: a concise follow-up, at twenty to twenty-eight years, of a previous report. J Bone Joint Surg Am 2011; 93(4):367-71.

[12] Callaghan JJ. Revision of the femoral component using cement fixation. In: Bono JV, McCarthy JC, Thornhil TS, Bierbaum BE, Turner RH. (eds.) Revision total hip arthroplasty. New York: Springer-Verlag; 1999. p. 204.

[13] Callaghan JJ, Salvati EA, Pellicci PM, Wilson PD Jr, Ranawat CS. Results of revision for mechanical failure after cemented total hip replacement, 1979 to 1982. A two to five-year follow-up. J Bone Joint Surg Am 1985; 67(7):1074-85.

[14] Cameron HU. Orthopaedic crossfire - Stem modularity is unnecessary in revision total hip arthroplasty: in opposition. J Arthroplasty 2003; 18(3 Suppl 1):101-3.

[15] Chandler H, Clark J, Murphy S, McCarthy J, Penenberg B, Danylchuk K, Roehr B. Reconstruction of major segmental loss of the proximal femur in revision total hip arthroplasty. Clin Orthop Relat Res 1994; 298:67-74.

[16] Chen WM, Engh CA Jr, Hopper RH Jr, McAuley JP, Engh CA. Acetabular revision with use of a bilobed component inserted without cement in patients who have acetabular bone stock deficiency. J Bone Joint Surg Am 2000; 82(2):197-206.

[17] Chiang PP, Burke DW, Freiberg AA, Rubash HE. Osteolysis of the pelvis. Evaluation and treatment. Clin Orthop Relat Res 2003; 417:164-74.

[18] Christie MJ, Barrington SA, Brinson MF, Ruhling ME, DeBoer DK. Bridging massive acetabular defects with the triflange cup: 2- to 9-year results. Clin Orthop Relat Res 2001; 393:216-27.

[19] Civinini R, Capone A, Carulli C, Villano M, Gusso MI. Acetabular revisions using a cementless oblong cup: five to ten year results. Int Orthop 2008; 32(2):189-93.

[20] Comba F, Buttaro M, Pusso R, Piccaluga F. Acetabular reconstruction with impacted bone allografts and cemented acetabular components: a 2- to 13-year follow-up study of 142 aseptic revisions. J Bone Joint Surg Br 2006; 88(7):865-69.

[21] Cook SD, Barrack RL, Thomas KA, Haddad RJ Jr. Tissue growth into porous primary and revision femoral stems. J Arthroplasty 1991; 6(Suppl):S37-46.

[22] Cummins F, Reilly PO, Flannery O, Kelly D, Kenny P. Defining the impaction frequency and threshold force required for femoral impaction grafting in revision hip arthroplasty. A human cadaveric mechanical study. Acta Orthop 2011; 82(4):433-7.

[23] D'Antonio J, McCarthy JC, Bargar WL, Borden LS, Cappelo WN, Collis DK, Steinberg ME, Wedge JH. Classification of femoral abnormalities in total hip arthroplasty. Clin Orthop Relat Res 1993; 296:133-39.

[24] D'Antonio JA. Periprosthetic bone loss of the acetabulum. Classification and management. Orthop Clin North Am 1992; 23:279-90.

[25] D'Antonio JA, Capello WN, Borden LS, Burgar WL, Bierbaum BE, Boettcher WG, Steinberg ME, Stulberg SD, Wedge JH. Classification and management of acetabular abnormalities in total hip arthroplasty. Clin Orthop Relat Res 1989; 243:126-37.

[26] Dearborn JT, Harris WH. Acetabular revision arthroplasty using so-called jumbo cementless components: an average 7-year follow-up study. J Arthroplasty 2000; 15(1): 8-15.

[27] Dearborn JT, Harris WH. High placement of an acetabular component inserted without cement in a revision total hip arthroplasty. Results after a mean of ten years. J Bone Joint Surg Am 1999; 81(4):469-80.

[28] DeBoer DK, Christie MJ, Brinson MF, Morrison JC. Revision total hip arthroplasty for pelvic discontinuity. J Bone Joint Surg Am 2007; 89(4):835-40.

[29] DeBoer DK, Christie MJ. Reconstruction of the deficient acetabulum with an oblong prosthesis: three- to seven-year results. J Arthroplasty 1998; 13(6):674-80.

[30] Della Valle CJ, Shuaipaj T, Berger RA, Rosenberg AG, Shott S, Jacobs JJ, Galante JO. Revision of the acetabular component without cement after total hip arthroplasty. A concise followup, at fifteen to nineteen years, of a previous report. J Bone Joint Surg Am 2005; 87(8):1795-800.

[31] Della Valle CJ, Berger RA, Rosenberg AG, Galante JO. Cementless acetabular reconstruction in revision total hip arthroplasty. Clin Orthop Relat Res 2004; 420:96-100.

[32] Della Valle CJ, Paprosky WG. Classification and an algorithmic approach to the reconstruction of femoral deficiency in revision total hip arthroplasty. J Bone Joint Surg Am 2003; 85:(Suppl. 4):1-6.

[33] Dennis DA. Management of massive acetabular defects in revision total hip arthroplasty. J Arthroplasty 2003; 18(3 Suppl 1):121-5.

[34] Deirmengian C, Hallab N, Tarabishy A, et al. Synovial fluid biomarkers for periprosthetic infection. Clin Orthop Relat Res 2010; 468(8):2017-23.

[35] Duncan WW, Hubble MJW, Howell JR, Whitehouse SL, Timperley AJ, Gie GA. Revision of the femoral stem using a cement-in-cement technique: a five- to 15-year review. J Bone Joint Surg Br 2009; 91(5):577-82.

[36] Eftekhar NS. Principles of total hip arthroplastv. St Louis : CV Mosby Co; 1978.

[37] Eisler T, Svensson O, Iyer V, Wejkner B, Schmalholz A, Larsson H, Elmstedt E. Revision total hip arthroplasty using third-generation cementing technique. J Arthroplasty. 2000 Dec;15(8):974-81.

[38] Eldridge JD, Smith EJ, Hubble MJ, Whitehouse SL, Learmonth ID. Massive early subsidence following femoral impaction grafting. J Arthroplasty 1997; 12(5):535-40.

[39] Engelbrecht DJ, Weber FA, Sweet MBE, Jakim I. Long term results of revision total hip arthroplasty. J Bone Joint Surg Br 1990; 72:41-5.

[40] Engelbrecht E, Siegel A. Komplikationen nach Hüftgelenks-endoprothesen. Radiologe 1989; 29(10): 508-18.

[41] Engh CA Jr, Hopper RH Jr, Engh CA Sr. Distal ingrowth components. Clin Orthop Relat Res 2004; 420:135-41.

[42] Engh CA, Glassman AH, Griffin WL, Mayer JG. Results of cementless revision for failed cemented total hip arthroplasty. Clin Orthop Relat Res 1988; 235:91-110.

[43] Estok DM 2nd, Harris WH. Long-term results of cemented femoral revision surgery using second-generation techniques. An average 11.7-year follow-up evaluation. Clin Orthop Relat Res 1994; 299:190-202.

[44] Etienne G, Bezwada HP, Hungerford DS, Mont MA. The incorporation of morselized bone grafts in cementless acetabular revisions. Clin Orthop Relat Res 2004; 428:241-46.

[45] Farfalli GL, Buttaro MA, Piccaluga F. Femoral fractures in revision hip surgeries with impacted bone allograft. Clin Orthop Relat Res 2007; 462:130-6.

[46] Fink B, Grossmann A, Schulz MS. Bone regeneration in the proximal femur following implantation of modular revision stems with distal fixation. Arch Orthop Trauma Surg 2011; 131(4):465-70.

[47] Fink B, Grossmann A. Modified transfemoral approach to revision arthroplasty with uncemented modular revision stems. Oper Orthop Traumatol 2007; 19(1):32-55.

[48] Flannery OM, Britton JR, O'Reilly P, Mahony N, Prendergast PJ, Kenny PJ. The threshold force required for femoral impaction grafting in revision hip surgery. Acta Orthop 2010; 81(3):303-7.

[49] Franzén H, Toksvig-Larsen S, Lidgren L, Onnerfält R. Early migration of femoral components revised with impacted cancellous allografts and cement. A preliminary report of five patients. J Bone Joint Surg Br 1995; 77(6):862-4.

[50] Garbuz D, Morsi E, Gross AE. Revision of the acetabular component of a total hip arthroplasty with a massive structural allograft. Study with a minimum five-year follow-up. J Bone Joint Surg Am 1996 May;78(5):693-7.

[51] Garcia-Cimbrelo E, Cruz-Pardos A, Garcia-Rey E, Ortega-Chamarro J. The survival and fate of acetabular reconstruction with impaction grafting for large defects. Clin Orthop Relat Res 2010; 468(12):3304-13.

[52] Gerber SD, Harris WH: Femoral head autografting to augment acetabular deficiency in patients requiring total hip replacement. J Bone Joint Surg 1986; 68:1241-8.

[53] Gie GA, Linder L, Ling RS, Simon JP, Slooff TJ, Timperley AJ. Impacted cancellous allografts and cement for revision total hip arthroplasty. J Bone Joint Surg Br 1993; 75:14-21.

[54] Gokhale S, Soliman A, Dantas JP, Richardson JB, Cook F, Kuiper JH, Jones P. Variables affecting initial stability of impaction grafting for hip revision. Clin Orthop Relat Res 2005; 432:174-80.

[55] Goodman S, Saastamoinen H, Shasha N, Gross A. Complications of ilioischial reconstruction rings in revision hip surgery. J Arthroplasty 2004;19:436-46.

[56] Greenwald AS, Narten NC, Wilde AH. Points in the technique of recementing in the revision of an implant arthroplasty. J Bone Joint Surg Br 1978; 60(1):107-10.

[57] Gross AE. Restoration of acetabular bone loss 2005. J Arthroplasty 2006; 21(4 Suppl 1):117-20.

[58] Gross AE, Duncan CP, Garbuz D, Mohamed EM. Revision arthroplasty of the acetabulum in association with loss of bone stock. Instr Course Lect 1998;48:57-66.

[59] Gross AE, Hutchison CR, Alexeeff M, Mahomed N, Leitch K, Morsi E. Proximal femoral allografts for reconstruction of bone stock in revision arthroplasty of the hip. Clin Orthop Relat Res 1995; 319:151-8.

[60] Gustilo RB, Pasternak HS. Revision total hip arthroplasty with titanium ingrowth prosthesis and bone grafting for failed cemented femoral component loosening. Clin Orthop Relat Res 1988; 235:111-9.

[61] Haddad FS, Spangehl MJ, Masri BA, Garbuz DS, Duncan CP. Circumferential allograft replacement of the proximal femur. A critical analysis. Clin Orthop Relat Res 2000; 371:98-107.

[62] Haentjens P, De Boeck H, Opdecam P. Proximal femoral replacement prosthesis for salvage of failed hip arthroplasty: complications in a 2-11 year follow-up study in 19 elderly patients. Acta Orthop Scand 1996; 67(1):37-42.

[63] Haentjens P, de Boeck H, Handelberg F, Casteleyn PP, Opdecam P. Cemented acetabular reconstruction with the Müller support ring. A minimum five-year clinical and roentgenographic follow-up study. Clin Orthop Relat Res 1993; 290:225-35.

[64] Halliday BR, English HW, Timperley AJ, Gie GA, Ling RS Femoral impaction grafting with cement in revision total hip replacement. Evolution of the technique and results. J Bone Joint Surg Br 2003; 85(6):809-17.

[65] Harris WH, Krushell RJ, Galante JO. Results of cementless revisions of total hip arthroplasties using the Harris-Galante prosthesis. Clin Orthop Relat Res 1988; 235:120-6.

[66] Herberts P, Malchau H. Long-term registration has improved the quality of hip replacement: a review of the Swedish THR Register comparing 160,000 cases. Acta Orthop Scand. 2000 Apr;71(2):111-21.

[67] Holt G, Hook S, Hubble M. Revision total hip arthroplasty: the femoral side using cemented implants. Int Orthop 2011; 35(2):267-73.

[68] Hooten JP Jr, Engh CA Jr, Engh CA. Failure of structural acetabular allografts in cementless revision hip arthroplasty. J Bone Joint Surg Br 1994; 76(3):419-22.

[69] Hunter GA, Welsh RP, Cameron HU, Bailey WH. The results of revision of total hip arthroplasty. J Bone Joint Surg Br 1979; 61:419-21.

[70] Huo MH, Salvati EA. Revision total hip arthroplasty using cement. Tech Orthop1993; 7:58-64.

[71] Iorio R, Healy WL, Presutti AH. A prospective outcomes analysis of femoral component fixation in revision total hip arthroplasty. J Arthroplasty 2008; 23:662-9.

[72] Issack PS, Nousiainen M, Beksac B, Helfet DL, Sculco TP, Buly RL. Acetabular component revision in total hip arthroplasty. Part II: management of major bone loss and pelvic discontinuity. Am J Orthop 2009; 38(11):550-6.

[73] Issack PS, Nousiainen M, Beksac B, Helfet DL, Sculco TP, Buly RL. Acetabular component revision in total hip arthroplasty. Part I: cementless shells. Am J Orthop 2009; 38(10):509-14.

[74] Jamali AA, Dungy DS, Mark A, Schule S, Harris WH. Isolated acetabular revision with use of the Harris-Galante Cementless Component. Study with intermediate-term follow-up. J Bone Joint Surg Am 2004; 86(8):1690-7.

[75] Joshi AB, Lee J, Christensen C. Results for a custom acetabular component for acetabular deficiency. J Arthroplasty 2002;17:643-8.

[76] Kang MN, Huddleston JI, Hwang K, Imrie S, Goodman SB. Early outcome of a modular femoral component in revision total hip arthroplasty. J Arthroplasty 2008; 23: 220-5.

[77] Karrholm J, Hultmark P, Carlsson L, Malchau H. Subsidence of a non-polished stem in revisions of the hip using impaction allograft: evaluation with radiostereometry and dual-energy x-ray absorptiometry. J Bone Joint Surg Br 1999; 81:135-42.

[78] Katz RP, Callaghan JJ, Sullivan PM, Johnston RC. Long-term results of revision total hip arthroplasty with improved cementing technique. J Bone Joint Surg Br 1997; 79:322-6.

[79] Kavanagh BF, Wallrichs S, Ilstrup D, Berry D, Fitzgerald RH. Ten year follow up of cemented revision total hip replacement. Orthop Trans 1993; 17:943.

[80] Kavanagh BF, Fitzgerald RH Jr. Multiple revisions for failed total hip arthroplasty not associated with infection. J Bone Joint Surg Am 1987; 69(8):1144-9.

[81] Kavanagh BF, Ilstrup DM, Fitzgerald RH Jr. Revision total hip arthroplasty. J Bone Joint Surg Am 1985; 67(4):517-26.

[82] Kelly MP, Bozic KJ. Cost drivers in total hip arthroplasty: effects of procedure volume and implant selling price. Am J Orthop 2009; 38(1):E1-4.

[83] Kershaw Ci, Atkins RM, Dodd CAF, Bulstrode CJK. Revision total hip arthroplasty for aseptic failure: a review of 276 cases. J Bone Joint Surg Br 1991; 73:564-8.

[84] Kinov P. Aseptic loosening of hip arthroplasty. PhD thesis. Medical University of Sofia; 2007.

[85] Kinov P, Bukarev D, Dimov V, Kazakov K, Tivchev P. Revision total hip arthroplasty with cementing technique-five-year results. Chir Narzadow Ruchu Ortop Pol 2007; 72(4):293-6.

[86] Knight JL, Helming C. Collarless polished tapered impaction grafting of the femur during revision total hip arthroplasty: pitfalls of the surgical technique and follow-up in 31 cases. J Arthroplasty 2000; 15(2):159-65.

[87] Kosashvili Y, Backstein D, Safir O, Lakstein D, Gross AE. Krishnamurthy AB, MacDonald SJ, Paprosky WG. 5- to Acetabular revision using an anti-protrusion (ilio-ischial) cage and trabecular metal acetabular component for severe acetabular bone loss associated with pelvic discontinuity. J Bone Joint Surg Br 2009; 91(7):870-6.

[88] Krishnamurthy AB, MacDonald SJ, Paprosky WG. 5-13-year follow-up study on cementless femoral components in revision surgery. J Arthroplasty 1997; 12(8):839-47.

[89] Kurtz S, Mowat F, Ong K, Chan N, Lau E, Halpern M. Prevalence of primary and revision total hip and knee arthroplasty in the United States from 1990 through 2002. J Bone Joint Surg Am 2005; 87:1487-97.

[90] Kwong LM, Jasty M, Harris WH. High failure rate of bulk femoral head allografts in total hip acetabular reconstructions at 10 years. J Arthroplasty 1993; 8:341-6.

[91] Lachiewicz PE, Hussamy OD. Revision of the acetabulum without cement with use of the Harris-Galante porous-coated implant: two to eight-year results. J Bone Joint Surg Am 1994; 76:1834-9.

[92] Lakstein D, Kosashvili Y, Backstein D, Safir O, Lee P, Gross AE. Revision total hip arthroplasty with a modular tapered stem. Hip Int 2010; 20(2):136-42.

[93] Lakstein D, Backstein D, Safir O, Kosashvili Y, Gross AE. Trabecular Metal cups for acetabular defects with 50% or less host bone contact. Clin Orthop Relat Res 2009; 467(9):2318-24.

[94] Langlais F, J. C. Lambotte, P. Collin, and H. Thomazeau, Long-term results of allograft composite total hip prostheses for tumors. Clin Orthop Relat Res 2003; 414:197-211.

[95] Lawrence JM, Engh CA, Macalino GE. Revision total hip arthroplasty. Long-term results without cement. Orthop Clin North Am 1993; 24(4):635-44.

[96] Li PL, Ingle PJ, Dowell JK. Cement-within-cement revision hip arthroplasty: should it be done? J Bone Joint Surg Br 1996; 78(5):809-11.

[97] Lieberman JR, Moeckel BH, Evans BG, Salvati EA, Ranawat CS. Cement-within-cement revision hip arthroplasty. J Bone Joint Surg Br 1993; 75(6):869-71.

[98] Malkani AL, F. H. Sim, and E. Y. S. Chao. Custom-made segmental femoral replacement prosthesis in revision total hip arthroplasty. Orthop Clin North Am 1993; 24(4): 727-33.

[99] Mallory TH. Preparation of the proximal femur in cementless total hip revision. Clin Orthop Relat Res 1988; 235:47-60.

[100] Masterson S, Lidder S, Scott G. Impaction femoral allografting at revision hip arthroplasty: uncemented versus cemented technique using a Freeman femoral component. J Bone Joint Surg Br 2012; 94(1):51-5.

[101] Masterson EL, Masri BA, Duncan CP. The cement mantle in the Exeter impaction allografting technique. A cause for concern. J Arthroplasty 1997; 12(7):759-64.

[102] McAuley JP, Engh CA Jr. Femoral fixation in the face of considerable bone loss: cylindrical and extensively coated femoral components. Clin Orthop Relat Res 2004; 429:215-21.

[103] Meding JB, Ritter MA, Keating EM, Faris PM. Impaction bonegrafting before insertion of a femoral stem with cement in revision total hip arthroplasty: a minimum two-year follow-up study. J Bone Joint Surg Am 1997; 79:1834-41.

[104] Miner TM, Momberger NG, Chong D, Paprosky WL. The extended trochanteric osteotomy in revision hip arthroplasty: a critical review of 166 cases at mean 3-year, 9-month follow-up. J Arthroplasty 2001; 16(Suppl 1):188-94.

[105] Moreland JR, Moreno MA. Cementless femoral revision arthroplasty of the hip: minimum 5 years followup. Clin Orthop Relat Res 2001; 393:194-201.

[106] Moreland JR, Bernstein ML. Femoral revision hip arthroplasty with uncemented, porous-coated stems. Clin Orthop Relat Res 1995; 319:141-50.

[107] Morsi E, Garbuz D, Gross AE. Revision total hip arthroplasty with shelf bulk allografts. A long-term follow-up study. J Arthroplasty 1996;11(1):86-90.

[108] Moskal JT, Higgins ME, Shen J. Type III acetabular defect revision with bilobed components: five-year results. Clin Orthop Relat Res 2008; 466(3):691-5.

[109] Mulroy WF, Harris WH. Revision total hip arthroplasty with use of so-called second-generation cementing techniques for aseptic loosening of the femoral component. A fifteen-year-average follow-up study. J Bone Joint Surg Am 1996; 78:325-30.

[110] Nadaud MC, Griffin WL, Fehring TK, Mason JB, Tabor OB Jr, Odum S, Nussman DS. Cementless revision total hip arthroplasty without allograft in severe proximal femoral defects. J Arthroplasty 2005; 20(6):738-44.

[111] Nehme A, Lewallen DB, Hanssen AD. Modular porous metal augments for treatment of severe acetabular bone loss during revision hip arthroplasty. Clin Orthop Relat Res 2004; 429:201-8.

[112] Nelson CL. Cemented cup revisions. Am J Orthop 2002; 31(8):479-80.

[113] Obenaus C, Winkler H, Girtler R, Huber M, Schwägerl W. Extra-large press-fit cups without screws for acetabular revision. J Arthroplasty 2003; 18(3):271-7.

[114] Ornstein E, Linder L, Ranstam J, Lewold S, Eisler T, Torper M. Femoral impaction bone grafting with the Exeter stem - the Swedish experience: survivorship analysis of

1,305 revisions performed between 1989 and 2002. J Bone Joint Surg Br 2009; 91(4): 441-6.

[115] Paprosky W G, Greidanus N V, Antoniou J. Minimum 10-year-results of extensively porous-coated stems in revision hip arthroplasty. Clin Orthop Relat Res 1999; 369:230-42.

[116] Paprosky WG, Perona PG, Lawrence JM. Acetabular defect classification and surgical reconstruction in revision arthroplasty. A 6-year follow-up evaluation. J Arthroplasty 1994; 9(1):33-44.

[117] Park DK, Della Valle CJ, Quigley L, Moric M, Rosenberg AG, Galante JO. Revision of the acetabular component without cement. A concise follow-up, at twenty to twenty-four years, of a previous report. J Bone Joint Surg Am 2009; 91:350-5.

[118] Parvizi J, Jacovides C, Antoci V, Ghanem E. Diagnosis of periprosthetic joint infection: the utility of a simple yet unappreciated enzyme. J Bone Joint Surg Am 2011; 93(24):2242-48.

[119] Parvizi J, Della Valle CJ. AAOS Clinical Practice Guideline: diagnosis and treatment of periprosthetic joint infections of the hip and knee. J Am Acad Orthop Surg 2010; 18(12):771-2.

[120] Parvizi J, Tarity TD, Slenker N, Wade F, Trappler R, Hozack WJ, Sim FH. Proximal femoral replacement in patients with non-neoplastic conditions. J Bone Joint Surg Am 2007; 89(5):1036-43.

[121] Pellicci PM, Wilson Jr PD, Sledge CB, Salvati EA, Ranawat CS, Poss R, Callaghan JJ.. Long-term results of revision total hip replacement. A follow-up report. J Bone Joint Surg Am 1985; 67:513-6.

[122] Pellicci PM, Wilson PD Jr, Sledge CB, Salvati EA, Ranawat CS, Poss R. Revision total hip arthroplasty. Clin Orthop Relat Res 1982; 170:34-41.

[123] Pekkarinen J, Alho A, Lepistö J, Ylikoski M, Ylinen P, Paavilainen T. Impaction bone grafting in revision hip surgery. A high incidence of complications. J Bone Joint Surg Br 2000; 82(1):103-7.

[124] Piccaluga F, González Della Valle A, Encinas Fernández JC, Pusso R. Revision of the femoral prosthesis with impaction allografting and a Charnley stem. A 2- to 12-year follow-up. J Bone Joint Surg Br 2002; 84(4):544-9.

[125] Pollock FH, Whiteside LA. The fate of massive allografts in total hip acetabular revision surgery. J Arthroplasty 1992; 7:271-6.

[126] Pulido L, Rachala SR, Cabanela ME. Cementless acetabular revision: past, present, and future. Revision total hip arthroplasty: the acetabular side using cementless implants. Int Orthop 2011; 35(2):289-98.

[127] Raut VV, Siney PD, Wroblewski BM. Cemented Charnley revision arthroplasty for severe femoral osteolysis. J Bone Joint Surg Br 1995; 77(3):362-5.

[128] Raut VV, Siney PD, Wroblewski BM: Cemented revision for aseptic acetabular loosening: a review of 387 hips. J Bone Joint Surg Br 1995; 77:357-61.

[129] Regis D, Sandri A, Bonetti I, Bortolami O, Bartolozzi P. A minimum of 10-year follow-up of the Burch-Schneider cage and bulk allografts for the revision of pelvic discontinuity. J Arthroplasty 2012; 27(6):1057-63.

[130] Ritter MA, Thong AE. The role of cemented sockets in 2004: is there one? J Arthroplasty 2004; 19(4 suppl 1):92-4.

[131] Rogers BA, Sternheim A, Backstein D, Safir O, Gross AE. Proximal femoral allograft for major segmental femoral bone loss: a systematic literature review. Adv Orthop 2011; 2011:257572.

[132] Roque PJ, Mankin HJ, Malchau H. Proximal femoral allograft: prognostic indicators. J Arthroplasty 2010; 25(7):1028-33.

[133] Rosenstein A, MacDonald W, Iliadis A, McLardy-Smith P. Revision of cemented fixation and cement-bone interface strength. Proc Inst Mech Eng (H) 1992; 206(1):47-9.

[134] Rubash HE, Harris WH. Revision of nonseptic, loose, cemented femoral components using modem cementing techniques. J Arthroplasty 1988; 3:241-8.

[135] Russotti GM, Harris WH. Proximal placement of the acetabular component in total hip arthroplasty. A long-term follow-up study. J Bone Joint Surg Am 1991; 73(4): 587-92.

[136] Safir O, Kellett CF, Flint M, Backstein D, Gross AE. Revision of the deficient proximal femur with a proximal femoral allograft. Clin Orthop Relat Res 2009; 467(1):206-12.

[137] Saleh KJ, Holtzman J, Gafni A, Saleh L, Davis A, Resig S, Gross AE. Reliability and intraoperative validity of preoperative assessment of standardized plain radiographs in predicting bone loss at revision hip surgery. J Bone Joint Surg Am 2001; 83:1040-6.

[138] Saleh KJ, Jaroszynski G, Woodgate I, Saleh L, Gross AE. Revision total hip arthroplasty with the use of structural acetabular allograft and reconstruction ring: a case series with a 10-year average follow-up. J Arthroplasty 2000; 15(8):951-8.

[139] Schreurs BW, Luttjeboer J, Thien TM, de Waal Malefijt MC, Buma P, Veth RP, Slooff TJ. Acetabular revision with impacted morselized cancellous bone graft and a cemented cup in patients with rheumatoid arthritis. A concise follow-up, at eight to nineteen years, of a previous report. J Bone Joint Surg Am 2009; 91(3):646-51.

[140] Schreurs BW, Arts JJ, Verdonschot N, Buma P, Slooff TJ, Gardeniers JW. Femoral component revision with use of impaction bone-grafting and a cemented polished stem. Surgical technique. J Bone Joint Surg Am 2006; 88(Suppl 1 Pt 2):259-74.

[141] Schreurs BW, Arts JJ, Verdonschot N, Buma P, Slooff TJ, Gardeniers JW. Femoral component revision with use of impaction bone-grafting and a cemented polished stem. J Bone Joint Surg Am 2005; 87(11):2499-507.

[142] Schreurs BW, Bolder SB, Gardeniers JW, Verdonschot N, Slooff TJ, Veth RP. Acetabular revision with impacted morsellised cancellous bone grafting and a cemented cup. A 15- to 20-year follow-up. J Bone Joint Surg Br 2004; 86(4):492-7.

[143] Schreurs BW, Slooff TJ, Buma P, Gardeniers JW, Huiskes R. Acetabular reconstruction with impacted morsellised cancellous bone graft and cement. A 10- to 15-year follow-up of 60 revision arthroplasties. J Bone Joint Surg Br 1998; 80(3):391-395.

[144] Shinar AA, Harris WH. Bulk structural autogenous grafts and allografts for reconstruction of the acetabulum in total hip arthroplasty. Sixteen-year-average follow-up. J Bone Joint Surg Am 1997; 79(2):159-68.

[145] Silverton CD, Rosenberg AG, Sheinkop MB, Kull LR, Galante JO. Revision of the acetabular component without cement after total hip arthroplasty. A follow-up note regarding results at seven to eleven years. J Bone Joint Surg Am 1996; 78(9):1366-70.

[146] Slooff TJ, Huiskes R, van Horn J, Lemmens AJ. Bone grafting in total hip replacement for acetabular protrusion. Acta Orthop Scand 1984; 55: 593-6.

[147] Sporer SM, Paprosky WG. Acetabular revision using a trabecular metal acetabular component for severe acetabular bone loss associated with a pelvic discontinuity. J Arthroplasty 2006; 21(6 Suppl 2):87-90.

[148] Sporer SM, O'Rourke M, Paprosky WG. The treatment of pelvic discontinuity during acetabular revision. J Arthroplasty 2005; 20(4 Suppl 2):79-84.

[149] Sternheim A, Rogers BA, Kuzyk PR, Safir OA, Backstein D, Gross AE. Segmental proximal femoral bone loss and revision total hip replacement in patients with developmental dysplasia of the hip: the role of allograft prosthesis composite. J Bone Joint Surg Br 2012; 94(6):762-7.

[150] Sutherland AG, D'Arcy S, Smart D, Ashcroft GP. Removal of the subchondral plate in acetabular preparation. Int Orthop 2000; 24(1):19-22.

[151] Sutherland CJ. Early experience with eccentric acetabular components in revision total hip arthroplasty. Am J Orthop 1996; 25:284-9.

[152] Tanzer M, Drucker D, Jasty M, McDonald M, Harris WH. Revision of the acetabular component with an uncemented Harris-Galante porous-coated prosthesis. J Bone Joint Surg Am 1992; 74(7):987-94.

[153] Templeton JE, Callaghan JJ, Goetz DD, Sullivan PM, Johnston RC. Revision of a cemented acetabular component to a cementless acetabular component. A ten to fourteen-year follow-up study. J Bone Joint Surg Am 2001; 83(11):1706-11.

[154] van Egmond N, De Kam DC, Gardeniers JW, Schreurs BW. Revisions of extensive acetabular defects with impaction grafting and a cement cup. Clin Orthop Relat Res 2011; 469(2):562-73.

[155] Vastel L, Lemoine CT, Kerboull M, Courpied JP. Structural allograft and cemented long-stem prosthesis for complex revision hip arthroplasty: use of a trochanteric claw plate improves final hip function. Int Orthop 2007; 31(6):851-7.

[156] Wagner H, Wagner M. Cone prosthesis for the hip joint. Arch Orthop Trauma Surg 2000; 120(1-2):88-95.

[157] Wedemeyer C, Neuerburg C, Heep H, von Knoch F, von Knoch M, Löer F, Saxler G. Jumbo cups for revision of acetabular defects after total hip arthroplasty: a retrospective review of a case series. Arch Orthop Trauma Surg 2008; 128:545-50.

[158] Weeden SH, Paprosky WG. Minimum 11-year follow up of extensively porous coated stems in femoral revision total hip arthroplasty. J Arthroplasty 2002; 17(Suppl 1): 134-7.

[159] Whaley AL, Berry DJ, Harmsen WS. Extra-large uncemented hemispherical acetabular components for revision total hip arthroplasty. J Bone Joint Surg Am 2001; 83(9): 1352-7.

[160] Winter E, Piert M, Volkmann R, Maurer F, Eingartner C, Weise K, Weller S. Allogeneic cancellous bone graft and a Burch-Schneider ring for acetabular reconstruction in revision hip arthroplasty. J Bone Joint Surg Am. 2001 Jun;83-A(6):862-7.

[161] Wraighte PJ, Howard PW. Femoral impaction bone allografting with an Exeter cemented collarless, polished, tapered stem in revision hip replacement: a mean follow-up of 10.5 years. J Bone Joint Surg Br 2008; 90(8):1000-4.

[162] Wysocki RW, Della Valle CJ, Shott S, Rosenberg AG, Berger RA, Galante JO. Revision of the acetabulum with a contemporary cementless component. J Arthroplasty 2009; 24(6 Suppl):58-63.

[163] Zehntner MK, Ganz R. Midterm results (5.5-10 years) of acetabular allograft reconstruction with the acetabular reinforcement ring during total hip revision. J Arthroplasty 1994; 9:469-79.

[164] Zehr RJ, Enneking WF, Scarborough MT. Allograft-prosthesis composite versus megaprosthesis in proximal femoral reconstruction. Clin Orthop Relat Res 1996; 322:207-23.

Chapter 15

# Total Joint Arthroplasty for Hemophilia

Hideyuki Takedani

Additional information is available at the end of the chapter

## 1. Introduction

Hemophilia is hereditary x-chromosomal recessive disorders. Hemophilia A is caused by deficiency or absence of coagulation factor VIII and hemophilia B is caused by that of coagulation factor IX. The prevalence is reported as one in 5000 in the male population and one in 10000 overall. These diseases are classified into three categories according to serum coagulation factor activity; severe (<1%), moderate (1-5%), or mild (>5%). The particular hemophilic manifestation is intra-articular bleeding. Intra-articular bleeding is usually occurred by trauma but also often spontaneously. Approximately 5% of first bleeding episodes in hemophilic boys are into a joint. The average age of first intra-articular bleeding is 1.91±0.91 years old and the median age of that is 1.63 years old [1]. A joint in which four or more recurrent bleedings have occurred in the prior 6 months is defined as target joint. In the United States, 2.3% of children 2-5 years of age enrolled in the Universal Data Collection Project have target joints [2]. Most of target joints have hemophilic synovitis, which is characterized by inflammation, angiogenesis and fibrosis [3] and develop hemophilic arthroplasty which is characterized by cartilage and bone destruction.

The average annual intra-articular bleeding number were higher in the episodic-therapy group than in the prophylaxis group and the relative risk of MRI-detected joint damage with the episodic was 6-fold greater compared with prophylactic group [4]. Therefore, it is a clear the relationship between intra-articular bleeding and hemophilic arthropathy. However, the number and volume of intra-articular bleedings which result in target joint and arthropathy is not understood. Experimental pathgenetic studies were reported and many points of the pathogenesis are still remained as poorly understood points [2,5,6].

As for radiological evaluation methods of hemophilic arthropathy, there are three major systems. De Palma classification is classical progressive system and popular in Japan. This system classified hemophilic arthropathy from grade 0 (normal) to grade IV (end-stage) [7].

Arnold-Hilgartner classification is also classical progressive system and classified from stage 0 (normal) to stage V (end-stage) [8]. Pettersson score is recommend additive scoring system by World Federation of Hemophilia (WFH) [9]. 8 categories in this system have 0 (normal) to 2 (worse) points and totally scored from 0 (normal) to 13 points (worst). There are classical and authorized good systems but it may need to improve them, because their inter-observer reliabilities were poor [10].

As for MRI evaluation methods, there were several reports since 2000 [11-13], and WFH recommended MRI scale and modified version were published from the international prophylaxis study group [14, 15].

The causative mechanism of hemophilia was recognized in the 1950s [16], and concentrates for coagulation factor replacement became generally available since 1960s, however the easy administration of the concentrates resulted in transmission of viral infection including hepatitis C (HCV) and Human immunodeficiency virus infection (HIV) during the 1980s [17]. Also, the appearance of allo-immune antibody (inhibitor) against deficient coagulation factor is severe adversity. Product development such as recombinant concentrates has especially improved therapeutic safety and availability [18], resulting in the possibility of performing elective orthopedic surgery and prevention of bleeding episodes. The routine administration of prophylactic treatment has undoubtedly resulted in a greatly improvement in the quality of life and life expectancy of hemophilic patients. However, many of young hemophilic adults still have severe destructive joints as a result of repeated intra-articular bleeding during their early years.

For hemophilic arthropathy, there are two major surgical options which are synovectomy for early stage (hemophilic synovitis) and total joint arthroplasty (TJA) for end stage. At progressive stage, there are not good surgical options so that several usual orthopedic options are tried: anti-inflammatory drugs, corticosteroids, joint infusion of hyaluronic acid or corticosteroids, braces and rehabilitation. However many of them are progressed to end-stage. Total joint arthroplasty (TJA) is effective procedure in the management of hemophilic arthropathy for them [19].

## 2. Major surgery for hemophilia

In our hospital, 126 major surgeries for 80 patients have been performed between June 2006 and June 2012 in which were 96 surgeries for 63 hemophilia A, 28 surgeries for 16 hemophilia B, and 2 surgeries for 2 other coagulation disorders. 18 surgeries with inhibitor were included. The average age at operation was 39.03 years (13 ~ 60 years). As for virus infection, HBs antigen positive ratio was 1.5% (2/126 surgeries), HCV antibody positive ratio was 89.7% (113/126), HIV antibody positive ratio was 33.3% (42/126) and both HCV and HIV antibody positive ratio was 31.7% (41/126).

Major surgery such as TJA is never easily undertaking in hemophilic patients. It required bleeding control at peri-operative periods, management for viral infection and inhibitor, and treatment for complication subsequently to bleeding.

As for bleeding control, guidelines were published[20, 21], in which the aim serum factor level at peri-operative period is explained clearly. However it is difficult without the support of hematologists so that major surgeries are usually performed at hemophilia centers.

As for HIV infection, CD4 cell counts had been important factor as major influence factor on bacterial infection in the early literatures [22-25]. HIV medical treatment has drastically improved during the last decade. In the recent literatures [26-29] and our experience, there was no evidence to suggest that bacterial deep infection at surgical site was influenced on the decline of CD4 cell counts. However HIV-positive patients whose CD4 cell counts is less than 50 cell/mm3 have a considerable risk of the occurrence of opportunistic infection at peri-operaive periods.

Most hemophilia adult patients infected hepatitis C virus at 1980s and long period of the virus carrier results in hepatic insufficiency and hepatoma. The treatment for chronic hepatitis has also improved, however it was not good enough to control it. According to our clinical experiences, severe hepatic insufficiency has been influenced on the fatal ratio after major surgery.

Between 10-30% of patients with hemophilia A and 2-5% of patients with hemophilia B develop an inhibitor to FVIII or FIX [30]. Intra-articular bleedings in inhibitor patients have a more negative impact on their joint function and daily life. They desire to reduce the pain and improve function at affected joint. However surgical treatments may be deferred until patients suffer from increasingly severe pain and progressive physical incapacity find no other options, due to the higher bleeding risks associated with surgery [31]. In fact, there are some surgical reports for inhibitors, but many of them are a few cases reports [32]. Guidelines for inhibitor [33] were also published, but bleeding control plan at peri-operative periods is not established. We believe surgical treatments for inhibitor should be performed at hemophilic center.

Delayed wound healing is the major complication subsequently to bleeding. In hemophilia B mice, dermal wound healing is delayed and can be treated with factor IX replacement therapy to restore thrombin generation. This delay is associated with bleeding into granulation tissue [34]. In our hospital, there were 3.3% delayed wound healings.

## 3. Total joint arthroplasty

TJA has been available as a final option in the end-stage hemophilic arthropathy with significantly reduced quality of life. The major objectives of TJA are to reduce the pain in the affected joint and improve the joint function. These effects are influenced on the adjacent joints beneficially. In addition, the frequency and number of the intra-articular bleeding is significantly reduced. Thereby, their life-style and quality of life significantly improved. The indications are adult hemophilia patients with severe destructive arthropathy and subjective dysfunction. Adult means the patient's epiphyses are closed. We have performed total hip arthroplasty for 18 years boy. Their dysfunction have been started from childhood and made worse gradually. They are satisfied to live on their ability even if they have severe destructive arthropathies. These cases are not indication subjectively. Total knee or hip arthroplasty (TKA, THA) are generally performed and total elbow and ankle arthroplasty (TEA, TAA) are rarely performed. However the most common affected joints are elbow, knee and ankle. The average of operation is around forty [35, 36]. In our hospital, 81 total joint arthroplasty were performed included 59 TKAs, 20 THAs, 1TEA and 1TAA and average age were 44.5. (figure 1, 2)

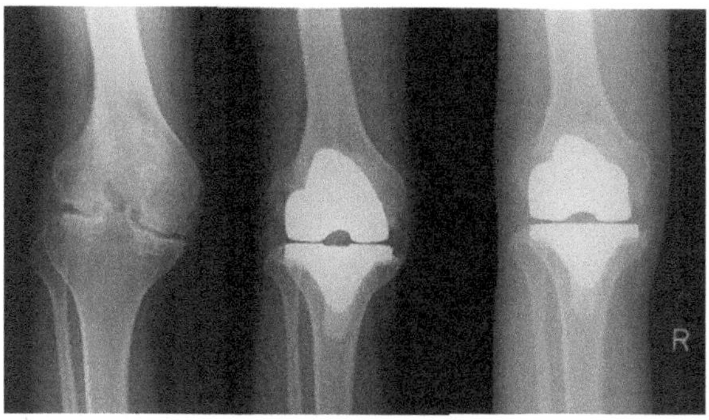


a b c

**Figure 1.** A 18-year-old hemophilia A patient without inhibitor. No virus infection. Severe hemophilic arthropathy of the right knee. His knee range of motion was improved at four years after surgery: extension was -30 degrees to 0 degrees and flexion was 90 degrees to 110 degrees. (a): pre-operative radiography; (b) at one month radiography (c) at four year radiography

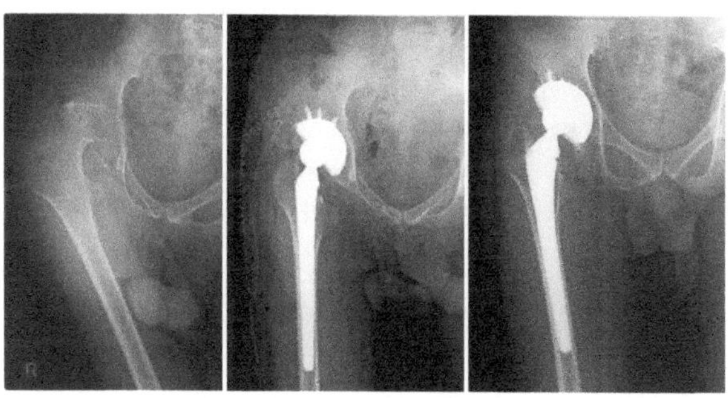

a b c

**Figure 2.** A 23-year-old hemophilia A patient with inhibitor. HCV is positive. Severe hemophilic arthropathy of the right hip. His back pain and tilted pelvis are improved after surgery. (a): pre-operative radiography; (b) just operative radiography (c) at five year radiography

As for surgical technique, we believe orthopedic surgeons do not need special skills when deficient factor level is kept with concentrate adequately. However, there are some careful points on TJA for hemophilia, in addition to the aforementioned surgical risks for hemophilia, which are higher infection rate, higher revision rate or shorter durability (table 1), and the occurrence of deep venous thrombosis (DVT).

| Authers | Year | Number of TJA | Average of Follow-up (years) | Infection rate (%) | Aseptic loosening rate (%) |
|---|---|---|---|---|---|
| Cohen et al | 2000 | 21 TKAs | 5.6 | 10 | 0 |
| Norian et al | 2002 | 53 TKAs | 5 | 13.2 | 9.4 |
| Sheth et al | 2004 | 14 TKAs | 6.4 | 0 | 0 |
| Goddard et al | 2010 | 70 TKAs | 9.2 | 1.5 | 8.6 |
| Habermann et al | 2007 | 15 THAs | 11 | 6.7 | 6.7 |
| Miles et al | 2008 | 34 THAs | 6.3 | 3 | 9 |
| Yoo et al | 2009 | 23 THAs | 7.7 | 0 | 4.8 |
| Powell et al | 2005 | 35 TKAs<br>16 THAs | 6.9 | TKA:14.3<br>THA:6.3 | 0 |
| Wang et al | 2012 | 40 TKAs<br>18 THAs | 10.7 | TKA:13<br>THA:0 | TKA:2.5<br>THA:5.6 |

**Table 1.** Infection and aseptic loosening rate after TJA in hemophilia including current study [35-38,40-44]

As for the infection after TJA, most reports show a deep infection rate of 10-16% [35-41], and our result shows much lower infection rate of 2.5 (2/81). However, these rates are higher than infection rate of 1-2% consistently reported in the literatures in the general population [45]. HIV infection had been important factor as major influence factor on bacterial infection, however the recent clinical results suggest there is no difference in the infection rate between HIV positive and negative. It is unclear why the ratio after TJA for hemophilia is much higher than that for non-hemophilia. The hypothesis that much frequent venous self-infusion is influenced on highly infection rate [40] is one of possibilities, but there is no evidence as yet.

As for durability, there are a few long clinical reports. When revision for aseptic mechanical failure was considered as endpoint, the survival rate for 40 TKAs at 10 years was 93%. The survival rate for 18 THAs at 8.5 years was 89% [36]. According to clinical result for 60 TKAs at a mean follow-up of 9.2 years, Kaplan-Meier analysis using infection and aseptic loosening as endpoint showed the survival rate at 20 years to be 94.0% [35]. These survival rates were similar to that in young non-hemophilia patients [46,47], however we believe it is not good enough rate for young hemophilic patients who have multi-arthropathy.

Hemophilia patients are often considered that their risk of DVT is lower by virtue of their bleeding disorder. However, they have as same risk of DVT as non-hemophilic patients, because the coagulation factor level is normalized by administration of concentrates at peri-operative periods. In our hospital, all patients use compression devices and not administrate drugs such as heparin or aspirin. Thrombosis has been checked by ultrasound and not detected at pre- and post-operation. Subclinical DVT was observed in 10% of hemophilia patients undergoing major orthopedic surgery [48]. According to the simple questionnaires survey at hemophilia treatment center in the United States, 78% provided thrombo-prophylaxis to selected patients. Of those providing of thrombo-prophylaxis, 67% used compression stocking or devices, 24% used low molecular weight heparin, 1% fondaparinux, 3% unfractionated heparin. 4% warfarin and 1% aspirin [49].

Finally, the cost of hemophilia treatment is major economical concern. The concentrate cost is occupied of major part of TJA cost and it is depended on the patient body weight. And the price of concentrates and insurance situation are quite differences internationally, so that we introduced our situation in this chapter. The cost is too expensive to performed surgery without insurance coverage, however Japanese general health insurance is covered with most of the cost, fortunately. The cost of TJA at peri-operative periods about two weeks is forty to fifty thousand dollars for average Japanese hemophilic patients without inhibitor (50-70kg). The cost for inhibitor cases is about 5 to 10-folds.

Total joint arthroplasty for hemophilia is a challenging surgery and never a simple undertaking, however hemophilia patient need to improve their life style and release severe pain. We believe it is a safe and effective procedure in the management of hemophilic arthropathy at hemophilia centers.

## Author details

Hideyuki Takedani*

Address all correspondence to: takedani@ims.u-tokyo.ac.jp

Department of Joint Surgery Research Hospital of the Institute of Medical Science The University of Tokyo 4-6-1 Shiroganedai, Minato-ku, Tokyo 108-8639, Japan

## References

[1] Pollmann, H., Richter, H., Ringkamp, H., & Jurgens, H. (1999). When are children diagnosed as having severe haemophilia and when do they start to bleed? A 10 -year single-centre PUP study. *Eur J Pediatr.*, Dec, 158(3), S166-170.

[2] Valentino, L. A., Hakobyan, N., Enockson, C., et al. (2012). Exploring the biological basis of haemophilic joint disease: experimental studies. *Haemophilia.*, May, 18(3), 310-318.

[3] Stein, H., & Duthie, R. B. (1981). The pathogenesis of chronic haemophilic arthropathy. *J Bone Joint Surg Br*, 63B(4), 601-9.

[4] Manco-Johnson, M. J., Abshire, T. C., Shapiro, A. D., et al. (2007). Prophylaxis versus episodic treatment to prevent joint disease in boys with severe hemophilia. *N Engl J Med*, Aug 9, 357(6), 535-544.

[5] Valentino, L. A., Hakobyan, N., Rodriguez, N., & Hoots, W. K. (2007). Pathogenesis of haemophilic synovitis: experimental studies on blood-induced joint damage. *Haemophilia*, Nov, 13(3), 10-13.

[6] Roosendaal, G., & Lafeber, F. P. (2006). Pathogenesis of haemophilic arthropathy. *Haemophilia*, Jul, 12(3), 117-121.

[7] De Palma, A. F., & Cotler, J. M. (1956). Hemophilic arthropathy. *AMA Arch Surg*, Feb, 72(2), 247-250.

[8] Arnold, W. D., & Hilgartner, M. W. (1977). Hemophilic arthropathy. Current concepts of pathogenesis and management. *J Bone Joint Surg Am*, Apr, 59(3), 287-305.

[9] Pettersson, H., Ahlberg, A., & Nilsson, I. M. (1980). A radiologic classification of hemophilic arthropathy. *Clin Orthop Relat Res.* [149], Jun, 153-9.

[10] Takedani, H., Fujii, T., Kobayashi, Y., Haga, N., Tatsunami, S., & Fujii, T. (2011). Inter-observer reliability of three different radiographic scores for adult haemophilia. *Haemophilia.*, Jan, 17(1), 134-138.

[11] Nuss, R., Kilcoyne, R. F., Rivard, G. E., & Murphy, J. (2000). Late clinical, plain X-ray and magnetic resonance imaging findings in haemophilic joints treated with radiosynoviorthesis. *Haemophilia.*, Nov, 6(6), 658-663.

[12] Funk, M. B., Schmidt, H., Becker, S., et al. (2002). Modified magnetic resonance imaging score compared with orthopaedic and radiological scores for the evaluation of haemophilic arthropathy. *Haemophilia.*, Mar, 8(2), 98-103.

[13] Kilcoyne, R. F., & Nuss, R. (2003). Radiological assessment of haemophilic arthropathy with emphasis on MRI findings. *Haemophilia*, 9(1), 57-63, discussion 63-54.

[14] Lundin, B., Babyn, P., Doria, AS, et al. (2005). Compatible scales for progressive and additive MRI assessments of haemophilic arthropathy. *Haemophilia*, Mar, 11(2), 109-115.

[15] Lundin, B., Manco-Johnson, M. L., Ignas, D. M., et al. (2012). An MRI scale for assessment of haemophilic arthropathy from the International Prophylaxis Study Group. *Haemophilia*, Jul 5

[16] Biggs, R., Douglas, AS, Macfarlane, R. G., Dacie, J. V., & Merskey, Pitney W. R. (1952). Christmas disease: a condition previously mistaken for haemophilia. *Br Med J.*, Dec 27, 2(4799), 1378-1382.

[17] Mannucci, P. M., & Tuddenham, E. G. (2001). The hemophilias--from royal genes to gene therapy. *N Engl J Med.*, Jun 7, 344(23), 1773-1779.

[18] Key, N. S., & Negrier, C. (2007). Coagulation factor concentrates: past, present, and future. *Lancet.*, Aug 4, 370(9585), 439-448.

[19] Takedani, H., Mikami, S., Abe, Y., Kin, H., & Kawasaki, N. (2000). [Total hip and knee arthroplasty for arthropathy in a hemophiliac]. *Rinsho Ketsueki.*, Feb;, 41(2), 97-102.

[20] Kasper, C. K. (2000). Protocols for the treatment of haemophilia and von Willebrand disease. *Haemophilia.*, Jul;, 6(1), 84-93.

[21] Guidelines for the management of hemophilia. (2005). Montreal: World Federation of Hemophilia.

[22] Goddard, N. (2010). Joint replacement. *In Lee CA, Berntop EE, Hoots WK. (ed.) Textbook of Hemophilia second edition.Cornwall: Wiley-Blackwell*, 176-181.

[23] Gregg-Smith, S. J., Pattison, R. M., Dodd, C. A., Giangrande, P. L., & Duthie, R. B. (1993). Septic arthritis in haemophilia. J Bone Joint Surg Br. May , 75(3), 368-370.

[24] Wiedel, J. D., Luck, J. V., & Gilbert, M. S. (1989). Total knee arthroplasty in the patient with haemophilia; evaluation and long term results. *Gilbert MS, Greene WB. (ed.) Musculo-skeltal problems in Hemophilia. New York National: Hemophilia foundation*, 152-157.

[25] Ragni, M. V., Crossett, L. S., & Herndon, J. H. (1995). Postoperative infection following orthopaedic surgery in human immunodeficiency virus-infected hemophiliacs with CD4 counts < or = 200/mm3. *J Arthroplasty.*, Dec, 10(6), 716-721.

[26] Birch, N. C., Ribbans, W. J., Goldman, E., & Lee, CA. (1994). Knee replacement in haemophilia. *J Bone Joint Surg Br.*, Jan, 76(1), 165-166.

[27] Phillips, A. M., Sabin, C. A., Ribbans, W. J., & Lee, C. A. (1997). Orthopaedic surgery in hemophilic patients with human immunodeficiency virus. *Clin Orthop Relat Res.* [343], Oct, 81-87.

[28] Hicks, J. L., Ribbans, W. J., Buzzard, B., et al. (2001). Infected joint replacements in HIV-positive patients with haemophilia. *J Bone Joint Surg Br.*, Sep, 83(7), 1050-1054.

[29] Rodriguez-Merchan, E. C., & Wiedel, J. D. (2002). Total knee arthroplasty in HIV-positive haemophilic patients. *Haemophilia.*, May, 8(3), 387-392.

[30] Valentino, L. A., Cooper, D. L., & Goldstein, B. (2011). Surgical experience with rFVIIa (NovoSeven) in congenital haemophilia A and B patients with inhibitors to factors VIII or IX. *Haemophilia*, Jul, 17(4), 579-589.

[31] Jimenez-Yuste, V., Rodriguez-Merchan, E. C., Alvarez, M. T., Quintana, M., Fernandez, I., & Hernandez-Navarro, F. (2008). Controversies and challenges in elective orthopedic surgery in patients with hemophilia and inhibitors. *Semin Hematol.*, Apr, 45(2, 1), S64-67.

[32] Takedani, H., Kawahara, H., & Kajiwara, M. (2010). Major orthopaedic surgeries for haemophilia with inhibitors using rFVIIa. *Haemophilia*, Mar, 16(2), 290-295.

[33] Gringeri, A., & Mannucci, P. M. (2005). Italian guidelines for the diagnosis and treatment of patients with haemophilia and inhibitors. *Haemophilia*, Nov, 11(6), 611-619.

[34] Monroe, D. M., Mackman, N., & Hoffman, M. (2010). Wound healing in hemophilia B mice and low tissue factor mice. *Thromb Res.*, Apr, 125(1), S74-77.

[35] Goddard, N. J., Mann, H. A., & Lee, C. A. (2010). Total knee replacement in patients with end-stage haemophilic arthropathy: 25-year results. *J Bone Joint Surg Br.*, Aug, 92(8), 1085-1089.

[36] Wang, K., Street, A., Dowrick, A., & Liew, S. (2012). Clinical outcomes and patient satisfaction following total joint replacement in haemophilia--23-year experience in knees, hips and elbows. *Haemophilia.*, Jan, 18(1), 86-93.

[37] Cohen, I., Heim, M., Martinowitz, U., & Chechick, A. (2000). Orthopaedic outcome of total knee replacement in haemophilia A. *Haemophilia.*, Mar, 6(2), 104-109.

[38] Powell, D. L., Whitener, C. J., Dye, C. E., Ballard, J. O., Shaffer, M. L., & Eyster, M. E. (2005). Knee and hip arthroplasty infection rates in persons with haemophilia: a 27 year single center experience during the HIV epidemic. *Haemophilia.*, May, 11(3), 233-239.

[39] Silva, M., & Luck, J. V. Jr. (2005). Long-term results of primary total knee replacement in patients with hemophilia. *J Bone Joint Surg Am.*, Jan, 87(1), 85-91.

[40] Sheth, DS, Oldfield, D., Ambrose, C., & Clyburn, T. (2004). Total knee arthroplasty in hemophilic arthropathy. *J Arthroplasty.*, Jan, 19(1), 56-60.

[41] Norian, J. M., Ries, MD, Karp, S., & Hambleton, J. (2002). Total knee arthroplasty in hemophilic arthropathy. *J Bone Joint Surg Am.*, Jul, 84A(7), 1138-1141.

[42] Habermann, B., Eberhardt, C., Hovy, L., Zichner, L., Scharrer, I., & Kurth, AA. (2007). Total hip replacement in patients with severe bleeding disorders A 30 years single center experience. *Int Orthop.*, Feb, 31(1), 17-21.

[43] Miles, J., Rodriguez-Merchan, E. C., & Goddard, N. J. (2008). The impact of haemophilia on the success of total hip arthroplasty. *Haemophilia*, Jan, 14(1), 81-84.

[44] Yoo, M. C., Cho, Y. J., Kim, K. I., Ramteke, A., & Chun, Y. S. (2009). The outcome of cementless total hip arthroplasty in haemophilic hip arthropathy. *Haemophilia*, May, 15(3), 766-773.

[45] Bengtson, S., & Knutson, K. (1991). The infected knee arthroplasty. A 6-year follow-up of 357 cases. *Acta Orthop Scand.*, Aug, 62(4), 301-311.

[46] Pospischill, M., & Knahr, K. (2005). Cementless total hip arthroplasty using a threaded cup and a rectangular tapered stem. Follow-up for ten to 17 years. *J Bone Joint Surg Br.*, Sep, 87(9), 1210-1215.

[47] Seyler, T. M., Bonutti, P. M., Shen, J., Naughton, M., & Kester, M. (2006). Use of an alumina-on-alumina bearing system in total hip arthroplasty for osteonecrosis of the hip. *J Bone Joint Surg Am.*, Nov, 88(3), 116-125.

[48] Hermans, C., Hammer, F., Lobet, S., & Lambert, C. (2010). Subclinical deep venous thrombosis observed in 10% of hemophilic patients undergoing major orthopedic surgery. May. *J Thromb Haemost.*, 8(5), 1138-1140.

[49] Pradhan, S. M., Key, N. S., Boggio, L., & Pruthi, R. (2009). Venous thrombosis prophylaxis in haemophilics undergoing major orthopaedic surgery: a survey of haemophilia treatment centres. *Haemophilia.*, Nov, 15(6), 1337-1338.

Chapter 16

# Ankle Osteoarthritis and Arthroplasty

Nadr M. Jomha, Angela Scharfenberger,
Gordon Goplen and M. Elizabeth Pedersen

Additional information is available at the end of the chapter

## 1. Introduction

The World Health Organization estimates that 10% of the world's population over the age of 60 suffers from osteoarthritis (OA) [1]. The majority of these cases involve the hip and knee. Symptomatic osteoarthritis of the ankle with radiographic changes is seen in approximately 11% of patients seeking treatment for "arthritis" [1]. Idiopathic arthritis, as seen in the hip and knee, is rare in the ankle joint. The majority of ankle arthritis is secondary to trauma (70%), with a smaller percentage being attributed to inflammatory arthropathies such as RA (12%) and only 7% attributed to primary OA [2]. Ankle arthritis can be a debilitating disease. In fact, the mental and physical disability associated with end-stage arthritis of the ankle is at least as severe as that associated with end stage hip arthritis [3].

### 1.1. Anatomy

The ankle joint consists of the tibio-talar joint incorporating articular surfaces between the talar dome with the tibial plafond, and the medial talus with the medial malleolus. In addition, there is an articulation between the lateral talus with the lateral malleolus. It is mainly a rolling joint with congruent surfaces at high loads, allowing it to withstand large pressures [1]. The ankle carries 5 times body weight during normal walking activities [4]. The majority of the load (75%) is distributed across the tibio-talar joint but some force is transmitted through the medial and lateral sides [5]. Pathological conditions such as a mal-united ankle fracture results in changes in the contact stresses and the overall contact area [5].

### 1.2. History

Patients with arthritic changes to the ankle have the typical "arthritic" complaints as seen in other affected joints. Patients often present with pain, swelling and stiffness. The pain may be worse with weight bearing/impact activities, with weather changes, and may wake them at night. Painful symptoms may be worse with initiation of activities (especially first thing in the morning) but may improve during the activity. The pain usually intensifies with prolonged activity and after the activity is completed. Stiffness can be present, usually worse first thing in the morning or after a prolonged rest. Swelling can be particularly bothersome and is usually intermittent. Patients complain of pain in the anterior talo-crural area and have difficulty with reciprocal stair climbing and hills. Subfibular or lateral foot pain is not common and is more typical for patients with subtalar arthritis which may be seen in combination with ankle arthritis. Patients with subtalar arthritis complain of difficulties with walking on uneven ground.

Given that most ankle arthritis is post-traumatic, a history of previous trauma should be determined including a history of severe or repetitive ankle sprains [6]. History of previous infection is important to ascertain as it can be a contraindication to joint arthroplasty and current infection should be treated immediately with antibiotics and possibly debridement. Systemic illness such as rheumatoid arthritis, gout, and hemophilia should be noted. Patients with diabetes mellitus can present with Charcot deformity including arthritis.

### 1.3. Physical exam

Patients should be inspected for general lower limb alignment, including the knees, ankle, hindfoot, midfoot and forefoot, paying particular attention to varus/valgus mal-alignment of the hindfoot and dorsiflexion/plantarflexion mal-alignment of the ankle. Inspection should note any swelling about the ankle, wasting of the calf musculature and previous surgical incisions. Gait should be observed. Patients generally have a foreshortened stance phase, and may walk with their foot externally rotated. Patients with ankle arthritis walk with a shorter stride length, reduced walking speed, and a shorter stance phase of the affected limb [4, 5, 7, 8]. Active and passive range of motion should be compared to the other side for ankle dorsi/plantar flexion and subtalar eversion/inversion. In severe ankle arthritis, it is important to differentiate range of motion coming from the ankle joint as opposed to the hindfoot and midfoot joints. Heel eversion and inversion may also show restrictions of movement. Palpation should include all bone prominences and the anterior margin of the ankle joint looking for areas of tenderness or synovitis. Sensory changes or motor dysfunction should be noted for possible neurological abnormalities. Both dorsalis pedis and posterior tibial pulses should be assessed along with capillary refill and any abnormalities may require further vascular investigations with ABI and/or CT angiogram.

### 1.4. Imaging

Standard radiographs should include WEIGHTBEARING AP/Lateral and mortise views of both ankles, and AP and lateral views of the foot. Radiographs can be reviewed for the classic signs of OA including loss of joint space, subchondral sclerosis, cyst formation and osteophyte formation. CT scan can be useful to determine arthritic changes in adjacent joints, or to look at the surrounding bone stock when considering arthroplasty but this technique is compromised for diagnosing early OA with cartilage loss because it is not done in the weightbearing position; therefore it can be misleading regarding joint space maintenance and overall joint alignment. MRI is not required when assessing ankle arthritis. If there is a past history of infection, quiescent infection should be ruled out with a bone/gallium scan combination or a white blood cell scan.

## 2. Conservative treatment

### 2.1. Medications

Non-steroidal anti-inflammatories drugs (NSAIDs) have long been the mainstay for symptomatic treatment of arthritic joint pain. These drugs control the pain of arthritis but are not disease modifying agents. Current classes of drugs include standard NSAIDs (eg. Ibuprofen, Naproxen, Indomethacin). The newer Cox 2 inhibitors [eg. Celecoxib (Celebrex) and Rofecoxib (Vioxx)] have less gastrointestinal side effects [9, 10]; however, concern about higher risks of myocardial infarction, thrombosis and stroke lead to withdrawl of Rofecoxib (Vioxx) from the market in 2004 Patients with long term NSAID use are counseled to have blood pressure and kidney function checked regularly with their family physicians as all NSAIDS still put patients at risk for renal-related complications.

Nutraceuticals such as glucosamine sulphate and chondroitin sulphate are popular non-prescription remedies. There have been a multiple studies on these products, the vast majority done in the arthritic knee population. Findings include pain modification similar to NSAIDS with a similar side effect profile, although the onset is slower [11, 12]. Other studies suggest actual disease modification with long term glucosamine use, as seen by NON progression of joint space narrowing [13, 14]. More recent authors have found no difference between glucosamine and placebo [15] and no evidence of disease modification or pain relief [16]. Popular dosing for glucosamine is 1.5 grams per day.

### 2.2. Injections

Corticosteroids demonstrate both anti-inflammatory response and immunosuppressive effect. After intra-articular administration, there is a decrease in erythema, swelling, heat and tenderness. This may be secondary to altered movement and function of leucocytes, reduced micro vascular dilation and permeability, and reduced prostaglandin synthesis. Side effects can include septic arthritis, tendon rupture, post injection wheal and flare, facial flushing, atrophic skin changes, toxic effect on cartilage (at large doses) and possible systemic absorption. Standard limit of injections in weight bearing joints is 3-4 injections per year [17].

Hyaluronic acid (HA) is a major component of synovial fluid, and comprises part of the structure of hyaline cartilage. Viscosupplementation by injection of HA derivatives (as available in pharmaceutical components) has multiple proposed mechanisms of action. Biologic effects include an anti-inflammatory as well as anti-oxidant effect, and restoration of endogenous synthesis via positive feedback loop. Viscoelastic properties include a "mechanical spongy" trapping of immune complexes and inflammatory cells and restoration of synovial fluid viscosity and elasticity. Multiple versions of HA exist from multiple pharmaceutical companies. Not all are available in all countries [18]. Some examples of currently available products include Hyalgan (sodium hyaluronate; Sanofi-Aventis, Bridgewater, NJ, USA), Synvisc (hylan GF-20; Genzyme Corportation, Cambridge, MA, USA), Supartz (sodium hyaluronate; Smith & Nephew, London, UK), Orthovisc (high molecular weight hyaluronan; Anika Therapeutics, Inc., Bedford, MA, USA), Euflexxa (1% sodium hyaluronate; Ferring Pharmaceuticals, Inc., Saint-Prex, Switzerland), and Durolane (stabilize hyaluronic acid; Smith & Nephew, York, UK). Most require multiple injections although newer ones (eg Durolane) are coming to market that require only one injection. Side effect of HA injections are rare but include anaphylaxis, pseudogout type reaction, and Severe Acute Inflammatory Reaction (SAIR) which presents like septic arthritis.

The effectiveness of hyaluronic acid derivatives in the ankle joint has not been determined due to poorly conducted studies with mixed results from the few good studies performed [19, 20] although a recent randomized control trial article comparing HA to saline in the ankle showed no therapeutic benefit from the HA injection. Both HA and Saline injection resulted in similar changes in VAS, AOS and AOFAS scores [21]. Further high quality studies need to be completed before a definitive recommendation for HA derivatives in the ankle can be given.

### 2.3. Bracing

There is a paucity of any literature on bracing and shoe modifications. Practically, bracing progresses from a simple lace-up ankle brace to a more elaborate rigid Ankle Foot Orthosis (AFO) (Figure 1). A rigid AFO works by restricting painful ankle range of motion.

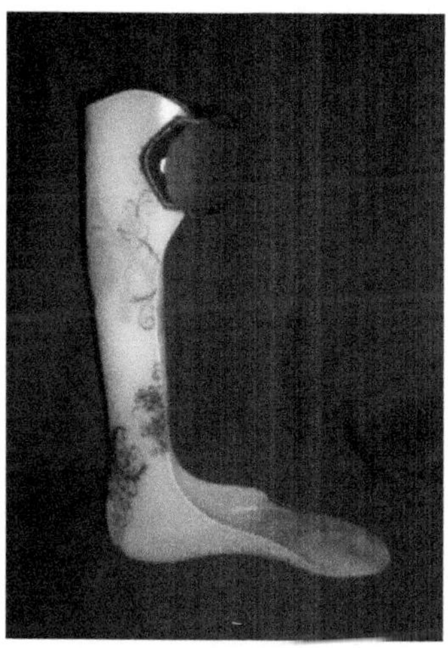

**Figure 1.** Photograph of a rigid AFO.

More severely affected joints may be helped by a clamshell AFO (offloading AFO) (Figure 2). This type of orthosis works by transferring weight from the ankle to the calf using the clamshell portion that wraps around the calf (similar in principle to a patellar-tendon brace). This type of AFO can have a hinge to maintain ankle range of motion or can be rigid to restrict motion as well as off-load the joint.

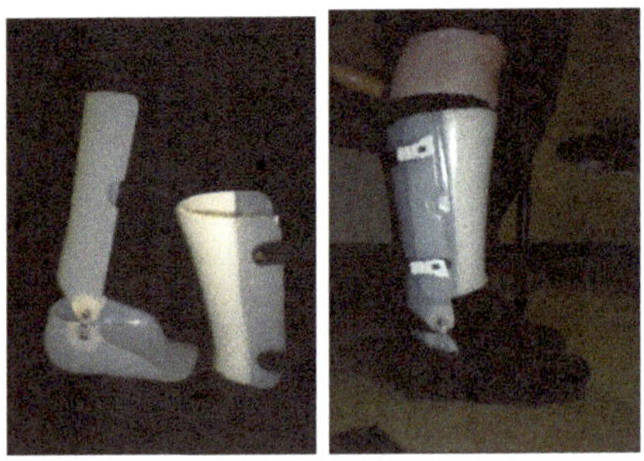

**Figure 2.** Offloading AFO with a hinge. Picture on the left demonstrates the AFO in a separated condition while the right picture shows it applied to the patient.

Some patients may benefit from shoe modifications such as a rocker bottom shoe (Figure 3). This provides increased toe-off, thereby stressing the ankle joint less.

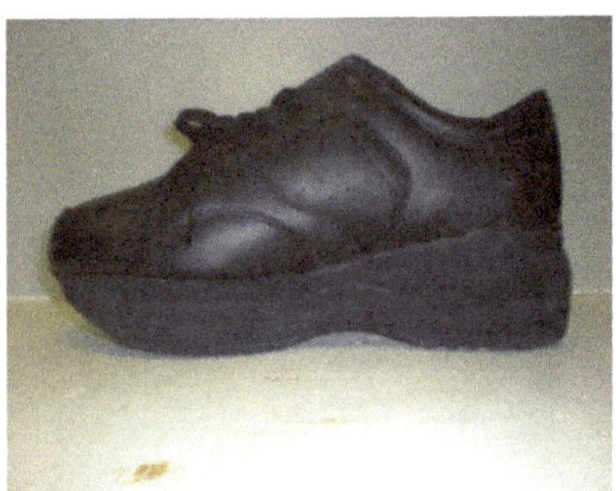

**Figure 3.** Forefoot rocker bottom shoe.

## 3. Surgical options

After non-operative treatments have been exhausted, surgical treatments can be considered. These options will depend on the location and extent of the arthritis.

### 3.1. Focal joint abnormalities

Localized lesions within the ankle joint can progress to generalized osteoarthritis. As documented in the knee, larger lesions have a worse prognosis than smaller lesions [22, 23]. Smaller lesions (usually considered 1cm$^2$ or less can be asymptomatic or often are dealt with by arthroscopic debridement of loose cartilage with or without microfracture technique. If there is underlying bone necrosis, removal of this bone and overlying damaged cartilage can provide symptomatic relief. For larger lesions, the surgical options become more complicated and less predictable. There are a variety of techniques that can be used but no specific technique has been shown to superior to the rest. The most basic and economical procedure is microfacture. This technique can be used to induce local mesenchymal stem cells to influx to the defect and produce a fibrocartilage repair surface that can function well, particularly in the short to medium term [24, 25],. Although most research has been performed in the knee, this can be successful in the ankle as well [26, 27]. Of the more complicated procedures, perhaps the most publicized is autologous chondrocyte implantation (ACI) first described in 1994 in the knee [28]. It is also performed in the ankle [29]. Although there is a lot of literature published on this technique in the knee, the inability to reproduce the complex nature of the articular matrix has led to further investigation into variations of the technique including matrix-associated chondrocyte implantation (MACI) [30, 31] and characterized chondrocyte implantation (CCI) [32]. Both of these techniques attempt to improve on the quality of matrix formed during the procedure. Other techniques utilize intact matrix to replace damaged matrix. This ensures the complex structure of the matrix is maintained. These techniques include osteochondral autograft transplantation (OATS) [33, 34] and mosaicplasty [35]) [36, 37], and bulk osteochondral allografts [38-41]. Finally, other more experimental techniques such as synthetic scaffolds and mesenchymal stem cells have been tried with variable success [42-45].

#### *3.1.1. Cell-based techniques*

*Microfracture* – Microfracture is a well-established technique for full thickness cartilage defects with an intact subchondral bone plate. The cartilage is debrided to form a well-contained defect with stable margins. The underlying bone is perforated with a sharp awl or pick at 3-4mm intervals while ensuring a stable subchondral plate remains intact to support the incoming cells. The perforations should penetrate deep enough to allow mesenchymal stem cells from the underlying spongy bone to enter the defect. The blood that emerges from the bone forms a clot and the stem cells differentiate into chondrocytes and fibrochondrocytes to produce a fibrocartilage that fills the defects.

Post-operatively, the patient is allowed early ROM but should be non-weight bearing for a period of time to allow some tissue formation. The length of time depends on the size and location of the lesion. Advantages of this technique include that it is one operation with low cost. Disadvantages include that fibrocartilage instead of hyaline cartilage is formed, filling of the defect is unpredictable and often incomplete [46]. That said, if good results can be obtained, the results in the ankle may not deteriorate over time [27]. This is considered a first line treatment by many surgeons, especially those that do not have access to the more complicated and expensive exogenous cell- or tissue-based therapies.

*Autologous Chondrocyte Implantation (ACI and its analogues)* – ACI is the most publicized technique for repairing/regenerating pure cartilage defects in the knee joint. First popularized by Brittberg in 1994 [28], thousands of patients have been treated using this technique in the knee joint but far fewer in the ankle joint. Studies in the ankle have reported good intermediate- and long-term results [47, 48]. Despite the historical background and extensive use, the technique has been modified to incorporate a matrix (MACI) or utilizing specific chondrocytes from the harvest (CCI) in an attempt to improve results. This suggests that the results from ACI are not optimal. ACI is a complicated technique that entails removing a portion of cartilage from a relative non-weight bearing portion of the joint and sending it to a lab for processing. Typically the donor cartilage is harvested from the ipsilateral knee joint [47, 48]. The ankle joint is typically not used as no specific safe area has been clearly defined [49]. During processing, the cells are removed from the matrix and expanded up to 20 million cells over a period of 3-4 weeks. The cells are then re-implanted at a second surgical procedure. This entails opening the joint, preparing the defect by making sure it has well-defined margins with an intact subchondral plate to prevent the intrusion of mesenchymal stem cells from the bone. A periosteal flap is harvested from a nearby area and sutured over the defect leaving a small area for injection of the expanded cells. The cells are injected under that flap that is then closed and sealed with fibrin glue. Often, a malleolar osteotomy is required to gain access to areas of the talar dome.

MACI is the next generation of ACI that incorporates the use of a scaffold [50-52]. The procedure is similar to that of ACI except that a matrix is used instead of a periosteal flap. The matrix is impregnated with the cells and shaped to the size of the defect. It is inserted and fixed by different mechanisms. Advantages of this technique include that it can be done arthroscopically in some cases and does not require the extra step of harvesting and suturing the periosteal flap. Thus it is less invasive. It has not been shown to be conclusively better than ACI. CCI (characterized chondrocyte implantation) is almost exactly the same as ACI except that the laboratory preselects specific cells that the company believes are predisposed to form articular cartilage out of all those that are harvested. These are the cells that are then expanded and re-implanted with the theory that the identified subpopulation of chondrocytes will produce a more physiologically intact matrix. The disadvantage of this technique is some patients do not have sufficient cells that meet the criteria for an enhanced population and, therefore, are not candidates for this procedure.

The results for these procedures have generally been good. Concerns with these procedures include that two separate surgical procedures are required and the cell processing can be prohibitively expensive. These major concerns limit their availability, especially when they have not been conclusively shown to be superior to other techniques [53]. The uncertainties of these techniques have led some researchers to investigate the use of mesenchymal stem cells instead of chondrocytes. This would allow the surgery to be completed at one time and may produce young chondrocytes that could potentially produce a more robust cartilage. These techniques are in the more experimental stage and 5
more commonly used in the knee joint.

### 3.1.2. Tissue-based techniques

Osteochondral autograft transplantation is a technique developed for small to medium sized defects. It consists of harvesting osteochondral plugs from less weight bearing portions of the same joint (or a different joint such as the knee when dealing with the ankle) and implanting them into the defect. This is accomplished by using 6mm diameter reamers to a depth of 10-15mm into the subchondal bone. A corresponding osteochondral core is harvested from another area and gently impacted into the newly formed defect attempting to achieve a press-fit while maintaining the contour of the articular surface. With lesions larger than 6mm diameter (ie most lesions that require treatment), multiple cores are required and press-fit with an interdigitating method and termed mosaicplasty. Once again, there are some reported good results using this technique [33, 36, 37, 54] but this is a complicated technique with multiple drawbacks. Harvesting cores from the ankle is usually not possible, therefore another joint must be violated and the harvest sites are not without possible complications such as knee pain and instability [35, 55]. Typically an osteotomy is required to gain access to the talar dome because the plugs must be inserted perpendicular to the surface of the joint. Alignment of the multiple plugs is difficult to ensure a smooth surface and the cartilage from the harvest often is of different thickness compared to the insertion site resulting in a variable underlying subchondral bone. Obtaining precise contour matching for lesions on the "shoulder" of the talus can be extremely difficult. Bone plugs of only 6mm diameter are susceptible to fracture resulting in unstable fixation and the boundary between the transplanted cartilage and native cartilage heals with fibrocartilage.

Osteochondral allografts can be done orthotopically and can be used for partial or whole joint replacement procedures. Popularized by Gross in the 1970's, these allografts were typically fresh and used for all types of defects in many joints including those defects due to tumours and trauma. Historically, these grafts were used in defects that consisted of bone and cartilage but can be used for cartilage-only defects as well. Good to excellent medium- and long-term results have been reported [38-41, 56] but the use of this technique became restricted as concerns regarding transmission of infectious diseases became more prevalent. Considering that this is not a life threatening disorder, the risk of transmission of infectious diseases does not seem warranted (although disease transmission has been very rarely reported) and this method is rarely used. To decrease the risk by allowing more time for testing, hypothermic storage at 4°C was developed and allows the tissues to be stored for 28-42 days prior to transplantation. Unfortunately, cellular deterioration tends to begin after 7-14 days [57, 58]. Given that regulatory clearance takes about 14 days, the viability of the cells within the tissue may not be as healthy as those in fresh allograft or in autograft. Investigations have been ongoing to develop storage techniques that eliminate the possibility of infectious disease transmission and tissue deterioration over time while enabling the creation of a large tissue bank for ready access. Recently we have developed a cryopreservation technique that can store the tissue indefinitely without deterioration and this may improve access to the tissue required for this technique [59]. Despite the limitations of hypothermic storage, there has been a resurgence of osteochondral allografting in recent years. This is the only biologic technique that can resurface whole joints [60, 61] and has been quite successful for partial joint replacements [40, 62]. Bugbee et al [60] have published promising results in total ankle arthroplasty using osteochondral allografts and similar procedures have been performed in Europe [61] but further improvements are required.

### 3.2. Early osteoarthritic changes

Once osteoarthritic changes become evident, cell based cartilage resurfacing techniques become less relevant due to the generalized nature of the process. There are some surgical techniques that can be used to palliate symptoms depending on the location and severity of the arthritis.

*Exostectomies* – Occasionally impingement symptoms can be a significant component of arthritis pain. This usually occurs with anterior osteophytes off the distal tibia or talar neck. Occasionally these osteophytes can form around the malleoli. When impingement pain is a prominent feature, removal of the osteophytes, either open or arthroscopically, can be performed with significant improvement of symptoms. The exostectomy can include only the osteophytes itself or also part of the arthritic articular surface leaving only healthier cartilage tissue (Figure 4).

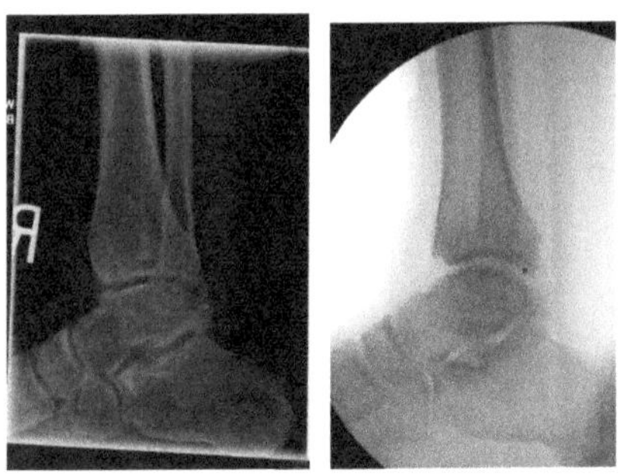

**Figure 4.** Left image shows preoperative lateral radiograph demonstrating anterior tibial and talar neck osteophytes. Right image shows intraoperative fluoroscopic image after anterior tibial and talar neck exostectomies.

*Osteotomies* – Occasionally the osteoarthritis is more severe in one portion of the joint. This is often medial or lateral. Offloading the arthritic portion of the joint with a closing (Figure 5), opening wedge osteotomy (Figure 6) or a dome osteotomy (Figure 7) can also provide some symptomatic relief [63-65].

*Distraction arthroplasty* – Recently, some investigation has gone into determining the effect of distraction arthroplasty. Joint distraction using an external fixator can alter the internal joint environment and possibly improve joint function. Early results are promising, even with more advanced osteoarthritis, but much more work needs to be completed [66].

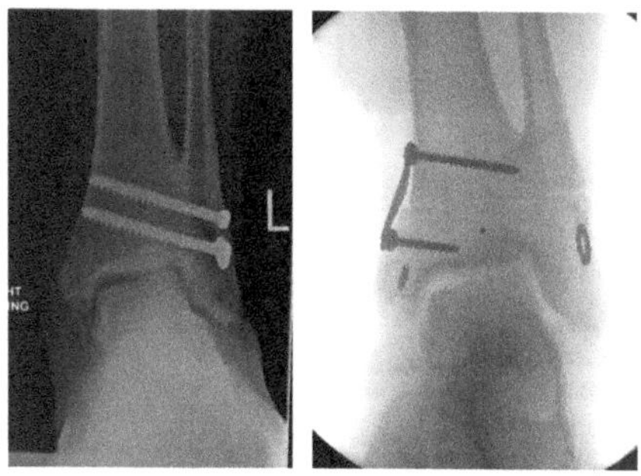


**Figure 5.** Radiographic images of medial closing wedge osteotomy after a distal tibial-fibular fusion resulted in lateral joint overload. Right image is an intraoperative fluoroscopic view after fixation with a compression staple.

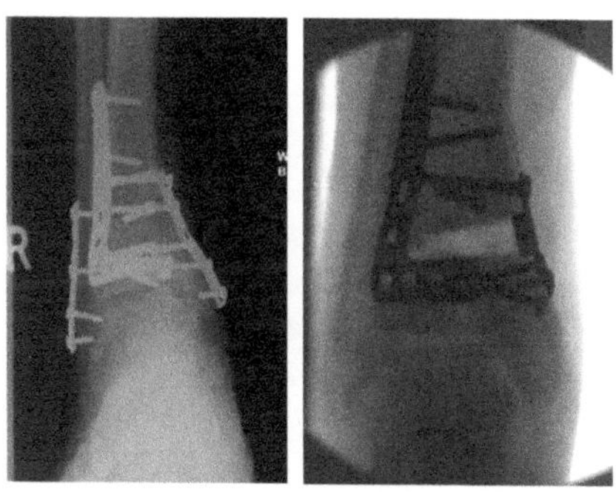


**Figure 6.** Radiographic images of a medial opening wedge osteotomy after open reduction and internal fixation resulted in a varus malunion. The distal screws were removed from the original plate and an opening wedge osteotomy was performed using an interposition plate.

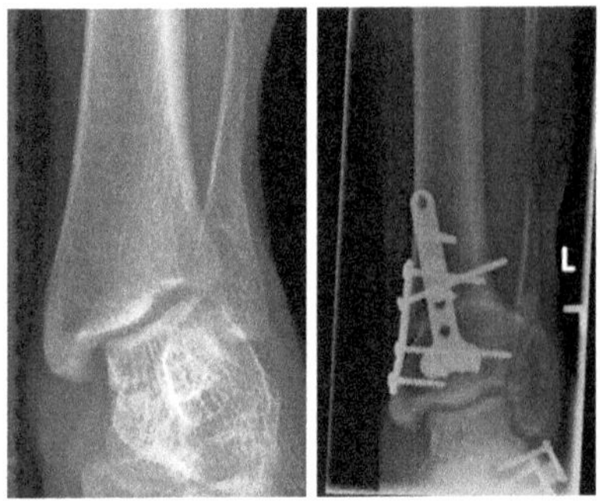


**Figure 7.** Dome osteotomy of the distal tibia. Original radiograph show severe valgus malunion due to a growth arrest after an open fracture as a child. The dome osteotomy was performed to incorporate the tibia and fibula and rotate the joint as a whole. Medial joint has been fully corrected while the lateral joint remains elevated due to intra-articular incongruity.

### 3.3. Global osteoarthritis

Once the osteoarthritis becomes global and more severe, the treatment options become more limited. The mainstay of treatment for end-stage ankle arthritis is ankle fusion although synthetic total joint arthroplasty is becoming more common as will be discussed. In addition, total ankle arthroplasty allografting is an experimental technique that has recently been developed that may be used in select cases.

Ankle fusion is the mainstay treatment for end-stage ankle arthritis. It has been performed for over 130 years [67] and there are research stucies that demonstrate the long-term effectiveness [68, 69]. Complications of ankle fusion include nonunion, malunion, infection, nerve injury, persisting pain, loss of ankle range of motion, limp, and arthritis of surrounding joints due to overload [70, 71]. Ankle fusion entails removing all of the remaining articular cartilage from the joint as well as the underlying subchondral bone leaving exposed cancellous bone. The surfaces are shaped so that there is excellent contact between the talar dome and the tibial plafond. Most techniques incorporate the medial malleolus as a medial buttress while some also include the lateral malleolus. Once the surfaces are prepared, internal fixation (occasionally external fixation) is applied. Postoperative splinting in either an aircast or plaster cast is employed for 6-12 weeks with non-weight bearing from 1-12 weeks depending on bone quality and rigidity of fixation and progression of fusion radiographically.

Over the years, many techniques have been described with increasing success with regards to fusion rates. Successful fusion rates can be expected to range from 86-100% depending on patient characteristics and surgical techniques [68, 72-83]. The most commonly used techniques utilize internal fixation. This can be completed using anterior, lateral or posterior approaches. Fixation can be achieved using crossed screws, plate and screws or an intramedullary nail. Another more recent method includes the joint debridement achieved arthroscopically with percutaneous screw fixation. Alternatively, external fixation using standard external fixation techniques or Ilizarov can be used after open joint debridement.

Traditionally, open techniques using an anterior approach going either medial or just lateral to the tibialis anterior tendon have been used. This approach typically provides access to the medial and superior aspects of the joint [75, 77]. This technique can be employed in ankles that do not have much structural deformity. Once the articular surfaces are properly prepared, the talus is compressed into the medial axilla and fixed by a variety of measures including crossed screws [76] (Figure 8), plate and screws [75, 77] or external fixation/Ilizarov [79, 80] (Figure 9). Less commonly, an intramedullary ankle arthrodesis nail can be used for fixation but this must also cross the subtalar joint [78, 83] (Figure 10).

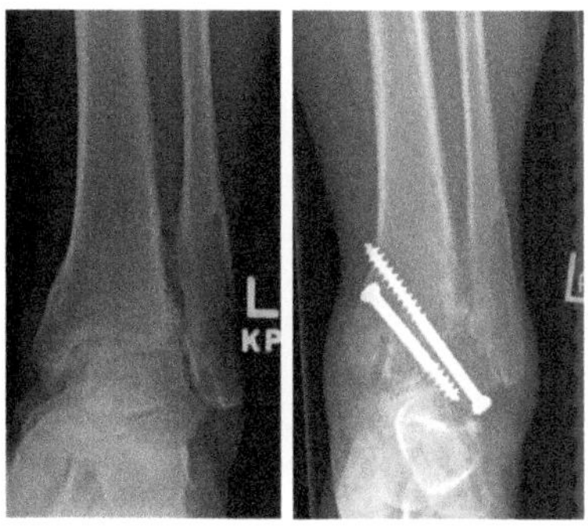


**Figure 8.** Left image showing severe OA changes but relatively normal structureal anatomy. Right image show fusion using crossed screws with the second screw entering the lateral process of the talus and crossing the joint pushing the talus into the medial axillay of the ankle mortice to achieve extra stability.

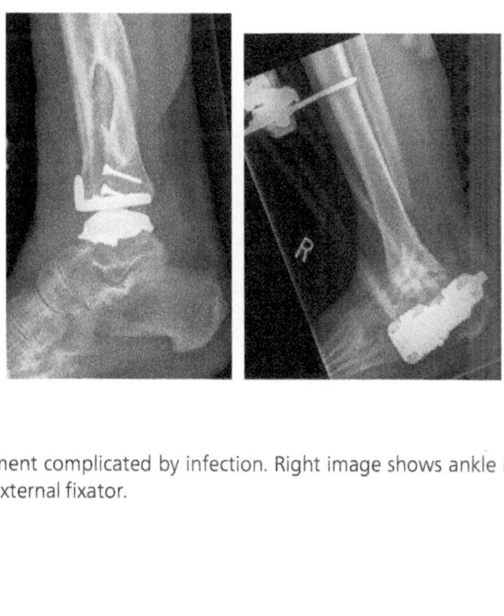


**Figure 9.** Total ankle replacement complicated by infection. Right image shows ankle replacement removed and attempt fusion using spanning external fixator.

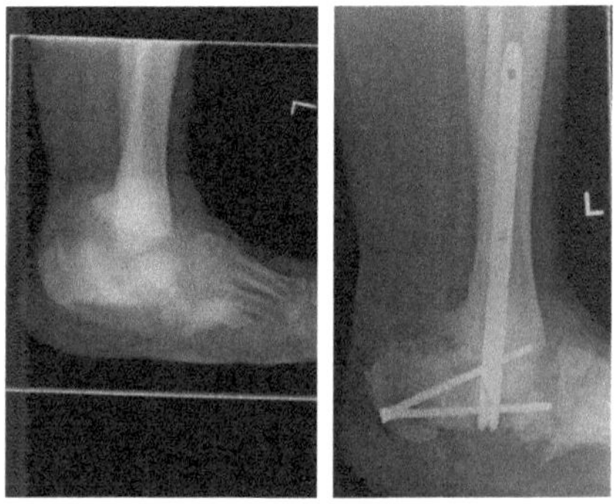


**Figure 10.** Severe Charcot arthropathy in an obese diabetic patient. Limb salvage ankle fusion using an ankle arthrodesis nail.

In ankles with more significant deformation, especially with bone loss, a more extensive approach may be considered. This entails a lateral approach and employs a fibular osteotomy approximately 5-6cm above the syndesmosis [72, 82] (Figure 11). The fibula is osteotomized obliquely over a 1cm distance and displaced from the tibia using anterior dissection while leaving an intact posterior hinge. The distal fibular segment is split sagitally and the inner ½ removed so that the other ½ (still attached by the posterior soft tissue hinge) can be used as a lateral buttress plate across the joint. Through this lateral incision, the surfaces of the talus and tibial plafond can be prepared for the fusion. This can be supplemented by a small anterior medial incision over the medial gutter for that surface preparation. This approach allows contouring of the fusion surfaces to achieve good bone apposition and to correct mal-alignment. Often supplemental bone graft is required to fill eroded defects. Fixation can be carried out by screws including two screws from the fibular strut into either the tibia and the talus or the tibia alone (to allow talar compression during weightbearing postoperatively).

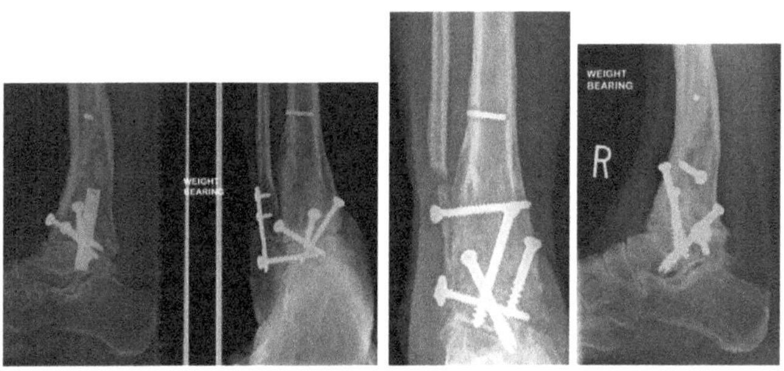


**Figure 11.** First 2 images on the left show attempted fusion using inadequate screw fixation with screws barely crossing the fusion site while the fibula was left intact despite screws inserted across it. Revision fusion demonstrating the use of the distal fibula as a strut plate graft with proper screw placement to achieve fusion.

Some surgeons prefer the posterior approach to the ankle for fusion [84-86]. This approach can be through or beside the Achilles tendon and can provide good exposure while minimizing risk to compromised anterior soft tissues when present. This approach can be extended to incorporate the subtalar joint in the fusion mass and a blade plate is often used for fixation.

In the circumstances of infection or soft tissue compromise, alternative approaches should be considered. The ankle joint can be adequately debrided with minimal invasiveness using arthroscopy [79, 87, 88] potentially decreasing soft tissue complications. Alternative fixation such as external fixators [78] or the Ilzarov [83] can be used to limit the issues of hardware insertion during ongoing infection. These devices may also be able to correct deformity over time.

As noted, ankle fusion can provide excellent relief of pain with significant improvement of function [89]. Surgical techniques have advanced such that it should be expected to have a 90-100% fusion rate in uncomplicated cases. Meticulous soft tissue handling and intraoperative care can mitigate complications. Despite these results, ongoing concerns of limitations of ankle motion and the increased stress on surrounding joints resulting in increased incidence of arthritis has led to the development of the total ankle arthroplasty as will be discussed in the next section.

## 4. Arthroplasty implants

### 4.1. Historical perspective

Total ankle arthroplasties were first introduced in the 1970s [90]. The first prosthesis, created by Lord and Marotte, was designed as an inverted total hip replacement [91]. Although Lord and Marotte's primary results were failures, over the next 20 years, more than 23 designs were developed using that generation's technology from hip and knee replacements characterized by cemented, two component, constrained implants [92]. Despite good initial results using this technology, there were problems with component loosening, severe osteolysis, infection, impingement and soft tissue breakdown [93, 94]. Kitaoka reviewed results of the first generation TAR that included three studies with greater than 5 year follow-up and found a 41% revision rate [95]. The high rate of failure for these first generation implants and difficult salvage procedures tempered enthusiasm and led to questions as to whether the ankle joint could be replaced successfully [92, 95-97]. Hintermann accurately stated, "in an era of joint replacement surgery, ankle procedures have failed to achieve what has been accomplished with other joints" [98].

The first generation implants were designed without proper understanding of ankle biomechanics [99, 100]. The ankle was assumed to be a hinge joint and the rotational and translational motions were not recreated which lead to loosening [97, 101]. These implants were either highly constrained or unconstrained. The highly constrained implants led to large shear and rotational forces that were distributed through a small joint surface and even smaller prosthesis interface [94, 102, 103]. The unconstrained implants were unstable due to lack of attention to soft tissue balancing and failure to address soft tissue impingement [94, 104, 105].

In general, ankle arthroplasties were implanted through an anterior approach to the ankle but the importance of the soft tissue envelope was underestimated and excess traction on the skin led to wound complications [92, 93]. The guides, jigs and instruments were not well designed and sizing was inaccurate so implants were mal-positioned and malleolar fractures were common [92]. Patients were left with mal-aligned implants either because the angular deformity was not corrected at the time of surgery [5] or because the ligaments were ignored leading to problems with functional mal-alignment despite good intraoperative positioning [94, 102]. Finally, most implants were cemented and required large bone resection including up to 17mm on the tibial side and 7mm on the talar side. This caused the implant to be cemented into soft cancellous bone which was unable to support the bone cement interface [92, 106]. Subsidence was further exacerbated by non-anatomically shaped, undersized implants [5, 92, 93, 107]. The aggressive bone resection of the tibia also changed the level of the ankle axis causing alterations in the ankle biomechanics [5]. When function was assessed via gait analysis, there was not as much improvement as had been anticipated. Gait analyses of the first generation implants revealed that patients were subconsciously protecting the joint by not bearing weight normally across the ankle despite denying pain and were not using normal ankle dorsiflexion in the stance phase despite adequate passive dorsiflexion on physical exam [4, 5, 106].

### 4.2. Biomechanical considerations

In order to understand the reasons for failure and to design a better total ankle arthroplasty, it was important to understand the biomechanics of the foot and ankle. The ankle is a highly constrained joint that does not function as a simple hinge joint because the axis is oblique extending further plantar and posterior on the lateral side. This creates eversion with dorsiflexion and inversion with plantarflexion [108]. Further, the axis of rotation changes throughout the range of motion so that when the ankle moves from a plantarflexed to a dorsiflexed position there is a combination of distraction, sliding and compression [108, 109]. Finally, there are rotational and translational movements that also need to be recreated with a replacement arthroplasty [94, 110].

The most important concepts in the design of an ankle arthroplasty are constraint and congruency. Constraint can be defined as the resistance of an implant to a particular degree of freedom of motion such as anterior-posterior translation or axial rotation [94]. In highly constrained implants such as a hinged ankle replacement, all axial torque forces are translated through the bone-prosthesis interface as shear forces that can lead to component loosening [92, 111]. Congruency or conformity can be defined as the closeness of fit of the various components of the implant [92, 94]. In a fully conforming implant, the articular surface of the tibia has the same radius of curvature as the articulating surface of the talus in both anterior-posterior and medial-lateral directions. This decreases the wear rate because the polyethylene contact stress remains below the fatigue threshold for delamination and pitting [92]. In a partially conforming or incongruent implant the round talus articulates with a flat tibia or there are differences in the radius of curvature of the 2 surfaces [92]. The optimal design for a total ankle replacement is with bearing surfaces that are not only highly conforming to ensure contact throughout the bearing surface thus reducing wear but also sufficiently constrained to give the implant sufficient inherent stability to minimize shear stresses at the prosthesis-bone interface [94, 112].

Second generation implants used these two concepts to improve the design of total ankle arthroplasties. In general, the two primary alternatives were 1) a two component, partially conforming ankle replacement which replaced all three articulations by changing the ankle into a two bone joint by fusing the distal tibia-fibular joint [5, 92] or 2) a three component design which resurfaced the tibio-talar joint and the talar side of the lateral and medial gutters [5, 92]. Third generation implants are more anatomically designed and rely on ligament support as well as hindfoot "balancing" to allow the components to recreate the ankle biomechanics [113].

Gait studies of the newer implants show a satisfactory recovery of the natural overall mobility of the ankle joint in all three planes of motion [114]. Further, in three component designs, there may be some movement of the polyethylene separate from the other components which helps to restore normal biomechanics [114]. Functional motion and muscle-generated moments during walking improved at the ankle joint after arthroplasty – especially plantar flexor muscle function. This function is important because it restrains the forward movement of the tibia during the first half of the gait cycle and brings about plantarflexion of the ankle during the propulsive phase of gait [99]. Brodsky has shown significant improvement in velocity, step length for operated side, total ankle ROM during gait, and maximum sagittal ankle joint power at push-off [115].

### 4.3. Current implants

Lewis has described key aspects for a successful ankle joint arthroplasty based on careful review of the first and second generation implants [97]. It is important that implant size be designed to balance the need for minimal bone resection with the requirement for sufficient implant to distribute stresses over a large area to decrease the risk of subsidence [97]. The anatomical axis needs to be recreated while also understanding that there is large variability in the axis between individuals [97, 116]. It is also important to recreate all the motions at the ankle joint instead of just plantar flexion and dorsiflexion [97]. This includes talar tilt as the ankle is coupled to the subtalar joint to accommodate to uneven ground, and the rotational motion of internal rotation coupled to plantar flexion and external rotation coupled to dorsiflexion. Failure to understand and recreate these motions will place abnormal stress through the implant-bone interface [97]. It is critical to understand the necessity of ligament support for ankle stability [5]. An implant designed to be sufficiently stable to negate the need for ligament support will transfer abnormal stress to the bone-implant interface leading to loosening [94, 102, 103]. In contrast, an implant designed with low stability that is implanted into an ankle without sufficient ligamentous support will fail due to component mal-alignment or dislocation of the polyethylene [94, 97, 104, 105]. The requirement to withstand high loads means that ultra-high molecular weight polyethylene is generally recommended [97, 117].

Third generation ankle arthroplasties are now in use. The new designs show better understanding of ankle biomechanics and allow for sliding and rotational movements [92]. There are many different third generation implants used across the world and the following discussion provides a representative sample of those commonly used in the Western world but is not inclusive of all implants. The implants will be discussed in relation to design rationale.

The common surgical approach, as will be discussed in further detail later, is an anterior approach in the interval between tibialis anterior tendon and extensor hallucis longus tendon. The neurovascular bundle is carefully protected under the extensor hallucis longus tendon. The major disadvantage of this approach is the high rate of wound healing complications [92, 118, 119]. The BOX ankle replacement (Finsbury Orthopaedics, Leatherhead, Surrey, UK) uses an anterolateral approach between the extensor digitorum longus tendon and the peroneal tertius tendon [112]. The Eclipse (Integra LifeSciences, Plaisboro, NJ) is inserted through either a medial (preferred) or lateral approach [112]. The disadvantage of this approach is the need for fixation of the disrupted medial or lateral malleolus.

The current implants are either mobile (3 component design) or fixed (2 component design) bearing [101]. Mobile bearing designs allow for greater congruence, which can increase the risk of dislocation, but they share the stress through 2 articular surfaces, which may increase weardue to "back side wear" [101, 120]. There is also the potential for "overstuffing" the joint with three component designs in an attempt to reduce the chance of polyethylene dislocation [121]). Overstuffing tightens the joint, increases ligament strain, decreases range of motion and increases the shear stress at the bone-prothesis interface [5, 121]. Fixed bearing designs increase the constraint so they may have higher rates of loosening but have decreased back side wear if the locking mechanism is intact [94, 101]. Current mobile bearing designs include the STAR (Waldemar Link, Hamburg, Germany; 1978)(Figure 12), Buechel-Pappas (Endotec, South Orange, NJ; 1989), Salto (Tornier, Saint Ismier, France; 1997), Hintegra (Integra LifeSciences/Newdeal, Lyon, France; 2002)(Figure 12), Mobility (DePuy International, Leeds, UK; 2005)(Figure 12), BOX (Finsbury Orthopaedics, Leatherhead, Surrey, UK; 2005), CCI Evolution (Van Straten Medical, The Netherlands, 2007), and Zenith (Corin, Cirencester, UK; 2009). Two component designs include the Agility (DePuy/Ace, Warsaw, IN; 1985)(Figure 13), TNK (Kyocera, Kyoto, Japan; 1996), INBONE (Wright Medical Technologies, Arlington, TN; 2005)(Figure 13), Salto Talaris (Tornier, Saint Ismier, France; 2006), and Eclipse (Integra LifeSciences, Plainsboro, NJ; 2007).

Most ankle arthroplasty implants are constructed from cobalt-chromium alloys which are hard, corrosion resistant and biocompatible (Hintegra, Agility, Mobility, Inbone talus, BOX, Salto and Salto-Talaris, and Buechel-Pappas). The CCI Evolution adds molybdenum to the alloy to increase strength (Van Straten Medical, The Netherlands, 2007). The STAR and Inbone (tibia only) use titanium implants which are softer but can be more porous to allow for better ingrowth. The TNK is a ceramic implant (Kyocera, Kyoto, Japan; 1996).

Initial implants were cemented; however, due to the high rate of failure, most implants today are uncemented relying on bone ingrowth stimulated by hydroxyapatite coating, sintered metal beads, plasma spray metals or fiber metals [101]. The different methods to encourage bony ingrowth include ensuring the metal is porous such as the Hintegra which is 20% porous [92]. Some implants, like the STAR, use a single or dual plasma spray. Others use a thin film ceramic coating. The Buechel-Pappas and CCI Evolution use a porous coating covered by a titanium nitride thin-film ceramic [92] which also improves the smoothness of the surface. The Zenith uses the trademarked "BONIT" coating which is the application of a thin calcium phosphate layer to the titanium plasma spray. The last common technique is the use of hydroxyapatite incorporated in the Hintegra [92].

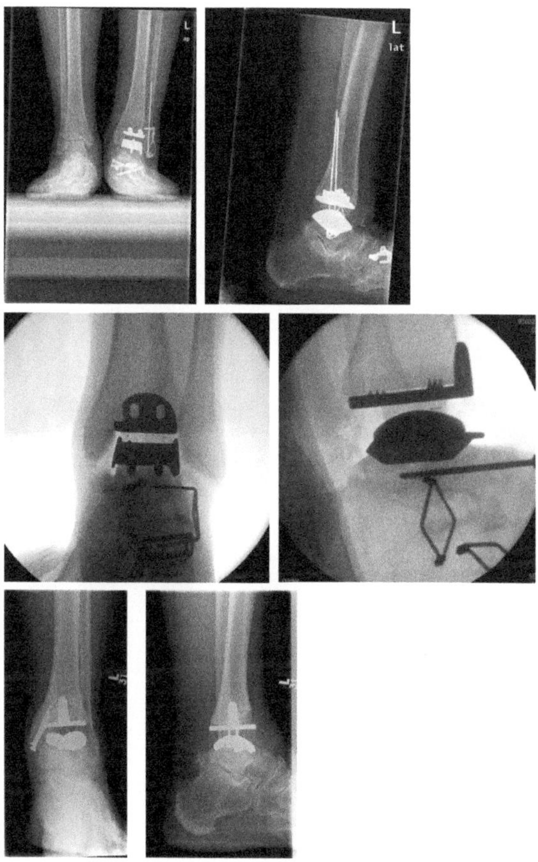

**Figure 12.** Radiographic images of three currently used mobile bearing total ankle arthroplasty designs. The top two images are STAR, middle two images are Hintegra and the bottom two images are Mobility.

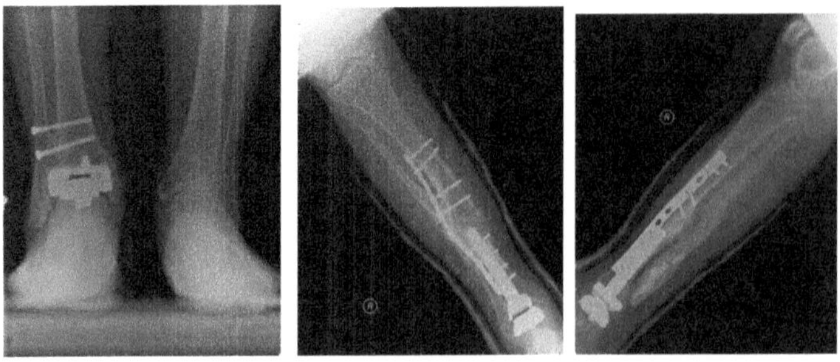

**Figure 13.** Radiographic images of two currently used fixed bearing total ankle arthroplasty designs. The left image is Agility while the right two images are Inbone.

In most implants the tibial cut is made first. Unlike the knee, the ankle cannot be dislocated sufficiently to allow for intramedullary guides to make the tibial cuts so all ankle arthroplasties, with the exception of the Inbone, use extramedully tibial guides with or without a foot holder. The Inbone uses an external guide and radiographs to guide the insertion of an intramedullary reamer and combines it with a foot holder to place the tibial cutting guide [112]. After the tibial cut has been completed and the intramedullary canal has been reamed, the tibial stem and plate components are inserted one at a time into the joint and built inside the ankle and tibia. The downside of using this intramedullary technique is that the subtalar joint is violated as the tibial canal is reamed retrograde through the calcaneus, talus and then tibia.

Other implants, such as the Buechel-Pappas, Mobility and Agility use intramedullary posts on the tibia to provide fixation by creating an anterior cortical window to insert the tibial component which is then replaced and generally heals without incident. If the tibial component does not have an intramedullary stem, the fixation can be with a fin (CCI Evolution), a fin with a cylinder (Salto), double cylinders (STAR), bars (BOX) or an anterior shield which may or may not be augmented with screws (Hintegra).

Tibial components can either rely on support from the intramedullary stem (Inbone) or cortical bone anteriorly and posteriorly (Hintegra). Some tibial components are rectangular and others are trapezoidal designed to be larger anterior than posterior (STARand CCI Evolution). Finally, while most are flat, they can be designed with a curve (BOX).

The design of the talus implant can be with a symmetrical curve (STAR, Buechel-Pappas, INBONE, Mobility) or asymmetrical so that the radius of curvature for the medial side is less than that for the lateral side (Salto, Hintegra, BOX, CCI Evolution). Most implants resurface the talus (STAR, Buechel-Pappas, Salto, Hintegra, Mobility, BOX, CCI Evolution, and Zenith), but the Inbone and Agility use a flat talar cut. Some designs replace the medial and lateral talar articulations (STAR, Buechel-Pappas, TNK, Salto, and Hintegra) while others do not (Agility, BOX, Mobility, CCI Evolution, and Zenith,). Finally, the polyethylene is ultra-high molecular weight polyethylene in the STAR, Buechel-Pappas, Salto, Hintegra and Inbone.

In summary, the third generation implants have been designed using the knowledge gained from more indepth study of the anatomy and biomechanics of the ankle joint as well as the causes of the failures of the first and second generation implants. When choosing an implant, the surgeon should consider the approach, the need for intramedullary guides and fixation of the tibial component, the relative importance of preserving talar bone stock by resurfacing the talus as opposed to a flat cut, the need for replacing the medial and lateral articulations of the talus, and the role for ultra-high molecular weight polyethylene.

## 5. Surgical considerations

Clinical indications for total ankle arthroplasty include end stage ankle arthritis that has exhausted all non-operative and joint-sparing operative treatments in a patient willing to undertake the risks of a major surgical procedure. Contraindications to this procedure include:

- Active infection
- Compromised soft tissues
- Inadequate blood supply
- Peripheral neuropathy (including Charcot arthropathy)
- Significant lower extremity neuromuscular impairment
- Severe ligamentous laxity
- Excessive malalignment
- Avascular necrosis of a significant portion of the tibia or talus
- Severe osteoporosis
- Inadequate bone stock
- Skeletal immaturity
- High demand lifestyle
- Pertinent metal allergy
- Sensory or motor dysfunction

Age is not explicitly mentioned as a contraindication in the literature. The safe zone appears to be somewhere after skeletal maturity and in conjunction with the assumption of a low demand lifestyle. Excessive malalignment is a nebulous term. The commonly accepted range is from 15-20 degrees of varus or valgus to not surgically correctable. It would appear that excessive malalignment is relative to the surgeon's skill and experience. Obesity as a contraindication to total ankle arthroplasty is controversial and was not correlated to aseptic loosening in a recent article [122].

### 5.1. Surgical approach

There are several different types of ankle arthroplasty systems currently on the market as discussed. Each system has unique features best explained by the surgical technique manual provided by the company marketing that system. There are, however, certain common aspects and principles of all of the systems which we will outline in this section.

### 5.2. Preoperative planning

The condition of the soft tissue envelope including locations of scars and documentation of neurovascular status are important when planning a total ankle arthroplsty. Ankle arthroplasty may be contraindicated in some cases due to an impaired soft tissue envelope or inadequate blood supply to the foot.

Long leg weight-bearing views will help identify concurrent ipsilateral limb deformities which may affect ankle alignment. Anteroposterior and lateral views of the tibia are also important because intraoperative alignment is usually referenced off of the tibia. Weightbearing anteroposterior and lateral views of the ankle and foot are important to assess the joint being replaced but also to identify coexisting deformities and/or arthritis affecting the rest of the foot which may affect the surgical plan resulting in additional procedures that can be performed in a staged manner or concurrently depending on surgeon skill and preference.

### 5.3. Positioning

The patient is positioned supine on a radiolucent table to allow fluoroscopic guidance of the procedure. The ipsilateral hip is supported to prop the foot perpendicular to the floor to allow easy access to both the medial and lateral aspects of the joint and enable evaluation of alignment intraoperatively. Rotation of the foot relative to the leg on the contralateral side should be noted before prepping and draping to determine what is normal for that patient.

### 5.4. Prepping and draping

A thigh tourniquet is utilized to provide hemostasis during the procedure. The leg is prepped and draped as a free extremity right up to the tourniquet to provide access to the knee. Many total ankle arthroplasty systems use the length of the tibia and an external alignment device as a guide to proper alignment.

### 5.5. Surgical exposure

The most common surgical approach to the ankle for insertion of a total ankle arthroplasty is the anterior approach. Some systems that involve tibiofibular fusion as part of the procedure may require and an additional lateral incision but still utilize the anterior approach as well. An incision is made over the anterior aspect of the ankle midway between the malleoli (Figure 14). The incision needs to be long enough to allow placement of the distal tibial cutting block and visualization of the talar neck. Care is taken to minimize injury to the branches of the superficial and deep peroneal nerves. The retinaculum is then split to expose the underlying tendons. The extensor hallucis longus tendon will be retracted laterally to protect the underlying neurovascular structures which should be located deep and lateral to the extensor hallucis longus tendon (Figures 14 and 15). If possible, the sheath of the tibialis anterior should be left intact to prevent undue pressure on the wound post-operatively (Figure 16). The anterior capsule is incised vertically and then peeled away in a subperiosteal plane medially and laterally to expose the joint (Figure 17). One should be able to see the medial malleolus clearly but the lateral malleolus is more posterior and often is not as easily seen.

Distal tibial osteophytes are now removed taking note of a commonly occurring large osteophyte anterior to the fibula. Care should be taken to differentiate the osteophyte from the fibula itself. There will also be osteophytes on the neck of the talus which can be removed with a curette, rongeur or burr to reestablish its normal contour. This will help with cutting block placement and ankle positioning when cuts are made (Figure 18).

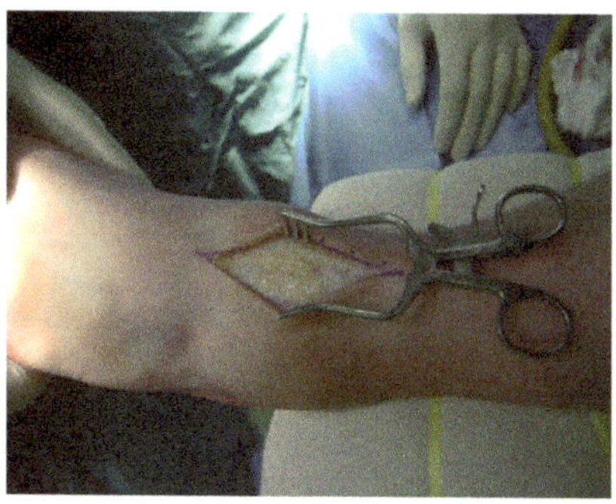

**Figure 14.** Anterior incision midway between the malleoli. Toes are to the left and knee is to the right. Blunt retractors and extreme soft tissue care are required.

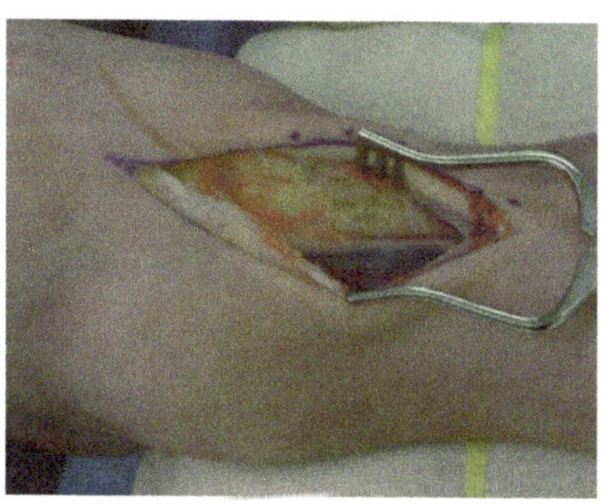

**Figure 15.** Exposure of the neurovascular bundle by retraction of the extensor hallucis longus tendon.

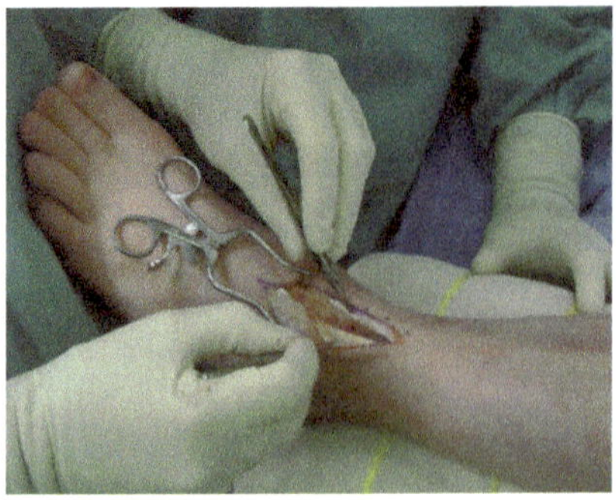

**Figure 16.** Tibialis anterior sheath.

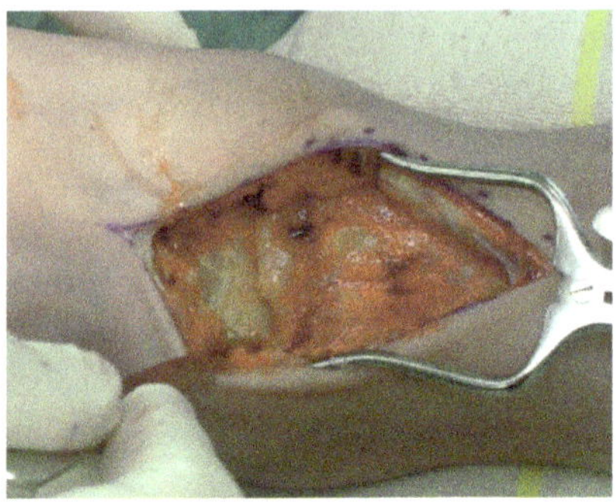

**Figure 17.** Exposure of the joint.

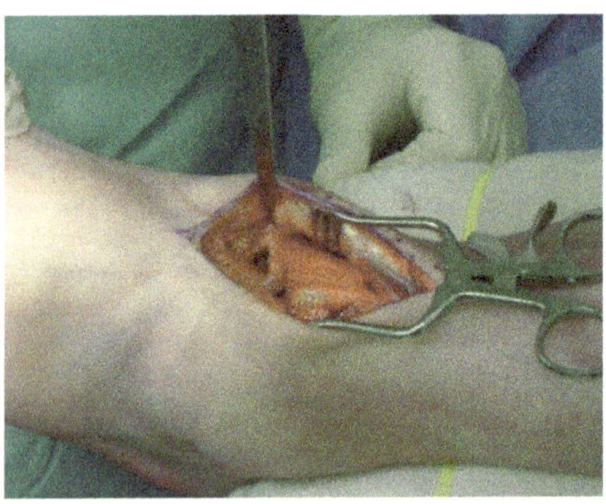

**Figure 18.** Anterior tibial osteophyte requires removal.

The soft tissues should be handled with extreme caution. Blunt self-retaining retractors should be repositioned periodically to prevent prolonged pressure on the soft tisse. Care should be taken with the bone as well. Levering on the medial malleolus may result in fracture. Notching the fibula during the distal tibial resection can result in fracture as well. Exposure can be facilitated by instruments such as laminar spreaders, distractors and various retractors. Performing the talar cuts can also facilitate removal of posterior malleolar fragments in systems that require this.

### 5.6. Alignment

The tibia is used to guide placement of the cutting blocks either with an external rod placed parallel to the shaft of the tibia by direct visualization or overlapped with the tibial canal fluoroscopically. The distal tibia is cut perpendicular to the anatomical axis of the tibia in the coronal plane. Most systems build in a posterior slope to the distal tibial cut in the sagittal plane and this can be adjusted in certain cases to allow more or less slope depending on the patient's needs. Longitudinal alignment of the talar component is usually in line with the second ray of the foot.

### 5.7. Ligamentous balancing

Ligamentous balancing is not yet as sophisticated as for total knee arthroplasty. The posterior capsule is resected during the removal of the posterior malleolus. Medially, the deltoid ligament can be released in a subperiosteal plane from the medial malleolus and/or talus, pie-crusted, released mid-substance or relatively lengthened through a medial malleolar osteotomy [123-126]. Laterally, the talofibular ligaments should be treated with care. Aggressive release from the talus can result in iatrogenic lateral instability. If there is a preexisting lateral instability, consent should be obtained for a lateral ligament reconstruction if required. Generally, stability is assessed after the bony cuts are made. A gastrocsoleus slide or Achilles tendon lengthening may be required if the ankle does dorsiflex past neutral after the ankle arthroplasty has been performed.

### 5.8. Closure

Repair of the extensor retinaculum during closure is very important. If left uncovered, the tibialis anterior may erode through the incision putting the arthroplasty and possibly even the leg at risk.

### 5.9. Post-op care

In the case of an uncomplicated ankle arthroplasty with no extra ligament reconstruction or fusion the patient has a short period of non-weight-bearing activity in a splint or cast followed by weight-bearing activity in a cast until the six week post-operative visit. Subsequently, physiotherapy to work on dorsiflexion and plantar flexion, gait retraining and leg strengthening is initiated.

There are no guidelines in regards to deep venous thrombosis (DVT) prophylaxis after total ankle arthroplasty but it would prudent to use propylaxis in patients with significant risk factors. Obesity, previous venous thromboembolism, and absence of full postoperative weightbearing were identified as risk factors for the development of DVT in a study on total ankle arthroplasty in the obese [122]. The importance of these risk factors was echoed by Barg et al in their article looking at risk factors for DVT in total ankle arthroplasty patients who were give thromboprophylaxis [127]. Other factors associated with increased incidence of DVTs include cancer, use of high dose estrogen replacement, and smoking.

### 5.10. Radiological follow-up

Ankle replacements should be followed radiologically as well as clinically in the post-operative period including weightbearing anteroposterior and lateral x-rays. One should look for changes in position which would indicate loosening of the components. Persistent periprosthetic lucencies should be followed for progression. There are a variety of angular measurements based on anatomical axes and component position as well as standardized distances from anatomical landmarks to component landmarks that can be used to assess technical success of prostheses implantation or subsequent subsidence [128].

### 5.11. Complications

The complications associated with total ankle arthroplasty would be familiar to any shoulder, hip or knee arthroplasty surgeon. and can be classified in different ways. Glazebrook et al recently published an evidence-based classification system that groups complications according to their correlation with failure of the prosthesis [3]. The goal of this classification system is to provide prognostic information to help surgeons deal with complications more effectively. To develop this classification system, the current literature on second and third generation prosthetic ankle arthroplasty outcomes were reviewed. Based on this information they were able to provide a summary of total ankle arthroplasty implant survival and complication rates. Twenty studies met their inclusion criteria with follow-up periods ranging from two to twelve years. In total 2,386 ankle arthroplasties were reviewed. They reported nine main complications including:

- Subsidence – 10.7%
- Aseptic loosening – 8.7%
- Intra-op fracture – 8.1%
- Wound healing problem – 6.6%
- Technical error – 6.0%
- Implant failure – 5.0%
- Non-union – 4.4%
- Post-op bone fracture – 2.0%

- Deep infection – 1.7%

These complications were compiled into three groups depending on how likely the complication would lead to failure of the arthroplasty. The three complications that lead to arthroplasty failure greater than 50% of the time were deep infection, aseptic loosening and implant failure. Other complications not included in this review that should be noted include tendon laceration, nerve injury, and instability (due to ligamentous imbalance). Impingement is another complication that is minor in terms of prosthesis survival but can have a significant effect in terms of patient satisfaction. It is usually medial and can be caused by osteophytes, scar tissue or tibialis posterior tendon degeneration.

### 5.12. Outcomes

In order to evaluate the outcomes of contemproary total ankle arthroplasty, it is instructive to look at the results published by joint registries from around the world. While not as common as registries for total hip and knee arthroplasty, there are at least four registries reported in the literature.

In 2007 the Norwegian registry reported on their experiences with total ankle arthroplasty [129]. This registry looked at 257 joints implanted between 1994 and 2005. This included a small number of cemented implants. The average age at the time of implantation was 58 for women and 60 for men. The The 5-year survival rate was 89% and the 10-year survival rate was 76%. There was no difference in the survival rates of the cemented and cementless prostheses.

The New Zealand registry reported on 202 joints in total also in 2007 [130]. This included both second and third generation prostheses. The average age of the patients at the time of implantation was 65. The most common diagnosis was primary osteoarthritis. The 5-year survival rate was 86%.

In 2010 the Finnish registry published their results on 573 total ankle arthroplasties [131]. These were all third-generation mobile-bearing designs. The average age of the patients was 55. The 5-year survival was 83%.

The Swedish Registry reported on the ten year survival of 780 third-generation total ankle arthoplasties in 2011 [132]. The registry included a variety of uncemented, three component implants. Revision rate was used as the primary outcome variable. The overall 10 year survival rate was 69% although this increased to 78% of the STAR prostheses were excluded. It is interesting to note that the other registries did include the STAR prostheses in their results.

Overall, age, sex, and diangosis did not affect survival in the Norwegian, New Zealand or Finnish registries. The Swedish registry, however, found that the risk for revision was higher in female patients under 60 years of age with a diagnosis of primary osteoarthritis or posttraumatic arthritis.

There have been a lot of outcome studies published in recent years but a disproportionate number have been published by the prostheses designers themselves according to Labek et al [133]. Approximately 50% of the publications reporting on total ankle arthroplasty outcomes have been produced by implant developers. Furthermore, the revision rates from the national registries (Swedish, Norwegian and New Zealand) have a much higher revision rate than those published in peer-reviewed scientific journals that include the manufacturers' reports [133].

That said, it is still worthwhile to look at all of the published data. There have been three relatively recent reviews of total ankle arthroplasty outcome study data [69, 134, 135]. The most recent one was published by Gougoulias et al in 2010 [134]. They included thirteen Level IV studies looking at 1105 total ankle arthroplasties. The most common diagnosis was posttraumatic arthritis. The overall failure rate was approximately 10% at 5 years. Range of motion did not change in one study and improved by 4-14 degrees in four others. In the studies reporting them, there were superficial wound complications in 0-14%, and deep infections in 0-4.6%. In seven studies, rates of residual pain in the hindfoot ranged from 23 to 60%. Interestingly, the most common sporting activities after total ankle arthroplasty were identified as swimming, cycling and fitness/weight training.

In an older review published in 2007 by Haddad et al, the intermediate outcomes of total ankle arthroplasty and ankle fusion were compared [69]. They looked at ten papers which evaluated total ankle arthroplasty and thirty-nine which looked at ankle fusion. The mean American Orthopaedic Foot and Ankle Society Ankle Hindfoot score was 78.2 for the arthroplasty group and 75.6 for the fusion group. The average age of patients undergoing arthroplasty was 58 and fusion 50. The majority of the fusion patients were male, while the major of the arthroplasty patients were female. Rheumatoid arthritis was the primary indication for total ankle arthroplasty, posttraumatic arthritis for fusion. The 5-year implant survival rate for the arthroplasty group was 90%, while the 10-year survival rate was 77%. They noted that a weakness of their review was that there were no direct comparisons of total ankle arthroplasty to ankle fusion.

Stengel et al's review in 2005 identified 10 adequate studies with a total of 497 ankle arthroplasties [135]. The total ankle arthroplasty patients showed a mean improvement in hindfoot scores of 45.2 points. Range of motion improved an average of 6.3%. Complications ranged from a 1.6% deep infection rate to a 14.7% impingement rate. The five year prosthesis survival rate was 90.6%.

Since the publication of the most recent of the above reviews, there have been some other publications of note. The long-term results of the United States STAR trial were published in 2011 [136]. They prospectively followed 80 patients treated with 84 STAR prostheses. The average age at implantation was 61 years. Their American Orthopaedic Foot and Ankle Society ankle-hindoot scores improved from an average of 42.7 to 81.9 points. Average range of motion was 39.5 degrees. Implant survival was 96% at 5 years and 90% at 10 years.

Bonnin et al recently published the long term follow-up of patients they had implanted with the SALTO total ankle arthroplasty and reported on previously [137]. They analyzed 98 prostheses with and average followup of 8.9 years. The mean American Foot and Ankle Society ankle-hindfoot score was 79. Range of motion was 27 degrees. The survival rate was

85% with an end point being the revision of a component. Limitations of this study included the series of patients being operated on by the implant designers and the implants and technique changed during the course of the study.

Wood et al compared the STAR implant to the Buechel-Pappas implant in a randomised trial [138]. The study involved 200 joint replacements. They were followed out for 6 years. The STAR survivorship was 95% and the Buechel-Pappas 79% with the end point being revision. The difference was not found to be statistically different.

Total ankle arthroplasty has been shown to improve ankle joint mechanics. Hahn et al demonstrated that both arthroplasty and fusion impoved gait function and reduced pain but that arthroplasty patients gained a more natural ankle joint function with increased range of motion [139]. Piriou et al were also interested in how gait was affected by total ankle arthroplasty [140]. They compared 12 arthroplasty patients to 12 fusion and 12 control patients. Neither the arthroplasty patients nor the fusion patients regained normal movement or walking speed, but the arthroplasty group had greater movement at the ankle, more symmetrical timing of gait and better restored ground reaction force patterns than the fusion group. The fusion group had a faster gait and longer step length than the arthroplasty group. Schuh et al compared 21 ankle fusion patients to 20 total ankle arthroplasty patients in regards to sport and recreational activities as well as functional outcome directly [89]. They found no signifcant difference between the groups concerning activity levels, participation in sports activities.

Finally, despite improved motion and decreased pain, total ankle arthroplasty does not result in weight loss. Penner at al investigated weight loss after total ankle arthroplasty and found that although pain and disability were reduced in overweight and obese patients after both ankle arthroplasty and fusion, the mean body mass index (BMI) remained unchanged [141].

## 6. Conclusion

Ankle arthritis can be a debilitating disorder as disabling mentally and physically as hip arthritis. There are a myriad of nonoperative and joint sparing operative treatments that can improved symptoms but do not arrest the disease process. When end-stage osteoarthritis develops, the gold standard has been ankle fusion. Some limitations to a successful ankle fusion such as stiffness and arthritic progression of surrounding joints as well as the successful replacements of the hip and knee joint led to the development of total ankle arthroplasty. Second and third generation prostheses have markedly improved function and long-term results compared to first generation prostheses. Although the procedure can be technically demanding and is associated with numerous potential complications, patients generally experience improved function and decreased pain. Based on current literature, it seems reasonable to expect an 80% prosthesis survival after 10 years. Further investigations into ankle joint mechanics, risk factors for implant failure and methods to minimize complications should lead to additional improvements in long-term outcomes. Finally, prospective, long-term direct comparison studies of ankle fusion versus total ankle arthroplasty are required to determine which procedure is best for which patient.

## Acknowledgements

Orthotic photographs provided by Orthotic Solutions, Edmonton, Alberta, Canada.

## Author details

Nadr M. Jomha, Angela Scharfenberger, Gordon Goplen and M. Elizabeth Pedersen

*Address all correspondence to: njomha@ualberta.ca

Division of Orthopaedic Surgery, Department of Surgery, University of Alberta, Edmonton, Alberta, Canada

## References

[1] Buckwalter JA, Saltzman C, Brown T. The impact of osteoarthritis: implications for research. Clin Orthop Relat Res. 2004 Oct(427 Suppl):S6-15.

[2] Saltzman CL. Ankle Arthritis. In: Coughlin M, Mann R, Saltzman C, eds. *Surgery of the foot and ankle.* 8th ed. Philadelphia, PA: Mosby Elselvier 2007:928.

[3] Glazebrook M, Daniels T, Younger A, Foote CJ, Penner M, Wing K, et al. Comparison of health-related quality of life between patients with end-stage ankle and hip arthrosis. J Bone Joint Surg Am. 2008 Mar;90(3):499-505.

[4] Stauffer RN, Chao EY, Brewster RC. Force and motion analysis of the normal, diseased, and prosthetic ankle joint. Clin Orthop Relat Res. 1977(127):189-96.

[5] Thomas RH, Daniels TR. Ankle arthritis. J Bone Joint Surg Am. 2003 May;85-A(5): 923-36.

[6] Valderrabano V, Horisberger M, Russell I, Dougall H, Hintermann B. Etiology of ankle osteoarthritis. Clin Orthop Relat Res. 2009 Jul;467(7):1800-6.

[7] Khazzam M, Long JT, Marks RM, Harris GF. Preoperative gait characterization of patients with ankle arthrosis. Gait & posture. 2006 Aug;24(1):85-93.

[8] Valderrabano V, Hintermann B, Dick W. Scandinavian total ankle replacement: a 3.7-year average followup of 65 patients. Clin Orthop Relat Res. 2004 Jul(424):47-56.

[9] Bombardier C, Laine L, Reicin A, Shapiro D, Burgos-Vargas R, Davis B, et al. Comparison of upper gastrointestinal toxicity of rofecoxib and naproxen in patients with

rheumatoid arthritis. VIGOR Study Group. The New England journal of medicine. 2000 Nov 23;343(21):1520-8, 2 p following 8.

[10] Silverstein FE, Faich G, Goldstein JL, Simon LS, Pincus T, Whelton A, et al. Gastrointestinal toxicity with celecoxib vs nonsteroidal anti-inflammatory drugs for osteoarthritis and rheumatoid arthritis: the CLASS study: A randomized controlled trial. Celecoxib Long-term Arthritis Safety Study. Jama. 2000 Sep 13;284(10):1247-55.

[11] Muller-Fassbender H, Bach GL, Haase W, Rovati LC, Setnikar I. Glucosamine sulfate compared to ibuprofen in osteoarthritis of the knee. Osteoarthritis Cartilage. 1994 Mar;2(1):61-9.

[12] Lopes Vaz A. Double-blind clinical evaluation of the relative efficacy of ibuprofen and glucosamine sulphate in the management of osteoarthrosis of the knee in out-patients. Current medical research and opinion. 1982;8(3):145-9.

[13] Reginster JY, Deroisy R, Rovati LC, Lee RL, Lejeune E, Bruyere O, et al. Long-term effects of glucosamine sulphate on osteoarthritis progression: a randomised, placebo-controlled clinical trial. Lancet. 2001 Jan 27;357(9252):251-6.

[14] Lee YH, Woo JH, Choi SJ, Ji JD, Song GG. Effect of glucosamine or chondroitin sulfate on the osteoarthritis progression: a meta-analysis. Rheumatology international. 2010 Jan;30(3):357-63.

[15] Hughes R, Carr A. A randomized, double-blind, placebo-controlled trial of glucosamine sulphate as an analgesic in osteoarthritis of the knee. Rheumatology (Oxford). 2002 Mar;41(3):279-84.

[16] Wandel S, Juni P, Tendal B, Nuesch E, Villiger PM, Welton NJ, et al. Effects of glucosamine, chondroitin, or placebo in patients with osteoarthritis of hip or knee: network meta-analysis. BMJ (Clinical research ed. 2010;341:c4675.

[17] Pekarek B, Osher L, Buck S, Bowen M. Intra-articular corticosteroid injections: a critical literature review with up-to-date findings. Foot (Edinburgh, Scotland). 2011 Jun; 21(2):66-70.

[18] Stitek T, Jong K, Gazzilo G, Lee C. *Injection procedures: Osteoarthritis and related conditions*. Newark, NJ: Springer Science and Business Media 2011:67-89.

[19] Abate M, Schiavone C, Salini V. Hyaluronic acid in ankle osteoarthritis: why evidence of efficacy is still lacking? Clin Exp Rheumatol. 2012 Mar-Apr;30(2):277-81.

[20] Migliore A, Giovannangeli F, Bizzi E, Massafra U, Alimonti A, Lagana B, et al. Viscosupplementation in the management of ankle osteoarthritis: a review. Arch Orthop Trauma Surg. 2011 Jan;131(1):139-47.

[21] DeGroot H, 3rd, Uzunishvili S, Weir R, Al-omari A, Gomes B. Intra-articular injection of hyaluronic acid is not superior to saline solution injection for ankle arthritis: a randomized, double-blind, placebo-controlled study. J Bone Joint Surg Am. 2012 Jan 4;94(1):2-8.

[22] De Smet AA, Ilahi OA, Graf BK. Untreated osteochondritis dissecans of the femoral condyles: prediction of patient outcome using radiographic and MR findings. Skeletal Radiol. 1997;26(8):463-7.

[23] Hughston JC, Hergenroeder PT, Courtenay BG. Osteochondritis dissecans of the femoral condyles. J Bone Joint Surg [Am]. 1984;66(9):1340-8.

[24] Apprich S, Trattnig S, Welsch GH, Noebauer-Huhmann IM, Sokolwski M, Hirschfeld C, et al. Assessment of articular cartilage repair tissue after matrix-associated autologous chondrocyte transplantation or the microfracture technique in the ankle joint using diffusion-weighted imaging at 3 Tesla. Osteoarthritis Cartilage. 2012 Jul;20(7): 703-11.

[25] Saxena A, Eakin C. Articular talar injuries in athletes: results of microfracture and autogenous bone graft. Am J Sports Med. 2007 Oct;35(10):1680-7.

[26] Doral MN, Bilge O, Batmaz G, Donmez G, Turhan E, Demirel M, et al. Treatment of osteochondral lesions of the talus with microfracture technique and postoperative hyaluronan injection. Knee Surg Sports Traumatol Arthrosc. 2012;20:1298-403.

[27] Becher C, Driessen A, Hess T, Longo UG, Maffulli N, Thermann H. Microfracture for chondral defects of the talus: maintenance of early results at midterm follow-up. Knee Surg Sports Traumatol Arthrosc. 2010 May;18(5):656-63.

[28] Brittberg M, Lindahl A, Nilsson A, Ohlsson C, Isaksson O, Peterson L. Treatment of deep cartilage defects in the knee with autologous chondrocyte transplantation. The New England journal of medicine. 1994;331(14):889-95.

[29] Battaglia M, Vannini F, Buda R, Cavallo M, Ruffilli A, Monti C, et al. Arthroscopic autologous chondrocyte implantation in osteochondral lesions of the talus: mid-term T2-mapping MRI evaluation. Knee Surg Sports Traumatol Arthrosc. 2011 Aug;19(8): 1376-84.

[30] Dixon S, Harvey L, Baddour E, Janes G, Hardisty G. Functional outcome of matrix-associated autologous chondrocyte implantation in the ankle. Foot Ankle Int. 2011 Apr;32(4):368-74.

[31] Giza E, Sullivan M, Ocel D, Lundeen G, Mitchell ME, Veris L, et al. Matrix-induced autologous chondrocyte implantation of talus articular defects. Foot Ankle Int. 2010 Sep;31(9):747-53.

[32] Saris DB, Vanlauwe J, Victor J, Haspl M, Bohnsack M, Fortems Y, et al. Characterized chondrocyte implantation results in better structural repair when treating symptomatic cartilage defects of the knee in a randomized controlled trial versus microfracture. Am J Sports Med. 2008 Feb;36(2):235-46.

[33] Liu W, Liu F, Zhao W, Kim JM, Wang Z, Vrahas MS. Osteochondral autograft transplantation for acute osteochondral fractures associated with an ankle fracture. Foot Ankle Int. 2011 Apr;32(4):437-42.

[34] Gobbi A, Francisco RA, Lubowitz JH, Allegra F, Canata G. Osteochondral lesions of the talus: randomized controlled trial comparing chondroplasty, microfracture, and osteochondral autograft transplantation. Arthroscopy. 2006 Oct;22(10):1085-92.

[35] Valderrabano V, Leumann A, Rasch H, Egelhof T, Hintermann B, Pagenstert G. Knee-to-ankle mosaicplasty for the treatment of osteochondral lesions of the ankle joint. Am J Sports Med. 2009 Nov;37 Suppl 1:105S-11S.

[36] Hangody L, Dobos J, Balo E, Panics G, Hangody LR, Berkes I. Clinical experiences with autologous osteochondral mosaicplasty in an athletic population: a 17-year prospective multicenter study. Am J Sports Med. 2010 Jun;38(6):1125-33.

[37] Hangody L, Kish G, Modis L, Szerb I, Gaspar L, Dioszegi Z, et al. Mosaicplasty for the treatment of osteochondritis dissecans of the talus: two to seven year results in 36 patients. Foot Ankle Int. 2001;22(7):552-8.

[38] El-Rashidy H, Villacis D, Omar I, Kelikian AS. Fresh osteochondral allograft for the treatment of cartilage defects of the talus: a retrospective review. J Bone Joint Surg Am. 2011 Sep 7;93(17):1634-40.

[39] Adams SB, Jr., Viens NA, Easley ME, Stinnett SS, Nunley JA, 2nd. Midterm results of osteochondral lesions of the talar shoulder treated with fresh osteochondral allograft transplantation. J Bone Joint Surg Am. 2011 Apr 6;93(7):648-54.

[40] Aubin PP, Cheah HK, Davis AM, Gross AE. Long-term followup of fresh femoral osteochondral allografts for posttraumatic knee defects. Clin Orthop. 2001(391 Suppl):S318-27.

[41] Tontz WL, Jr., Bugbee WD, Brage ME. Use of allografts in the management of ankle arthritis. Foot Ankle Clin. 2003 Jun;8(2):361-73, xi.

[42] Garcia EJ, Bear RR, Schoenfeld AJ, Owens BD. Treatment of osteochondral lesions of the talus with a biosynthetic scaffold: a report of four cases. J Bone Joint Surg Am. 2010 Jul 21;92(8):1774-9.

[43] Giannini S, Buda R, Vannini F, Cavallo M, Grigolo B. One-step bone marrow-derived cell transplantation in talar osteochondral lesions. Clin Orthop Relat Res. 2009 Dec; 467(12):3307-20.

[44] Barnewitz D, Endres M, Kruger I, Becker A, Zimmermann J, Wilke I, et al. Treatment of articular cartilage defects in horses with polymer-based cartilage tissue engineering grafts. Biomaterials. 2006 May;27(14):2882-9.

[45] Candrian C, Barbero A, Bonacina E, Francioli S, Hirschmann MT, Milz S, et al. A novel implantation technique for engineered osteo-chondral grafts. Knee Surg Sports Traumatol Arthrosc. 2009 Nov;17(11):1377-83.

[46] Lee KB, Bai LB, Yoon TR, Jung ST, Seon JK. Second-look arthroscopic findings and clinical outcomes after microfracture for osteochondral lesions of the talus. Am J Sports Med. 2009 Nov;37 Suppl 1:63S-70S.

[47] Nam EK, Ferkel RD, Applegate GR. Autologous chondrocyte implantation of the ankle: a 2- to 5-year follow-up. Am J Sports Med. 2009 Feb;37(2):274-84.

[48] Giannini S, Battaglia M, Buda R, Cavallo M, Ruffilli A, Vannini F. Surgical treatment of osteochondral lesions of the talus by open-field autologous chondrocyte implantation: a 10-year follow-up clinical and magnetic resonance imaging T2-mapping evaluation. Am J Sports Med. 2009 Nov;37 Suppl 1:112S-8S.

[49] Matricali GA, Bartels W, Labey L, Dereymaeker GP, Luyten FP, Vander Sloten J. Changes in contact area characteristics of the ankle after a cartilage biopsy at the postero-medial rim of the talar dome. Osteoarthritis Cartilage. 2009 Nov;17(11): 1477-84.

[50] Giannini S, Buda R, Vannini F, Di Caprio F, Grigolo B. Arthroscopic autologous chondrocyte implantation in osteochondral lesions of the talus: surgical technique and results. Am J Sports Med. 2008 May;36(5):873-80.

[51] Schneider TE, Karaikudi S. Matrix-Induced Autologous Chondrocyte Implantation (MACI) grafting for osteochondral lesions of the talus. Foot Ankle Int. 2009 Sep;30(9): 810-4.

[52] Thermann H, Driessen A, Becher C. [Autologous chondrocyte transplantation in the treatment of articular cartilage lesions of the talus]. Der Orthopade. 2008 Mar;37(3): 232-9.

[53] Lim HC, Bae JH, Song SH, Park YE, Kim SJ. Current treatments of isolated articular cartilage lesions of the knee achieve similar outcomes. Clin Orthop Relat Res. 2012 Aug;470(8):2261-7.

[54] Kilic A, Kabukcuoglu Y, Gul M, Ozkaya U, Sokucu S. [Early results of open mosaicplasty in osteochondral lesions of the talus]. Acta orthopaedica et traumatologica turcica. 2009 May-Jul;43(3):235-42.

[55] Reddy S, Pedowitz DI, Parekh SG, Sennett BJ, Okereke E. The morbidity associated with osteochondral harvest from asymptomatic knees for the treatment of osteochondral lesions of the talus. Am J Sports Med. 2007 Jan;35(1):80-5.

[56] Hahn DB, Aanstoos ME, Wilkins RM. Osteochondral lesions of the talus treated with fresh talar allografts. Foot Ankle Int. 2010 Apr;31(4):277-82.

[57] Williams SK, Amiel D, Ball ST, Allen RT, Wong VW, Chen AC, et al. Prolonged storage effects on the articular cartilage of fresh human osteochondral allografts. J Bone Joint Surg Am. 2003 Nov;85-A(11):2111-20.

[58] Ball ST, Amiel D, Williams SK, Tontz W, Chen AC, Sah RL, et al. The effects of storage on fresh human osteochondral allografts. Clin Orthop Relat Res. 2004 Jan(418): 246-52.

[59] Jomha NM, Elliott JA, Law GK, Maghdoori B, Fraser Forbes J, Abazari A, et al. Vitrification of intact human articular cartilage. Biomaterials. 2012 Sep;33(26):6061-8.

[60] Meehan R, McFarlin S, Bugbee W, Brage M. Fresh ankle osteochondral allograft transplantation for tibiotalar joint arthritis. Foot Ankle Int. 2005 Oct;26(10):793-802.

[61] Giannini S, Buda R, Grigolo B, Bevoni R, Di Caprio F, Ruffilli A, et al. Bipolar fresh osteochondral allograft of the ankle. Foot Ankle Int. 2010 Jan;31(1):38-46.

[62] Bugbee WD, Convery FR. Osteochondral allograft transplantation. Clinics in sports medicine. 1999;18(1):67-75.

[63] Mann HA, Filippi J, Myerson MS. Intra-articular opening medial tibial wedge osteotomy (plafond-plasty) for the treatment of intra-articular varus ankle arthritis and instability. Foot Ankle Int. 2012 Apr;33(4):255-61.

[64] Knupp M, Stufkens SA, van Bergen CJ, Blankevoort L, Bolliger L, van Dijk CN, et al. Effect of supramalleolar varus and valgus deformities on the tibiotalar joint: a cadaveric study. Foot Ankle Int. 2011 Jun;32(6):609-15.

[65] Lee WC, Moon JS, Lee K, Byun WJ, Lee SH. Indications for supramalleolar osteotomy in patients with ankle osteoarthritis and varus deformity. J Bone Joint Surg Am. 2011 Jul 6;93(13):1243-8.

[66] Saltzman CL, Hillis SL, Stolley MP, Anderson DD, Amendola A. Motion versus fixed distraction of the joint in the treatment of ankle osteoarthritis: a prospective randomized controlled trial. J Bone Joint Surg Am. 2012 Jun 6;94(11):961-70.

[67] Albert E. Zur resection des Kniegelenkes. Wein Med Press. 1879;20:705-8.

[68] Hendrickx RP, Stufkens SA, de Bruijn EE, Sierevelt IN, van Dijk CN, Kerkhoffs GM. Medium- to long-term outcome of ankle arthrodesis. Foot Ankle Int. 2011 Oct;32(10): 940-7.

[69] Haddad SL, Coetzee JC, Estok R, Fahrbach K, Banel D, Nalysnyk L. Intermediate and long-term outcomes of total ankle arthroplasty and ankle arthrodesis. A systematic review of the literature. J Bone Joint Surg Am. 2007 Sep;89(9):1899-905.

[70] Crosby LA, Yee TC, Formanek TS, Fitzgibbons TC. Complications following arthroscopic ankle arthrodesis. Foot Ankle Int. 1996 Jun;17(6):340-2.

[71] Cooper PS. Complications of ankle and tibiotalocalcaneal arthrodesis. Clin Orthop Relat Res. 2001 Oct(391):33-44.

[72] Akra GA, Middleton A, Adedapo AO, Port A, Finn P. Outcome of ankle arthrodesis using a transfibular approach. J Foot Ankle Surg. 2010 Nov-Dec;49(6):508-12.

[73] Gessmann J, Ozokyay L, Fehmer T, Muhr G, Seybold D. [Arthrodesis of the infected ankle joint: results with the Ilizarov external fixator]. Zeitschrift fur Orthopadie und Unfallchirurgie. 2011 Apr;149(2):212-8.

[74] Hollawell SM. Allograft cellular bone matrix as an alternative to autograft in hindfoot and ankle fusion procedures. J Foot Ankle Surg. 2012 Mar-Apr;51(2):222-5.

[75] Guo C, Yan Z, Barfield WR, Hartsock LA. Ankle arthrodesis using anatomically contoured anterior plate. Foot Ankle Int. 2010 Jun;31(6):492-8.

[76] Zwipp H, Rammelt S, Endres T, Heineck J. High union rates and function scores at midterm followup with ankle arthrodesis using a four screw technique. Clin Orthop Relat Res. 2010 Apr;468(4):958-68.

[77] Mohamedean A, Said HG, El-Sharkawi M, El-Adly W, Said GZ. Technique and short-term results of ankle arthrodesis using anterior plating. International orthopaedics. 2010 Aug;34(6):833-7.

[78] Boer R, Mader K, Pennig D, Verheyen CC. Tibiotalocalcaneal arthrodesis using a reamed retrograde locking nail. Clin Orthop Relat Res. 2007 Oct;463:151-6.

[79] Tang KL, Li QH, Chen GX, Guo L, Dai G, Yang L. Arthroscopically assisted ankle fusion in patients with end-stage tuberculosis. Arthroscopy. 2007 Sep;23(9):919-22.

[80] Eylon S, Porat S, Bor N, Leibner ED. Outcome of Ilizarov ankle arthrodesis. Foot Ankle Int. 2007 Aug;28(8):873-9.

[81] Gougoulias NE, Agathangelidis FG, Parsons SW. Arthroscopic ankle arthrodesis. Foot Ankle Int. 2007 Jun;28(6):695-706.

[82] Colman AB, Pomeroy GC. Transfibular ankle arthrodesis with rigid internal fixation: an assessment of outcome. Foot Ankle Int. 2007 Mar;28(3):303-7.

[83] Pelton K, Hofer JK, Thordarson DB. Tibiotalocalcaneal arthrodesis using a dynamically locked retrograde intramedullary nail. Foot Ankle Int. 2006 Oct;27(10):759-63.

[84] Didomenico LA, Sann P. Posterior approach using anterior ankle arthrodesis locking plate for tibiotalocalcaneal arthrodesis. J Foot Ankle Surg. 2011 Sep-Oct;50(5):626-9.

[85] Hanson TW, Cracchiolo A, 3rd. The use of a 95 degree blade plate and a posterior approach to achieve tibiotalocalcaneal arthrodesis. Foot Ankle Int. 2002 Aug;23(8): 704-10.

[86] Nickisch F, Avilucea FR, Beals T, Saltzman C. Open posterior approach for tibiotalar arthrodesis. Foot Ankle Clin. 2011 Mar;16(1):103-14.

[87] Collman DR, Kaas MH, Schuberth JM. Arthroscopic ankle arthrodesis: factors influencing union in 39 consecutive patients. Foot Ankle Int. 2006 Dec;27(12):1079-85.

[88] Cameron SE, Ullrich P. Arthroscopic arthrodesis of the ankle joint. Arthroscopy. 2000 Jan-Feb;16(1):21-6.

[89] Schuh R, Hofstaetter J, Krismer M, Bevoni R, Windhager R, Trnka HJ. Total ankle arthroplasty versus ankle arthrodesis. Comparison of sports, recreational activities and functional outcome. International orthopaedics. 2012 Jun;36(6):1207-14.

[90] Goldberg AJ, Sharp RJ, Cooke P. Ankle replacement: current practice of foot & ankle surgeons in the United kingdom. Foot Ankle Int. 2009 Oct;30(10):950-4.

[91] Lord G, Marotte JH. [Total ankle replacement (author's transl)]. Revue de chirurgie orthopedique et reparatrice de l'appareil moteur. 1980 Nov-Dec;66(8):527-30.

[92] Hintermann B, Valderrabano V. Total ankle replacement. Foot Ankle Clin. 2003 Jun; 8(2):375-405.

[93] Bolton-Maggs BG, Sudlow RA, Freeman MA. Total ankle arthroplasty. A long-term review of the London Hospital experience. J Bone Joint Surg Br. 1985 Nov;67(5): 785-90.

[94] Easley ME, Vertullo CJ, Urban WC, Nunley JA. Total ankle arthroplasty. The Journal of the American Academy of Orthopaedic Surgeons. 2002 May-Jun;10(3):157-67.

[95] Kitaoka HB, Patzer GL. Clinical results of the Mayo total ankle arthroplasty. J Bone Joint Surg Am. 1996 Nov;78(11):1658-64.

[96] Hamblen DL. Can the ankle joint be replaced? J Bone Joint Surg Br. 1985 Nov;67(5): 689-90.

[97] Lewis G. Biomechanics of and research challenges in uncemented total ankle replacement. Clin Orthop Relat Res. 2004 Jul(424):89-97.

[98] Hintermann B. Total ankle arthroplasty. St. Stefan, Austria: Springer Wein New York 2005.

[99] Dyrby C, Chou LB, Andriacchi TP, Mann RA. Functional evaluation of the Scandinavian Total Ankle Replacement. Foot Ankle Int. 2004 Jun;25(6):377-81.

[100] Michelson JD, Schmidt GR, Mizel MS. Kinematics of a total arthroplasty of the ankle: comparison to normal ankle motion. Foot Ankle Int. 2000 Apr;21(4):278-84.

[101] Yalamanchili P, Neufeld S, Lin S. Total ankle arthroplasty: A modern perspective. Curr Orthop Prac. 2009;20(2):106-11-.

[102] Neufeld SK, Lee TH. Total ankle arthroplasty: indications, results, and biomechanical rationale. American journal of orthopedics (Belle Mead, NJ. 2000 Aug;29(8):593-602.

[103] Pyevich MT, Saltzman CL, Callaghan JJ, Alvine FG. Total ankle arthroplasty: a unique design. Two to twelve-year follow-up. J Bone Joint Surg Am. 1998 Oct;80(10): 1410-20.

[104] Gould JS, Alvine FG, Mann RA, Sanders RW, Walling AK. Total ankle replacement: a surgical discussion. Part II. The clinical and surgical experience. American journal of orthopedics (Belle Mead, NJ. 2000 Sep;29(9):675-82.

[105] Gould JS, Alvine FG, Mann RA, Sanders RW, Walling AK. Total ankle replacement: a surgical discussion. Part I. Replacement systems, indications, and contraindications. American journal of orthopedics (Belle Mead, NJ. 2000 Aug;29(8):604-9.

[106] Demottaz JD, Mazur JM, Thomas WH, Sledge CB, Simon SR. Clinical study of total ankle replacement with gait analysis. A preliminary report. J Bone Joint Surg Am. 1979 Oct;61(7):976-88.

[107] Gill LH. Challenges in total ankle arthroplasty. Foot Ankle Int. 2004 Apr;25(4): 195-207.

[108] Inman VT. Inman's joints of the ankle. Baltimore, MD: Williams & Wilkins 1976.

[109] Sammarco J. Biomechanics of the ankle. I. Surface velocity and instant center of rotation in the sagittal plane. Am J Sports Med. 1977 Nov-Dec;5(6):231-4.

[110] Komistek RD, Stiehl JB, Buechel FF, Northcut EJ, Hajner ME. A determination of ankle kinematics using fluoroscopy. Foot Ankle Int. 2000 Apr;21(4):343-50.

[111] Saltzman CL. Perspective on total ankle replacement. Foot Ankle Clin. 2000 Dec;5(4): 761-75.

[112] Cracchiolo A, 3rd, Deorio JK. Design features of current total ankle replacements: implants and instrumentation. The Journal of the American Academy of Orthopaedic Surgeons. 2008 Sep;16(9):530-40.

[113] Chou LB, Coughlin MT, Hansen S, Jr., Haskell A, Lundeen G, Saltzman CL, et al. Osteoarthritis of the ankle: the role of arthroplasty. The Journal of the American Academy of Orthopaedic Surgeons. 2008 May;16(5):249-59.

[114] Cenni F, Leardini A, Belvedere C, Bugane F, Cremonini K, Miscione MT, et al. Kinematics of the three components of a total ankle replacement: in vivo fluoroscopic analysis. Foot Ankle Int. 2012 Apr;33(4):290-300.

[115] Brodsky JW, Polo FE, Coleman SC, Bruck N. Changes in gait following the Scandinavian Total Ankle Replacement. J Bone Joint Surg Am. 2011 Oct 19;93(20):1890-6.

[116] Barnett CH, Napier JR. The axis of rotation at the ankle joint in man; its influence upon the form of the talus and the mobility of the fibula. Journal of anatomy. 1952 Jan;86(1):1-9.

[117] Newton SE, 3rd. Total ankle arthroplasty. Clinical study of fifty cases. J Bone Joint Surg Am. 1982 Jan;64(1):104-11.

[118] Conti SF, Wong YS. Complications of total ankle replacement. Foot Ankle Clin. 2002 Dec;7(4):791-807, vii.

[119] Raikin SM, Kane J, Ciminiello ME. Risk factors for incision-healing complications following total ankle arthroplasty. J Bone Joint Surg Am. 2010 Sep 15;92(12):2150-5.

[120] Kobayashi A, Minoda Y, Kadoya Y, Ohashi H, Takaoka K, Saltzman CL. Ankle arthroplasties generate wear particles similar to knee arthroplasties. Clin Orthop Relat Res. 2004 Jul(424):69-72.

[121] Conti S, Lalonde KA, Martin R. Kinematic analysis of the agility total ankle during gait. Foot Ankle Int. 2006 Nov;27(11):980-4.

[122] Barg A, Knupp M, Anderson AE, Hintermann B. Total ankle replacement in obese patients: component stability, weight change, and functional outcome in 118 consecutive patients. Foot Ankle Int. 2011 Oct;32(10):925-32.

[123] Cornelis Doets H, van der Plaat LW, Klein JP. Medial malleolar osteotomy for the correction of varus deformity during total ankle arthroplasty: results in 15 ankles. Foot Ankle Int. 2008 Feb;29(2):171-7.

[124] Reddy SC, Mann JA, Mann RA, Mangold DR. Correction of moderate to severe coronal plane deformity with the STAR ankle prosthesis. Foot Ankle Int. 2011 Jul;32(7): 659-64.

[125] Shock RP, Christensen JC, Schuberth JM. Total ankle replacement in the varus ankle. J Foot Ankle Surg. 2011 Jan-Feb;50(1):5-10.

[126] Ryssman DB, Myerson MS. Total ankle arthroplasty: management of varus deformity at the ankle. Foot Ankle Int. 2012 Apr;33(4):347-54.

[127] Barg A, Henninger HB, Hintermann B. Risk factors for symptomatic deep-vein thrombosis in patients after total ankle replacement who received routine chemical thromboprophylaxis. J Bone Joint Surg Br. 2011 Jul;93(7):921-7.

[128] Bestic JM, Peterson JJ, DeOrio JK, Bancroft LW, Berquist TH, Kransdorf MJ. Postoperative evaluation of the total ankle arthroplasty. Ajr. 2008 Apr;190(4):1112-23.

[129] Fevang BT, Lie SA, Havelin LI, Brun JG, Skredderstuen A, Furnes O. 257 ankle arthroplasties performed in Norway between 1994 and 2005. Acta orthopaedica. 2007 Oct;78(5):575-83.

[130] Hosman AH, Mason RB, Hobbs T, Rothwell AG. A New Zealand national joint registry review of 202 total ankle replacements followed for up to 6 years. Acta orthopaedica. 2007 Oct;78(5):584-91.

[131] Skytta ET, Koivu H, Eskelinen A, Ikavalko M, Paavolainen P, Remes V. Total ankle replacement: a population-based study of 515 cases from the Finnish Arthroplasty Register. Acta orthopaedica. 2010 Feb;81(1):114-8.

[132] Henricson A, Nilsson JA, Carlsson A. 10-year survival of total ankle arthroplasties: a report on 780 cases from the Swedish Ankle Register. Acta orthopaedica. 2011 Dec; 82(6):655-9.

[133] Labek G, Klaus H, Schlichtherle R, Williams A, Agreiter M. Revision rates after total ankle arthroplasty in sample-based clinical studies and national registries. Foot Ankle Int. 2011 Aug;32(8):740-5.

[134] Gougoulias N, Khanna A, Maffulli N. How successful are current ankle replacements?: a systematic review of the literature. Clin Orthop Relat Res. 2010 Jan;468(1): 199-208.

[135] Stengel D, Bauwens K, Ekkernkamp A, Cramer J. Efficacy of total ankle replacement with meniscal-bearing devices: a systematic review and meta-analysis. Arch Orthop Trauma Surg. 2005 Mar;125(2):109-19.

[136] Mann JA, Mann RA, Horton E. STAR ankle: long-term results. Foot Ankle Int. 2011 May;32(5):S473-84.

[137] Bonnin M, Gaudot F, Laurent JR, Ellis S, Colombier JA, Judet T. The Salto total ankle arthroplasty: survivorship and analysis of failures at 7 to 11 years. Clin Orthop Relat Res. 2011 Jan;469(1):225-36.

[138] Wood PL, Sutton C, Mishra V, Suneja R. A randomised, controlled trial of two mobile-bearing total ankle replacements. J Bone Joint Surg Br. 2009 Jan;91(1):69-74.

[139] Hahn ME, Wright ES, Segal AD, Orendurff MS, Ledoux WR, Sangeorzan BJ. Comparative gait analysis of ankle arthrodesis and arthroplasty: initial findings of a prospective study. Foot Ankle Int. 2012 Apr;33(4):282-9.

[140] Piriou P, Culpan P, Mullins M, Cardon JN, Pozzi D, Judet T. Ankle replacement versus arthrodesis: a comparative gait analysis study. Foot Ankle Int. 2008 Jan;29(1):3-9.

[141] Penner MJ, Pakzad H, Younger A, Wing KJ. Mean BMI of overweight and obese patients does not decrease after successful ankle reconstruction. J Bone Joint Surg Am. 2012 May 2;94(9):e57.

# Permissions

The contributors of this book come from diverse backgrounds, making this book a truly international effort. This book will bring forth new frontiers with its revolutionizing research information and detailed analysis of the nascent developments around the world.

We would like to thank Plamen Kinov, MD, PhD, for lending his expertise to make the book truly unique. He has played a crucial role in the development of this book. Without his invaluable contribution this book wouldn't have been possible. He has made vital efforts to compile up to date information on the varied aspects of this subject to make this book a valuable addition to the collection of many professionals and students.

This book was conceptualized with the vision of imparting up-to-date information and advanced data in this field. To ensure the same, a matchless editorial board was set up. Every individual on the board went through rigorous rounds of assessment to prove their worth. After which they invested a large part of their time researching and compiling the most relevant data for our readers. Conferences and sessions were held from time to time between the editorial board and the contributing authors to present the data in the most comprehensible form. The editorial team has worked tirelessly to provide valuable and valid information to help people across the globe.

Every chapter published in this book has been scrutinized by our experts. Their significance has been extensively debated. The topics covered herein carry significant findings which will fuel the growth of the discipline. They may even be implemented as practical applications or may be referred to as a beginning point for another development. Chapters in this book were first published by InTech; hereby published with permission under the Creative Commons Attribution License or equivalent.

The editorial board has been involved in producing this book since its inception. They have spent rigorous hours researching and exploring the diverse topics which have resulted in the successful publishing of this book. They have passed on their knowledge of decades through this book. To expedite this challenging task, the publisher supported the team at every step. A small team of assistant editors was also appointed to further simplify the editing procedure and attain best results for the readers.

Our editorial team has been hand-picked from every corner of the world. Their multi-ethnicity adds dynamic inputs to the discussions which result in innovative outcomes. These outcomes are then further discussed with the researchers and contributors who give their valuable feedback and opinion regarding the same. The feedback is then collaborated with the researches and they are edited in a comprehensive manner to aid the understanding of the subject.

Apart from the editorial board, the designing team has also invested a significant amount of their time in understanding the subject and creating the most relevant covers. They scrutinized every image to scout for the most suitable representation of the subject and create an appropriate cover for the book.

The publishing team has been involved in this book since its early stages. They were actively engaged in every process, be it collecting the data, connecting with the contributors or procuring relevant information. The team has been an ardent support to the editorial, designing and production team. Their endless efforts to recruit the best for this project, has resulted in the accomplishment of this book. They are a veteran in the field of academics and their pool of knowledge is as vast as their experience in printing. Their expertise and guidance has proved useful at every step. Their uncompromising quality standards have made this book an exceptional effort. Their encouragement from time to time has been an inspiration for everyone.

The publisher and the editorial board hope that this book will prove to be a valuable piece of knowledge for researchers, students, practitioners and scholars across the globe.

# List of Contributors

**Hiran Amarasekera**
Orthopedic Research Fellow/ PhD Student, Warwick Medical School, University of Warwick, and University Hospital of Coventry and Warwickshire, UK

**Michelle M. Dowsey**
University of Melbourne, Department of Surgery, St. Vincent's Hospital Melbourne, Australia

**Peter F. M. Choong**
Department of Orthopedics, St. Vincent's Hospital Melbourne, Australia

**A.O. Erdogan, N.S. Gokay and A. Gokce**
Namik Kemal University School of Medicine, Department of Orthopedics and Traumatology, Tekirdag, Turkey

**Hamid Reza Seyyed Hosseinzadeh, Ali Sina Shahi, Mehrnoush Hassas Yeganeh, Gholam Reza Kazemian and Aidin Masoudi**
Shahid Beheshti Unversity of Medical Sciences, Tehran, Iran

**Usama Hassan Saleh and Samih Tarabichi**
American Hospital, Dubai, United Arab Emirates

**Hamid Reza Seyyed Hosseinzadeh, Mohammad Emami, Farivarabdollahzadeh Lahiji, Ali Sina Shahi, Aidin Masoudi and Sina Emami**
Akhtar Orthopaedic Hospital, Shahid Beheshti University of Medical Sciences, Iran

**Kálmán Tóth and Gellért Sohár**
Department of Orthopedics, University of Szeged, Faculty of Medicine, Szeged, Hungary

**Jean-Yves Lazennec and Marc Antoine Rousseau**
Department of orthopedic and trauma surgery, La Pitié-Salpétrière hospital. Paris, France

**Adrien Brusson**
Department of Anatomy, université Pierre ET Marie Curie, Paris, France

**Lee E. Rubin**
Division of Adult Reconstruction, Warren Alpert Medical School of Brown University, University Orthopedics, Inc. Providence, Rhode Island, USA

**Scott A. Ritterman**
Brown University and Rhode Island Hospital, Providence, Rhode Island, USA

**Timothy McTighe**
Joint Implant Surgery and Research Foundation (JISRF), Chagrin Falls, Ohio, USA

**Moby Parsons**
Seacoast Orthopedics & Sports Medicine, Somersworth, NH, USA

**Eun-Kyoo Song, Jong-Keun Seon, Jae-Young Moon and Yim Ji-Hyoun**
Department of Orthopedic Surgery, Chonnam National University Hwasun Hospital, Hwasun, Korea

**Jean-Yves Lazennec**
Department of Orthopedic and Trauma Surgery, La Pitié-Salpétrière Hospital, Paris, France Biomechanics Lab, Arts et Métiers Paritech, Paris, France Department of Anatomy, Universite´ Pierre ET Marie Curie, Paris, France

**Marc Antoine Rousseau**
Department of Orthopedic and Trauma Surgery, La Pitié-Salpétrière Hospital, Paris, France Biomechanics Lab, Arts ET Métiers Paritech, Paris, France

**Alain Aaron**
FH Orthopedics, Heimsbrunn, France

**Adrien Brusson**
Department of Anatomy, Universite´ Pierre et Marie Curie, Paris, France

**Jean Patrick Rakover**
Clinique du Pré, Le Mans, France

**Tsutomu Gomi**
School of Allied Health Sciences, Kitasato University, Japan

**Hiroshi Hirano**
Department of Radiology, Shinshu University Hospital, Japan

**Masahiro Nakajima**
Department of Radiology, Dokkyo Medical University Hospital, Japan

**Andrew Gordon and Hosam E. Matar**
Department of Orthopaedics the Northern General Hospital, Sheffield, United Kingdom

**J. Mark Wilkinson**
Academic Unit of Bone Metabolism, University of Sheffield, Sheffield, United Kingdom

**Plamen Kinov and Peter Tivchev**
Queen Giovanna - ISUL University Hospital, Department of Orthopedics and Traumatology, Medical University of Sofia, Bulgaria

**Hideyuki Takedani**
Department of Joint Surgery Research Hospital of the Institute of Medical Science the University of Tokyo 4-6-1 Shiroganedai, Minato-ku, Tokyo 108-8639, Japan

**Nadr M. Jomha, Angela Scharfenberger, Gordon Goplen and M. Elizabeth Pedersen**
Division of Orthopaedic Surgery, Department of Surgery, University of Alberta, Edmonton, Alberta, Canada